THE ENCYCLOPEDIA OF

SEXUALLY TRANSMITTED DISEASES

THE ENCYCLOPEDIA OF

SEXUALLY TRANSMITTED DISEASES

Jennifer Shoquist, M.D.
Diane Stafford

☑®
Facts On File, Inc.

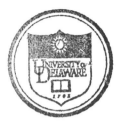

The Encyclopedia of Sexually Transmitted Diseases

Facts On File, Inc.
132 West 31st Street
New York NY 10001

Library of Congress Cataloging-in-Publication Data

Shoquist, Jennifer.
The encyclopedia of sexually transmitted diseases / Jennifer Shoquist, Diane Stafford.
p. cm.
Includes bibliographical references and index.
ISBN 0-8160-4881-9 (alk. paper)
1. Sexually transmitted diseases—Encyclopedias. I. Stafford, Diane. II. Title.
RC200.1.S525 2003
616.95'1'003—dc21
2003040813

Facts On File books are available at special discounts when purchased in bulk quantities for businesses, associations, institutions, or sales promotions. Please call our Special Sales Department in New York at (212) 967-8800 or (800) 322-8755.

You can find Facts On File on the World Wide Web at http://www.factsonfile.com

Text and cover design by Cathy Rincon

Printed in the United States of America

VB Hermitage 10 9 8 7 6 5 4 3 2 1

This book is printed on acid-free paper.

Disclaimer

This book contains the authors' ideas and accumulated facts/knowledge. It is intended to provide helpful information on the subject matter covered herein. It is sold with the understanding that the authors and the publisher are not engaged in rendering professional medical, health, or any other kind of personal professional services via this book. If the reader wants or needs personal advice or guidance, he or she should seek an in-person consultation with a competent medical professional. Furthermore, the reader should consult his or her medical, health, or other competent professional before adopting any of the suggestions in the book or drawing inferences from information that is included herein. This is a supplement, not a replacement, for medical advice from a reader's personal health care provider. Check with your doctor before following any suggestions in this book; consult your doctor before using information on any condition that may require medical diagnosis or treatment.

The authors and publisher specifically disclaim any responsibility for any liability, loss, or risk, whether personal or otherwise, that someone may incur as a consequence, direct or indirect, of the use and application of any contents of this book. In no way does reading this book replace the need for an evaluation by a physician. Also, the full responsibility for any adverse effects that result from the use of information in this book rests solely with the reader.

CONTENTS

ACKNOWLEDGMENTS

We would like to thank our editor at Facts On File, James Chambers, for his helpful suggestions, his answers, and his editorial guidance. We also thank Sarah Fogarty of Facts On File for her editing and hard work and copy editor Susan Thornton. Also, special thanks to Elizabeth Frost Knappman of New England Publishing Associates.

Also, we appreciate the efforts of countless people from national organizations, services, and government agencies who offered information, statistics, and support.

And, especially, our deepest thanks to family and friends for their patience and understanding while we were hard at work on this book.

Most important, we hope those of you who read this book will become more knowledgeable about sexually transmitted diseases and take a proactive approach to maintaining your health.

INTRODUCTION

Worldwide, sexually transmitted diseases (STDs) are among the most common causes of illness. Although prevention-and-education efforts have curbed the rise of certain STDs in the United States, the diseases continue to ravage sexually active people in the United States as well as other countries.

The Centers for Disease Control and Prevention (CDC) report that as of the year 2002, about 65 million Americans were living with sexually transmitted diseases, with millions more likely to become infected each year—and most of these diseases occur in people below the age of 25. Worldwide, at the end of 2002, about 42 million people were living with human immunodeficiency virus (HIV) or acquired immunodeficiency syndrome (AIDS); 28 million have died since the beginning of the epidemic, 75 percent of them in sub-Saharan Africa. AIDS deaths worldwide in 2002 were 3.1 million.

Year 2001 data from the Centers for Disease Control and Prevention show that about 16,000 Americans are dying of AIDS every year, and 40,000 more becoming HIV-infected annually—figures that have not changed much since 1998, the year when the epidemic in the United States stabilized somewhat. Women are increasingly affected by HIV: about 48 percent of new adult and adolescent HIV cases worldwide were women as of the end of 2002.

Most of those who have HIV—about 95 percent—live in the developing world, and sexually transmitted diseases are among the most common causes of illness globally.

Statistics and Demographics

One factor that complicates all forms of reporting demographics and statistics on sexually transmitted diseases is the private nature of sex—the means of transmission. Americans (and often even their doctors) do not like talking about STDs, and their reluctance makes tracking difficult.

Nevertheless, it is clear that millions of new sexually transmitted disease infections occur every year in the United States—as many as about 15 million—and this figure includes about 4 million cases of chlamydia, 800,000 cases of gonorrhea, 110,000+ cases of syphilis, several million cases of trichomonas vaginitis and nonspecific urethritis, 1 million to 2 million cases of human papillomavirus, 200,000 to 1 million cases of hepatitis B, 200,000–500,000 cases of genital herpes, and 40,000–80,000 new HIV infections. Many of these, however, are not reported to the CDC.

Estimates suggest that in the United States, there are about 1 million Americans infected with human immunodeficiency virus, 31 million to 50 million infected with herpes simplex virus, 24 million infected with human papillomavirus, and more than 1 million chronic hepatitis B carriers. Of the 15 million new cases of STDs in Americans each year, about 25 percent will be in the age group 15 to 19.

Increasing globally are molluscum contagiosum and condyloma acuminata, while herpes simplex has reached epidemic proportions, having increased by 30 percent from 1986 to 2001 in the United States.

Human papillomavirus is the most common viral sexually transmitted disease and probably the most common STD as of 2001. Since the 1960s, doctors have seen a dramatic rise in patient visits to clinics for diagnosis or treatment of clinical human papillomaviruses. At any given time, about 20 million people in the United States have genital human papillomavirus infections that are transmittable, and about 1 to 2 million more individuals are infected each year. There are more than 100 known types, varying in affinity for the genital tract (about 35 types), clinical expression, and oncogenic potential. Widely noted as the most common sexually transmitted disease in young people who are sexually active, human papillomavirus (HPV) can cause genital warts (a type of HPV that is often easy to treat), or it can result in subclinical infections that cannot be cured but are often cleared spontaneously by the body's immune system.

In 2001, chlamydia was the most reported bacterial infection in the United States and the most common bacterial (curable) sexually transmitted disease. Health care experts estimate that 4 million new cases of chlamydia occur in the United States every year, and almost half of these new cases occur in people below the age of 19.

Gonorrhea is a big problem in the United States. According to a report released December 5, 2000, although rates of STDs are declining in the United States, gonorrhea remains very troublesome.

Changes in Prevalence of Certain STDs

For the first time in two decades, doctors are seeing increases in gonorrhea rates in the United States; some increases are due to better screening and improved tests. Cities with the highest rates of gonorrhea and syphilis are Atlanta; Baltimore; Detroit; Indianapolis; Memphis; New Orleans; Newark, New Jersey; Norfolk, Virginia; Saint Louis; and Washington, D.C. Epidemiologists link the South's high rate of infections to poverty and inadequate treatment.

According to the CDC, in 2001, the rate of reported gonorrhea infections was 128.5 per 100,000 persons. After gonorrhea rates stabilized in the period from 1996 to 1997, they increased by 9 percent from 1997 to 1999, raising concerns that

the disease's decline of the past two decades may have been reversed, according to a biennial report from the CDC released at the National STD Prevention Conference in Milwaukee in December 2000. Highest rates of gonorrhea are seen in women ages 15 to 19 and men ages 20 to 24. About 75 percent of gonorrhea cases in the United States are in people 15 to 29, according to CDC statistics. Of the total cases of gonorrhea reported to the CDC in 1999, 77 percent were in African Americans.

The overall reported rate of syphilis in the United States in 2001 (2.2 cases per 100,000) was above the rate in 2000 (2.1 cases per 100,000). The rate of syphilis declined by 89.2 percent from 1990 through 2000. However, the rate increased slightly in 2001, an increase seen only in men. Between 2000 and 2001, CDC data also indicate that congenital syphilis decreased by 20.7 percent, from 14.0 to 11.1 per 100,000 live births. In 2000, the United States saw a 9.6 percent drop from 1999 in reported cases of syphilis, primary and secondary—the figure for 2000 was 5,979. According to the CDC, this marks an all-time low in syphilis rate and places this particular STD in reach of elimination. Experts attribute the decline to the National Campaign to Eliminate Syphilis in the United States. Half of syphilis cases in 2000 occurred in 21 counties and one city; of those, 11 reported more than 100 cases of syphilis, with the most in Chicago, Cook County, Illinois; Indianapolis, Marion County, Indiana; and Detroit, Wayne County, Michigan.

When syphilis cases in Indianapolis went up by nearly 475 percent from 1997 to 1999, this touched off aggressive prevention programs that cut in half the number of new cases of syphilis in that city. And although prevention programs have succeeded in curbing the growth rates of syphilis, gonorrhea, nongonococcal urethritis, chancroid, granuloma inguinale, and lymphogranuloma venereum in most parts of the United States, "hot spots" still exist in the South and in nonwhite and urban populations.

The "Why" behind the Problem

Ignorance of risk factors, denial of risk, and deliberate deception are three significant factors in the spread of sexually transmitted diseases. In particular, the sharp rise of STDs in the teen population reflects the perennial tendency of young people to perceive themselves as invulnerable. The startling news is that, according to the CDC, about three of five Americans living with HIV were infected as teens.

Some health experts attribute the rising rates of sexually transmitted diseases to an overblown sense of immortality in young people in particular, based on a lax attitude that one can embrace sexuality without worrying about health repercussions. In truth, no one can maintain good health by visually screening prospective sex partners; despite much wishful thinking, one simply cannot spot a person with an STD, in most cases. By the same token, an STD carrier may not even know that he or she is infected. In an era when an increasingly large number of young people regard oral sex as casual sexual activity, doctors see more cases of sexually transmitted diseases being spread via oral sex than in the past. Today, oral gonorrhea and oral herpes are increasingly prevalent.

Some studies present evidence that the current resurgence in HIV infections probably stems from complacency and a resulting increase in risky behavior of young gay and bisexual men. Physicians and health agencies nationwide partly attribute the increase in gonorrhea and syphilis infections in gay and bisexual men to an alarming trend toward looser attitudes toward safe-sex practices, because people have developed a reduced fear of HIV. This disturbing "complacency" has become prevalent in a new and improved HIV treatment era during which highly active antiretroviral therapy (HAART) has been shown to be effective in lengthening the lives of those with HIV infection.

Another problem that continues to keep HIV rates high is the transmission of the infection from intravenous drug users to fellow drug users and sex partners. The public health motto "One shot, one syringe" is clearly not being taken seriously by illicit drug users. Furthermore, availability of clean syringes by way of needle exchange programs has increased, but only very slowly. About a fourth of all AIDS cases can be attributed to injection drug use alone, but a frightening statistic is that intravenous (IV) drug use probably accounts for more than half of all new infections, according to research reported in the year 2000.

Health care authorities are also concerned about the "unenlightened" attitudes that still exist in the United States, despite widespread dissemination of information on sexually transmitted diseases. According to a 1999 survey, most of the female respondents reported very limited knowledge of common STDs, and fewer than one-fourth of those at highest risk—young women and women with multiple partners—actually believed they were at risk. Many people do not understand that a person with a sexually transmitted disease can be symptom-free—or have symptoms that can be easily mistaken for those of other illnesses. Others who are sexually active claim that they do not know about certain basic risks: that numerous partners multiply risk of infection, and that anyone—even someone using condoms—can become infected through sexual activity with an infected person.

Certainly, every proactive health consumer should arm himself or herself with information on STD symptoms and treatments. Those in the realm of health care should exercise increased vigilance; the discovery that a patient has a sexually transmitted disease should prompt physicians to check for other STDs, because occurrence of multiple concurrent infections is common.

The truth is, however, that one reason so many STDs are undiagnosed and untreated is that some doctors are reluctant to ask about exposure to sexually transmitted diseases. In an article in the *Wall Street Journal* (February 13, 2002), Jonathan Zenilman, a professor at Johns Hopkins School of Medicine, admitted: "It's embarrassing. People aren't trained to do this. It's not revenue-producing, and it takes time." In the article "Sexually Transmitted Diseases Appear Sharply Underreported," the reporter, Marilyn Chase, noted that a recent study of young adults in Baltimore found so many undiagnosed cases of chlamydia and gonorrhea in the 579 volunteers aged 18 to 35 that the researchers called into question the CDC's number of officially reported cases. It is estimated that in the year 2000 there were about 4 million new cases of chlamydia and almost 360,000 new cases of gonorrhea in the United States, both of which are diseases easily treated with antibiotics. The study's lead author, Charles Turner, recommended routine annual or biannual monitoring of these diseases in large metropolitan areas, and

J. Dennis Fortenberry of the University of Indiana Medical School suggested routine school-based urine testing for STDs, a recommendation that, of course, raises the controversial issues of cost, politics, and confidentiality. Nevertheless, he says, "The time has come." Judith Wasserheit, an expert in STDs and AIDS, believes that the wide prevalence of STDs reflects "how smart these bugs are—they spread almost like stealth bombs."

A message that cannot be ignored is this: people get sexually transmitted diseases by being infected via sex with someone who has an infection. Though typically passed on by intercourse, these diseases are also communicated through oral sex. Furthermore, any person who has ever been sexually active may have a sexually transmitted disease.

Fear should not prevent someone from seeing a doctor to find out whether he or she has a sexually transmitted disease. In most cases, a physician can diagnose this kind of disease via a physical exam, secretions culture, and/or a blood test. Anyone who believes he or she or a partner may have a disease should have an assessment because most sexually transmitted diseases lead to other, bigger problems when they are untreated.

The Majors

Chlamydia stealthily erodes one's health because the sufferer may have no symptoms at all, particularly in the case of women. In later stages, a woman may experience itchiness around her vagina; a yellow, odorless vaginal discharge; painful intercourse; and frequent urination. Some women have dull pain in the pelvic area, and others have intermittent bleeding. Men may have pain or burning when they urinate, and there can be a watery or milky-colored discharge from the penis. Unfortunately, chlamydia can result in pelvic inflammatory disease (PID) in women, and this disease makes many females infertile. In men, it can cause epididymitis—a painful swelling of the tubes that carry sperm from the testicles.

Syphilis has an early signal—the chancre, which is a painless, red sore that usually appears in places where an individual was touched during sex: genitals, anus, tongue, throat. Sometimes, glands near the chancre swell, and months later, the sufferer

experiences fever, sore throat, headache, and joint pain. Some people have a scaly rash on the soles of their feet and on their palms. After symptoms disappear, there may be no symptoms for years, but when these recur, the sinister infection can affect the brain, spinal cord, skin, and bone.

Gonorrhea, often called "the clap," manifests itself in a thick, yellow discharge from the penis and painful urination (in men), whereas women usually have no symptoms. When symptoms do appear in females, usually they are vaginal discharge (white, green, or yellow), painful urination, heavy bleeding during periods, and spotting between periods. Gonorrhea can also result in pelvic inflammatory disease. Those who participate in anal sex can have pain in the anus. Oral sex with a gonorrhea-infected individual can result in sore throat.

Herpes usually causes tingling or itching around the genitals, with small blisters that form and then burst open. There may be burning, especially during urination. Scabs form over these painful sores. The first herpes outbreak can also be accompanied by swollen glands, fever, and aching. Herpes sufferers can have outbreaks the rest of their lives; in many people, these becomes less frequent over time.

Hepatitis B sufferers have muscle aches, loss of appetite, fever, fatigue, headache, and dizziness. With progression of this disease, a person may have loose stools, yellow eyes and skin, dark urine, and tenderness in the liver area (just below the ribs on the right).

People who have human papillomavirus (HPV) may have soft, flesh-colored warts around the genital area or on the cervix; these warts are painless but can proliferate wildly. Sometimes the virus causes warts that are not visible. A huge downside is that HPV—the virus that causes genital warts—sometimes leads to cancer of the cervix or penis when it is untreated. A CDC research study showed that half of all cervical cancer cases can be attributed to human papillomavirus type 16. Another report says that HPV causes more than 95 percent of the 18,000 new cases of invasive cervical and anal cancer each year. Further, a study calls this percentage an underestimate, and researchers contend that HPV causes virtually all cases of cervical cancer, according to "Monitoring HPV Infection" (*Patient Care*, March 15, 2000).

Human immunodeficiency virus (HIV) causes acquired immunodeficiency syndrome (AIDS), which weakens the body's ability to fight off disease. With increased weakening of the immune system, the individual is blighted with illnesses until it is impossible to battle them successfully. Often, HIV symptoms—unexplained fatigue, night sweats, weight loss, and unusual infections—are slow to develop.

Scope of the STD Problem

The physical, psychological, and societal collateral damage due to sexually transmitted diseases is immense. Human papillomavirus infection accounts for more than one-third of the funds allocated annually in the United States for treating STDs. Since about one-third of new cases of STDs in the United States are genital warts, this is an enormous problem, leading to HPV infection costs of more than 42 percent of total direct medical STD-related expenditures in the United States, according to the American Social Health Association. The second most common disease reported to the CDC in 1999 was gonorrhea, with more than 360,000 official cases listed; the direct medical cost of treating gonorrhea in the United States is about $56 million yearly. The CDC estimates that the annual cost of chlamydia in the United States surpasses $2 billion. U.S. spending on HIV/AIDS for the fiscal year 2002 was $14.7 billion.

Considering the physical and emotional devastation of such diseases, it is impossible to overestimate their impact on individuals, couples, and families. For example, undiagnosed human papillomavirus may, in some individuals, lead to cervical cancer. A pregnant woman living with active herpes may require a cesarean section to prevent infection of her baby. A person with syphilis can suffer blindness, paralysis, heart damage, mental illness, and death. In some people, hepatitis B leads to liver failure or liver cancer, and thus death. Gonorrhea can lead to pelvic inflammatory disease. HIV leads to AIDS, a terminal illness.

Furthermore, people with sexually transmitted diseases are often ostracized because of prejudice or ignorance (some people still think they can contract HIV by hugging or touching people with this disease). Ostracism can have a devastating effect on the mental health of those who suffer from STDs, and the high incidence of depression in those who have HIV, AIDS, herpes, and other sexually transmitted diseases is not surprising.

The United States has federal laws that preclude discrimination against those with disabilities, but there are still cases of workplace and schoolhouse discrimination against those with HIV and AIDS. There are laws designed to protect those afflicted with disabilities from job loss, but courts continue to see cases in which people are harassed and fired. Other legal and social issues that cause difficulties for those with sexually transmitted diseases, especially HIV/AIDS, are home health care, managed care, care for the indigent, and care for those who are rendered incapable of employment as a result of illness.

Diagnosis and treatment guidelines in the *2002 Guidelines for Treatment of Sexually Transmitted Diseases* from the Centers for Disease Control and Prevention include new alternative regimens for scabies, bacterial vaginosis, early syphilis, and granuloma inguinale; expanded information on genital herpes diagnosis; new recommendations for treatment of recurrent genital herpes in those with HIV; expanded regimens for treating urethral warts; and inclusion of hepatitis C as a sexually transmitted infection.

Increasing Public Awareness

Many people do not even know that they have a sexually transmitted disease. Thus, these individuals may fail to seek treatment until the illnesses have advanced to the point that the diseases are already beginning to ravage their bodies. This underscores the importance of disseminating information in new and better ways. Consumers need an understanding of STDs and a feel for their own levels of susceptibility, given their own forms of sexual activity and partners. With knowledge in hand, people are more likely to seek evaluation for an STD even in the early stages, when symptoms are mild or even nonexistent but the individual knows he or she has participated in high-risk behavior.

It is hoped that a good fund of information will spur people to ask a doctor's advice if there is cause for concern. At the same time, this book is not meant to be a substitute for an in-person physical exam and evaluation by a physician.

A Look at the Global HIV/AIDS Picture

On November 28, 2001, Surgeon General David Satcher revisited the global HIV/AIDS picture—a health crisis that he had first described in April 1999. In 1999 and 2001 publications, he reiterated that "we know what works." Nevertheless, he still underscored the importance of educational efforts and emphasis on treatment, and he applauded the international community's increased display of commitment in the preceding two years. He stated that the base of the response to global HIV/AIDS is PPPs—public–private partnerships—such as the Accelerating Access Initiative (of United Nations [UN] agencies including UNAIDS and the World Health Organization [WHO] and seven research-based pharmaceutical companies); the Secure the Future Program in southern and West Africa; and the African Comprehensive HIV/AIDS Partnership in Botswana. Newest was the Global Fund to Fight AIDS, Tuberculosis, and Malaria.

Also, an unclassified version of a national intelligence estimate from the National Intelligence Council, "The Global Infectious Disease Threat and Its Implications for the United States," revealed that many people believe that new and reemerging infectious diseases will pose a rising global health threat and complicate U.S. and global security in this decade and the next. These diseases cause grave problems because they endanger U.S. citizens at home and abroad, threaten the armed forces deployed overseas, and worsen the social and political instability of key countries in which the United States has significant interests. Accounting for about one-fourth to one-third of an estimated 54 million deaths worldwide in 1998, infectious diseases remain a leading cause of death. Further, it is clear that infectious diseases are spread as much by human behavior (lifestyles, travel, inappropriate use of antibiotics) as by pathogen mutation.

Some of the key areas of difficulty are the following:

- Well-known diseases (200, including tuberculosis [TB], malaria, and cholera) have reemerged or spread geographically since 1973, and often the spread takes drug-resistant and/or more virulent forms.

- About 30 previously unknown disease agents have been identified since 1973; these include HIV, ebola, hepatitis C, and Nipah virus. There are no cures for these.
- Of the world's seven major killers, TB, malaria, hepatitis, and HIV/AIDS continue to surge. Experts predict that these four will cause the majority of deaths from infectious diseases by the year 2020.

And what is the impact of this news on the United States? Although the threat of infectious disease remains somewhat low compared to that of noninfectious diseases, the trend is definitely upward. The annual death rates in the United States of infectious diseases have almost doubled, to about 170,000, after hitting a historic low in 1980.

Some infectious diseases, such as West Nile virus, originate outside the United States and are ushered in by immigrants, travelers, military personnel, and animals or food. In fact, this route of transmission is viewed as such a threat that researchers at the U.S. Institute of Medicine contend that the next major infectious disease threat to the United States will be a previously unrecognized pathogen, as HIV was. Even if that eventually does not come to pass, HIV/AIDS, hepatitis C, TB, and more lethal variants of flu will pose major dangers in the United States in the next two decades. Here are some of the reasons—those that pertain to the role of sexually transmitted diseases in this picture:

- Emerging microbial resistance to drugs and continued new infections will sustain the HIV/AIDS problem—even though multidrug regimens have cut HIV/AIDS deaths by two-thirds, to about 16,000 a year, since 1995.
- About 4 million Americans are hepatitis C carriers, so the U.S. death toll from offshoots of hepatitis C, such as liver cancer and cirrhosis, may surpass that of HIV/AIDS by the year 2005.
- TB's comeback poses a huge health problem, one that creates a greater threat, which is due to multidrug-resistant strains and HIV/AIDS coinfection. Also, a large number of tuberculosis-infected illegal immigrants new to the United States will contribute to the spread.

Looking at the world picture, it is believed that the most vulnerable region is sub-Saharan Africa, where health care capacity is the poorest in the world, and death rates for many diseases, including HIV/AIDS and malaria, exceed those in all other regions. In the realm of HIV news, there is growing epidemiological evidence from sub-Saharan Africa that male circumcision reduces the risk of acquiring HIV.

Asia and the Pacific, with a huge spread of HIV/AIDS in South and Southeast Asia that is likely to spread to East Asia, could surpass Africa in number of HIV infections by 2010. In the Russian Federation, the number of HIV infections reached more than 200,000 by mid-2002—a large increase over the 10,993 reported in 1998. In Uzbekistan, there were almost as many new HIV infections in the first six months of 2002 as there were in the previous decade.

The Middle East and North Africa have a high prevalence of TB and hepatitis B and C. It is believed the low HIV infection rate is probably due to gross underreporting because of the stigma in Muslim societies associated with this disease.

Western Europe must deal with HIV/AIDS, TB, and hepatitis B and C, as well as some diseases of animal-to-human transmission origin.

In the National Intelligence Council report, three scenarios as to the course of infectious disease over the next two decades were studied. The "least likely" was one of steady progress—one that the report authors viewed as untenable, considering the ongoing demographic and socioeconomic challenges in developing countries, increasing microbial resistance to existing antibiotics, and tendency to underestimate the strength of the major killers, HIV/AIDS, TB, and malaria.

A second scenario was "progress stymied," meaning that we would see little or no progress in countering infectious diseases over the next two decades. This would mean that HIV/AIDS would reach catastrophic proportions as the virus spread through India, China, the former Soviet Union, and Latin America. On the other hand, this scenario could also be unlikely because it does not take into account prospects for socioeconomic development, international collaboration, and medical and health care advances that would restrain the spread of some diseases.

Finally, the third scenario is the one viewed most likely to occur. This would mean "deterioration, then limited improvement," whereby the infectious disease threat, especially from HIV/AIDS, would make the situation bleaker during the years up to 2010, when erratic improvements due to new drugs/vaccines, better prevention and control, and socioeconomic progress would occur. This improvement stage will occur only if a worst-possible scenario does not evolve; that would be one in which a deadly, highly infectious new disease takes hold; or there is a huge upward surge in the rate of HIV/AIDS; or a biological agent that is capable of rapid and widespread contagion is released.

The report also looked at implications for U.S. national security. Because the United States remains a major hub of commerce, immigration, and travel, the country and its interests abroad are always at risk from infectious diseases, and the following are pertinent issues:

- Infectious diseases will kill about 170,000 every year—unless that figure zooms up as a result of an epidemic of a yet-unknown disease or the HIV/AIDS drugs experience a huge decline in effectiveness.
- Infectious diseases will continue to account for more military hospital admissions than battlefield injuries. At highest risk are those soldiers in developing countries.
- The infectious disease burden will weaken the military capabilities of some countries because their armies and recruitment pools will experience HIV rates ranging from 10 to 60 percent.
- Infectious diseases will slow socioeconomic development in former communist countries and developing countries.
- Infectious disease–related embargoes and restrictions on travel and immigration will contribute to frictions between developed and developing countries.
- The probability of a bioterrorist attack against U.S. civilian and military personnel overseas or in the United States will grow as more groups and states develop biological warfare capabilities.

Note: All data on global disease incidence, including data from WHO, must be viewed as primarily indicative of trends rather than precise and accurate measures of disease prevalence. In developing countries, these diseases are unreported or underreported for several reasons: the stigma, the lack of adequate resources for reporting, and the reluctance of countries' governments to reveal real figures for fear of generating massive losses in trade and tourism. Another problem is that diagnosis and reporting are blurred because morbidity and mortality rates can be multicausal. For example, the ranking of AIDs mortality rate ahead of TB mortality rate can be attributed to the fact that HIV-positive individuals dying of TB were included in the AIDS mortality group in the most recent WHO survey.

London, England, posted the highest chlamydia infection rates in 1999. The figure was 155 per 100,000 men and 184 per 100,000 women. Furthermore, London doctors conjecture that these reported infections are only about 10 percent of all cases. From 1999 to 2000 in the United Kingdom, the incidence of chlamydia rose by 17 percent, and the number of cases doubled from 1994 to 2000. About 9 percent of sexually active U.K. women 25 and younger have chlamydia. With a higher incidence in teens and low socioeconomic groups, chlamydia is important because most infections exist in the absence of symptoms—and such infections have major consequences.

In Retrospect

To see how matters have changed in regard to sexually transmitted diseases, consider the contents of the article "Prophylaxis of Venereal Disease," which appeared in the *Journal of the American Medical Association,* December 7, 1901.

Citing their shock that "150,000 cases of venereal disease" were under treatment in the borough of Manhattan in 1900, the authors state that "legal regulation of prostitution seems inadvisable, not only because of the opposition that any question of even qualified toleration of vice arouses among English-speaking people, but especially because all methods of legal regulation hitherto attempted have proved failures." They add that "segregation of prostitutes in one part of the city smacks too much of quasi authorization, or at least toleration,

of vice," and they recommend "domiciliary segregation," adding that "immoral persons must not under any circumstances be allowed to live in the same house with those who lead moral lives." This can be accomplished, the authors contend, by suppressing all external prostitution signs: red lights, red curtains, street soliciting, window tapping, and so on. Doctors can use a prophylactic strategy of educating the public with regard to "risks of venereal diseases and the difficulty and uncertainty of their cure." Furthermore, family physicians are urged to express themselves "candidly," to tell "young men that sexual indulgence is not necessary to health and may involve serious infection with enduring disease." They advise requiring hospitals that receive state aid to make arrangements for treating venereal diseases; suppressing all advertisements of preventives, and so forth, that encourage vice by promising impunity; making transmission of syphilis an offense that would merit a jail sentence (adding that this probably could not be enforced but that its presence on the statute book would be "a striking educational measure"); and concluding that the "careful humane enforcement of existing laws is the best prophylaxis for venereal disease." Clearly, there was rising concern over the predicament that sexually transmitted diseases caused, but no one could agree on the proper answer. All ideas advanced were fraught with tinges of ethics and morals, and thus their wisdom was limited to pointing accusing fingers at prostitutes and randy young male customers. The buds of an education program were launched; as is clear from current statistics, it apparently failed miserably—or fell on deaf ears.

And, sadly, the major change in the spread of sexually transmitted diseases is that these have proliferated greatly and have become mainstream problems as they increased exponentially over the decades since 1901. Unfortunately, surveys and studies illustrate graphically the brass-tacks facts—that many people still do not understand the most basic information on STDs or consider them a matter of much concern. Whereas many people think HIV poses a risk to women primarily if they are needle sharing in IV drug use, the truth is, women are most likely today to contract HIV through heterosexual activity with an infected partner. Also, few people understand that the CDC recommends HIV testing six months after possible exposure—because antibodies take three to six months to appear. (Many people think they should have an HIV test a month after any suspected exposure.)

Many people do not know that having a sexually transmitted disease will increase the risk of contracting HIV; for example, genital sores enhance receptiveness to the virus via an immune response triggered by STDs.

Another little-known fact: some medical centers now offer postexposure HIV drug therapy for those who have had unsafe sex in the past few days; patients take multiple drugs daily for at least 30 days, but there is no guarantee that this treatment actually works.

Recent Findings

In the rapidly changing world of HIV and other sexually transmitted diseases, it is not easy to stay on top of the many new developments that researchers unveil on a regular basis. Some of the latest reports are the following:

- A report in *Science* (March 2002) tells of a gene in rats that appears to produce a compound that could be protective against sexually transmitted diseases. The gene seems to show great potential for fighting microbes, including HIV. Researchers hope to develop a drug that would be a microbicide and contraceptive.

- A study suggests that protection of a woman's cervix is very important in preventing the transmission of HIV. This is especially critical information for those in developing countries where women lack the power to control how sex occurs, because these females could for the first time be able to protect themselves from STDs by using a diaphragm, which does not requires a partner's knowledge or consent. Researchers view the cervix as a "hot spot" in its susceptibility to HIV infection, and this means that barrier protection by a diaphragm may have greater potential for disease protection than was previously believed. Researchers have seen that the upper genital tract is very vulnerable to sexually transmitted diseases. The

belief being advanced is that using a diaphragm with a topical microbicide would constitute prevention, especially since there is currently no vaccine or solution for all STDs. If these findings hold up in other research, many women in the United States may show a resurgence of interest in diaphragms.

- Once a person contracts HIV, he or she can pass on the virus to another person via sexual activity within a week or two. Documented in the *Journal of the American Medical Association* (October 10, 2001), a study conducted at the University of North Carolina at Chapel Hill and in Switzerland showed that in some cases, the transmission of the virus can take place before the infected individual experiences any of the flulike symptoms that are typical of early-stage HIV. This is noteworthy because for the first time it has been proved that sexual transmission can happen readily. This was suspected but never before confirmed. It has tremendous repercussions for those who are sexually active in that persons engaging in unsafe sex cannot assume that they are not HIV infected or infectious, even though they had a recent negative test finding for HIV.

- Researchers suggest that self-obtained vaginal swabs could help control the spread of sexually transmitted diseases. These can help detect treatable STDs in teens, and it appears that young people would be willing to use these swabs. Investigators looked at 512 African-American teenage women in a nonclinical program; the participants were offered a choice of STD screening method—pelvic exam or the use of vaginal swabs. None of the participants chose the first option. Most of the young women had no symptoms, whereas results showed that 28.7 percent had one or more STDs.

- In February 2002, there were news reports of transmission of HIV by a blood transfusion at a hospital in San Antonio, Texas. The donor had not had the infection long enough for its presence to show up in regular blood-screening procedures. This was the first such case in decades, since the inception of stringent blood screening was instituted in the United States.

- Scientists discovered high levels of HIV in the saliva, semen, vaginal fluid, and blood of people newly infected by the virus, and these levels were higher than or as high as levels in those people with long-standing infection. A second key finding in this University of North Carolina study was that virus levels (viral load) dropped quickly in all fluids after the patients were treated with drug therapy. Previously, the jury was out on whether drugs worked during primary infection. These are findings that suggest using combination antiretroviral therapy as an avenue of health intervention early on. The strategy would be to reduce shedding of HIV in semen and vaginal fluid with the goal of lowering the number of people contracting the virus. Medical scientists have been concentrating on primary HIV infection to understand the virus's mode of attacking the body. They had long been suspicious that primary infection with HIV was a time of high infectiousness.

- A study presented at the 2000 meeting of the Interscience Congress on Antimicrobial Agents and Chemotherapy in Toronto, Canada, showed better results for suppressive (daily-pill) therapy for herpes than for episodic therapy for those with recurring infections. The 225 patients, all of whom had three to 10 flare-ups a year, could use episodic treatment (drugs twice daily for five consecutive days used only when experiencing recurrences) or daily suppressive treatment. Results showed that recurrences were almost five times more frequent in the episodic treatment group. During the first 24-week period, 42 percent of patients on suppressive therapy had flare-ups, compared to 91 percent of those on episodic therapy. In the second 24-week period, the figures were 44 percent (suppressive) and 74.5 (episodic).

- Self-testing by teenage girls who provided vaginal samples they obtained during a two-year study revealed a high percentage of undiagnosed sexually transmitted diseases. This underscored the belief that self-testing can be very valuable in detecting undiagnosed sexually transmitted diseases and preventing their spread. Nearly 13 percent of women who had never previously had a gynecological exam had a positive test finding for an STD, and 51 percent of infected students would not have pursued STD testing by means of a traditional exam. The participants were 228 teenage women. Diseases were trichomoniasis, chlamydia, and gonorrhea.

- A study of 3,500 visitors to an STD clinic in Atlanta, Georgia, revealed that although many people have no idea how to protect themselves from STDs, counseling does make a difference. What most surprised investigators were the many basic misconceptions about the kinds of behavior that prevent infection. Upon initial interviews, about half said they thought douching protected them from STDs. About 20 percent believed use of birth control pills protected them from STDs. Some thought that washing and urinating after sex were both protective measures. Three months after their visit to the clinic, half of those who previously believed myths were found to be better informed in a retrospective survey.

- Researchers have found that one reason for the difficulties involved in developing vaccines against STDs is that these pose extremely different and formidable challenges because of the repetitive exposure to the infecting virus.

- Scientists are seeing much greater risk for HIV infection in women who have genital ulcers. Studies show a clear link between sexually transmitted diseases and the risk of sexual HIV transmission.

- On February 24, 2003, TV networks broadcast the news that the AIDSVAX vaccine had failed, but 20 other vaccines for HIV/AIDS are still in the works. VaxGen, maker of AIDSVAX, plans to continue to analyze the study data to determine the vaccine's effectiveness in preventing HIV transmission in some subgroups (blacks and Asians).

- A study points to anal cancer screening as a way to save lives at a reasonable cost. A simple procedure (much like a Pap smear) can result in detection of cancerous lesions among high-risk HIV-negative men, removal of lesions, and early treatment of anal cancer.

- Researchers cite HPV as a likely cause of certain head and neck cancers—but it is also associated with improved survival rates (more so than such cancers stemming from other causes). In findings reported in the May 2000 *Journal of the National Cancer Institute*, data showed that although HPV deoxyribonucleic acid (DNA) has been seen in head and neck cancers for some time, its role in cancer development and the means of transmission to the upper airway have been unclear.

- A new study shows that people with genital herpes but no symptoms still shed herpes simplex virus (HSV) in the genital area. Estimates suggest that one of four Americans has HSV-2, but most do not know it. It is believed that about one in five is actually aware of his or her infection. Doctors are being encouraged to pay more attention to asymptomatic HSV-2. Women and men without symptoms were equally likely to shed.

- In 2002, Dr. Steven Morin presented information on San Francisco trends that point to a new rise in HIV incidence over each successive quarter of 2000. Focus groups of men who have sex with men gathered to work on prevention plans to address the problem, and they looked at the reasons behind the increase in HIV infections, what has changed in the past decade that may have contributed to the problem, and what can be done. The groups came up with a list of factors contributing to HIV transmission: denial of risk, sense of inevitability of getting HIV, loneliness, low self-esteem, drug use, and greater opportunities for social services, assistance, and so on. The group felt that several conditions had changed in recent years: people were now less likely to perceive HIV as a health threat among those who were not HIV-positive; there was less media and friend communication about HIV; and the gay community's norms had changed, with increasing peer pressure to be unsafe and a celebration of "bareback" sex.

- A study showed that low blood levels of HIV appear to reduce risk of heterosexual transmission, according to results published in the *New England Journal of Medicine* (March 2000). Thus, it seems clear that using antiviral drug regimens will reduce viral load and therefore reduce likelihood of heterosexual transmission. Also, researchers saw that circumcision was associated with less likelihood of acquiring HIV.

- New research shows that small blips in HIV levels (termed intermittent viremia) may not be as ominous as was once believed. According to two studies published in the *Journal of the American Medical Association* in July 2001, the widely held belief was that blips in virus levels in an HIV patient on highly active antiretroviral therapy (HAART) indicated drug failure (detectable levels seemed to show that the doctor should change medications for this patient because the virus was exhibiting signs of drug resistance). Now it is believed that slight virus-level surges do not necessarily point to drug resistance.

- Researchers advanced a new belief that people with drug-resistant strains of HIV can still benefit from HAART treatment via a report in the February 2001 issue of the *New England Journal of Medicine*. The existing belief was that although a drug cocktail zaps HIV from the blood of some patients, another large group of HIV patients (as many as half or more) see the virus persist even with HAART treatment because, apparently, the virus is drug-resistant. In a small group (16 male volunteers with drug-resistant HIV), researchers saw two interesting results when 10 of the men stopped drug therapy for 12 weeks: (1) the HIV level in their blood rose quickly, suggesting that the drugs were managing to moderate virus levels even though they were not maximally effective; and (2) the number of disease-fighting CD4 cells dropped faster in the men not treated than in those treated. The suspicion now is that discontinuing treatment makes virus particles that are drug-susceptible more likely to proliferate and kill immune cells than their drug-resistant peers.

- Whereas casual contact (kissing, holding hands, etc.) has never been viewed as a viable means of HIV transmission, Argentine researchers are now suggesting the possibility that casual household contact could be the cause of a new case of HIV. Initially, it was believed that an HIV-infected man with open sores infected his child—a report discussed widely in Buenos Aires at the first International AIDS Society Conference on HIV Pathogenesis and Treatment (July 2001). The research scientist Ana Ceballos said that scientific data gave a strong indication that transmission was due to father–child contact. The three-year-old boy had an opportunistic infection seen chiefly in AIDS patients—cryptosporidium infection—and testing showed that he did indeed have HIV in a strain almost exactly like that of his parent. On the other hand, the report coauthor, Silvia Gonzalez Ayala, remained unconvinced that this was not a case of vertical transmission (mother-to-child). She hypothesized that the father's sperm, when fertilizing the egg from which the child developed, probably contained HIV. Also, from the time the child was only six months old, he had AIDS-like diseases, but the mother was not HIV-positive. Yet to be ruled out are drug-related needlestick transmission (the father is an IV drug user) and sexual contact. Ceballos and Gonzalez Ayala are now investigating three other Argentine cases that involve mothers without HIV but HIV-positive fathers and children.

- At the International AIDS Society Conference on HIV Pathogenesis and Treatment in July 2001, experts predicted a huge explosion of the AIDS epidemic in coming decades unless billions can be spent on education, prevention, and treatment. Stated were figures of 200 million with HIV in 20 years, 100 million of them dead by 2020.

- Boehringer Ingelheim launched two Phase III trials of tipranavir, a new protease inhibitor (PI) that bonds to the enzyme differently than do PIs now available. This was announced in February 2003. The U.S. study RESIST 1 addresses those HIV patients who have developed resistance to PIs. Early evidence suggests that tipranavir has shown activity against HIV with multiple protease resistance mutations. For information on RESIST trial sites, see www.clinicaltrials.gov.

- Reported at the 10th Annual Conference on Retroviruses and Opportunistic Infections in Boston in February 2003, a large study on structured treatment interruption (STI) revealed strong evidence that unsupervised STI can be dangerous for those with advanced HIV.

- In his January 2003 State of the Union speech, President George Bush unveiled a surprising new AIDS initiative including $15 billion for Africa and the Caribbean.

FREQUENTLY USED ABBREVIATIONS

ACTG	AIDS Clinical Trials Group
ACTU	AIDS Clinical Trial Unit
ACT UP	AIDS Coalition to Unleash Power
ADAPs	AIDS drug assistance programs
AIDS	acquired immunodeficiency syndrome
amFAR	American Foundation for AIDS Research
AMA	American Medical Association
ARC	AIDS-related complex
ARV	AIDS-associated retrovirus
ASCUS	atypical squamous cells of undetermined significance
AZT	azidothymidine
BV	bacterial vaginosis
CBC	complete blood count
CDC	Centers for Disease Control and Prevention
CID	Center for Infectious Diseases
CIN	cervical intraepithelial neoplasia
CIS	carcinoma in situ
CMV	cytomegalovirus
CNS	central nervous system
COBRA	Consolidated Omnibus Budget Reconciliation Act of 1985
CSF	cerebrospinal fluid
CT	computed tomography (CT scan)
DNA	deoxyribonucleic acid
DNR	do not resuscitate
EGWs	external genital warts
ELISA	enzyme-linked immunosorbent assay
EPSDT	Early and Periodic Screening, Diagnosis, and Treatment

EBV	Epstein-Barr virus
ESR	erythrocyte sedimentation rate
FDA	Food and Drug Administration (U.S.)
FTA-ABS	fluorescent treponemal antibody-absorption test
GLS	generalized lymphadenopathy syndrome
GMHC	Gay Men's Health Crisis
GRID	gay-related immunodeficiency disease
HAART	highly active antiretroviral therapy
HCFA	Health Care Financing Administration
HIV	human immunodeficiency virus
HPV	human papillomavirus
HRT	hormone replacement therapy
HSIL	high-grade squamous intraepithelial lesion
HSV	herpes simplex virus
HTLV I, II, III	Human T cell lymphotropic virus types I–III
IDU	injection drug user
ITP	idiopathic thrombocytopenic purpura
IND	Investigational new drug
IUD	intrauterine device
IV	intravenous
KS	Kaposi's sarcoma
LEEP	loop electrocautery excision procedure
LGV	lymphogranuloma venereum

LP	lumbar puncture		PID	pelvic inflammatory disease
LSIL	low-grade squamous intraepithelial lesion		PIs	protease inhibitors
			PLWA	Persons living with AIDS
MAC	*Mycobacterium avium* complex		PMS	premenstrual syndrome
MACS	Multicenter AIDS Cohort Study		PWA	Person with AIDS
MPC	mucopurulent cervicitis		RNA	ribonucleic acid
MRI	magnetic resonance imaging		RPR	rapid plasma reagin
NCI	National Cancer Institute		SAIDS	simian acquired immunodeficiency syndrome
NETSS	National Electronic Telecommunications System for Surveillance		SIL	squamous intraepithelial lesion
NGU	nongonococcal urethritis		STD	sexually transmitted disease
NHL	non-Hodgkin's lymphoma		TB	tuberculosis
NIAID	National Institute of Allergy and Infectious Diseases (U.S.)		TMP-SMX	trimethoprim-sulfamethoxazole
			UTI	urinary tract infection
NIH	National Institutes of Health		VAIN	vaginal intraepithelial neoplasia
NNRTIs	nonnucleoside reverse transcriptase inhibitors		VD	venereal disease
			VDRL	Venereal Disease Research Laboratory
NRTIs	nucleoside reverse transcriptase inhibitors		VIN	vulvar intraepithelial neoplasia
OI	opportunistic infection		WHO	World Health Organization
PCP	*Pneumocystis carinii* pneumonia		ZDV	zidovudine (AZT)

ENTRIES A–Z

abscess A localized collection of pus anywhere in the body, surrounded by damaged and inflamed tissues. An abscess can occur as a complication of pelvic inflammatory disease.

abstinence The act of refraining voluntarily from some form of indulgence: liquor, foods, or sexual activity. In the context of sexually transmitted diseases, as well as pregnancy, abstinence is touted as the only 100 percent safe means of prevention. Essentially, in sexual terms, *abstinence* is defined as absolute absence of sexual contact with a partner, thus eliminating any possibility of pregnancy or of contracting sexually transmitted diseases.

access to treatment Also referred to as "access to medical care," this is one criterion by which health care systems are measured as to quality and responsiveness to needs of the public. In respect to the treatment of HIV/AIDS, early accessing of drug therapies has sometimes been at odds with governmental agencies' lengthy processes required for approval of experimental drugs. Activist groups have taken up this issue in an effort to gain speedier approval of drugs needed for those with HIV/AIDS.

acidophilus These bacteria help maintain a healthy bacterial environment in the digestive system. Sold in concentrated form in health food stores, acidophilus consists of live bacteria taken to alter the flora of the digestive system and replace harmful organisms. Some AIDS patients find acidophilus supplements helpful in the management of diarrhea and thrush.

acquired immunodeficiency syndrome AIDS is the appropriate diagnosis for anyone 13 years or older who has HIV and has one of the Centers for Disease Control and Prevention–defined AIDS indicator illnesses—or an HIV-positive individual who has a specific CD4+ T cell count (less than 200 CD4+ cells per cubic millimeter of blood) that rates an AIDS diagnosis, even if this person has not experienced any serious illnesses. In children younger than 13, the definition of AIDS is similar except that lymphoid interstitial pneumonitis and recurrent bacterial infections are included in the list of AIDS-defining conditions.

Acquired immunodeficiency syndrome is the late stage of a serious disease that is caused by infection with human immunodeficiency virus (HIV), which attacks a person's immune system and decreases the number of CD4+ cells (or helper T cells), key elements in the immune defense of the body. As the number of these cells decreases in a person with HIV, the immune system becomes weaker and thus more susceptible to being ravaged by opportunistic infections and tumors. When the CD4+ count goes below 200 cells/mm3, or the person has one or more opportunistic infections or tumors, a diagnosis of AIDS is considered appropriate. This definition follows standards set by the Centers for Disease Control and Prevention (CDC). Healthy individuals have T cell counts of 600 to 1,000.

The rate of conversion from HIV to AIDS is a subject of extensive investigation, because it differs greatly from individual to individual. In some who contract HIV, AIDS develops very soon thereafter, but in others full-blown AIDS does not develop for 10 or more years. Highly active antiretroviral therapy (HAART) often slows the rate at which HIV weakens the immune system.

According to the CDC, dating from the beginning of the AIDS epidemic, 816,149 cases of AIDS had been reported in the United States through December 2001; this included 666,026 cases in men and 141,048 in women. In children 13 and below, there had been 9,075 AIDS cases. By race and ethnicity, whites had 343,889 reported cases; African Americans, 313,180; Hispanics, 149,752; Asians/Pacific Islanders, 6,157; American Indians/Alaska Natives, 2,537; and race/ethnicity unknown, 634.

AIDS deaths from the start of the epidemic through December 2001 totaled 467,910. Of these, those dying of HIV-related causes were 29 percent whites, 52 percent blacks, 18 percent Hispanics, and less than 1 percent Asians/Pacific Islanders and American Indians/Alaska Natives.

By the late 1990s, the United States saw a decline in AIDS deaths due to advances in treatments that slowed the progression of HIV. However, in recent years, the rate of decline for cases and deaths began to slow. In 1999, the number of new cases reported annually appeared to be leveling off. At the same time, the decline in AIDS deaths had slowed a great deal. The upshot has been that a larger number of people are now living with AIDS than ever before.

Another important figure is the dramatic reduction in vertical transmission of HIV, which appears to reflect the emphasis by various agencies of public health on routine counseling and voluntary testing for pregnant women. This shows the effect of many health services offering pregnant women with HIV the option of taking zidovudine and giving affected infants the medication after birth.

At the outset, AIDS was mainly a disease affecting gay men in the age range of 25 to 44, but as gay men began to see many of their friends die of AIDS, they started safe-sex practices, which resulted in a dramatic shift in demographics. Whereas about 68 to 78 percent of AIDS cases in 1985 were seen in male homosexuals, Americans witnessed an upsurge in female cases, especially Hispanic and black women, at the dawn of the new millennium. Many of these women contracted the disease through sex with an intravenous drug user. As of 2002, the rates of HIV in the black and His-

panic communities were much higher than among Caucasians.

In full-blown AIDS, opportunistic infections (OIs) can wreak havoc, devastating health. The immune system, already ravaged by HIV, has difficulty fighting off viruses, certain bacteria, and other microbes, and in many instances, these OIs prove fatal. The AIDS sufferer with OIs may be subject to symptoms such as coughing, shortness of breath, seizures, confusion and forgetfulness, severe diarrhea that is hard to resolve, fever, vision loss, severe headaches, weight loss, extreme fatigue, nausea, vomiting, decreased coordination, coma, stomach cramps, and difficult, sometimes painful swallowing. Children with AIDS also experience ear infections, tonsillitis, and eye infections.

Those who have AIDS also are vulnerable to virus-induced cancers: Kaposi's sarcoma, cervical cancer, and lymphomas. Furthermore, if an individual has AIDS, these diseases are harder to treat and usually very aggressive.

In light-skinned people with AIDS, the signs of Kaposi's sarcoma are round brown, reddish, or purple spots on the skin or in the mouth. These are more pigmented in dark-skinned people.

The crucial CD4+ T cells gradually decline as AIDS progresses. Some even experience dramatic dips in their counts. This disease is so variable that an individual who has a CD4+ T cell count above 200 cells/mm3 may experience early HIV symptoms, whereas others with counts below 200 remain free of symptoms.

As is obvious from reviewing the severe health effects of AIDS, this disease can be so debilitating that it forces an individual to quit his or her job. Some are unable to perform even simple household chores. There are AIDS sufferers who have periods in which they can function normally, interrupted by extremely ill periods.

See also HIV.

activism Vigorous and vocal action with the intent of achieving certain political goals. In respect to AIDS, this word has come to refer to united efforts to keep HIV and AIDS issues in the forefront of public consciousness so that those who have HIV/AIDS are empowered in accessing public services and rights and in fighting instances of discrimination.

ACT UP   See AIDS COALITION TO UNLEASH POWER.

acupressure   A popular Chinese technique that is included under the umbrella term *alternative medicine,* acupressure usually calls for using finger pressure on specific points of the body in order to relieve various forms of pain and tension. Some people also do acupressure by applying pressure with blunt needles; others use devices such as balls. Advocates assert that acupressure can relieve muscular tension by increasing blood flow to tissue. It is also believed that acupressure serves to trigger release of endorphins, which are neurochemicals that ease pain. Some people with HIV and AIDS try acupressure for pain relief. The most widely known form of needleless acupressure is shiatsu, in which practitioners use finger pressure on certain body points to stimulate *chi* (vital energy).

acupuncture   A traditional Chinese system of healing in which symptoms are relieved by pressing or puncturing with needles at specific body sites in order to relieve pain or tension. Viewed by the traditional medical establishment as alternative medicine, acupuncture has many advocates who swear by its effectiveness. An acupuncturist seeks to correct deficiencies of *chi,* or life energy, and thereby enhance the patient's health. The thrust of the treatment is helping the patient balance the *chi* energy among his or her organs. To this end, needles are used to direct *chi* to specific areas in the body and to drain excessive *chi.* In essence, what this boils down to is that the needling serves to activate deep sensory nerves, thus causing the brain to release endorphins, which are generally considered the brain's natural painkillers. Popular for use in smoking cessation and as part of drug-abuse rehabilitation, acupuncture is also used for pain management for those with cancer and with HIV/AIDS.

acute respiratory distress syndrome   The sudden onset of severe diffuse lung injury, which usually occurs within 24 to 72 hours of a predisposing event. Although there are many causes, infection and trauma are two of the most common. Patients with acute respiratory distress syndrome (ARDS) often require mechanical ventilation because of respiratory failure. ARDS was formerly known as adult respiratory distress syndrome.

acyclovir   An antiviral drug that is commonly used to treat herpes simplex virus infections.

adenopathy   Swelling or enlargement of lymph nodes.

adenovirus   One of a group of DNA-containing viruses that most commonly causes upper and lower respiratory tract infections but that can also cause other illnesses such as conjunctivitis (eye infection). Forty-nine types that cause human illness have been found. Certain types have been shown to cause malignancy in rodents.

adherence   Compliance or a patient's cooperation with a medical professional's recommendations concerning a specific therapy. In regard to HIV disease, adherence has been cited as an important determinant of degree and duration of virologic suppression. Studies have supported the belief that there is a strong association between poor adherence and failed virologic suppression. In several studies, nonadherence by patients on highly active antiretroviral therapy (HAART) was the strongest predictor of failure to achieve viral suppression below the level of detection. It has also been documented that 90 to 95 percent of doses must be taken for optimal suppression; lesser degrees of compliance are more often associated with virologic failure. In regard to HIV, imperfect adherence by patients is commonplace. When a study group of HIV patients was queried concerning their compliance with their medication regimens, one-third admitted to missing doses within three days of the survey. Reasons cited were forgetting, being busy or depressed, disliking adverse side effects, or being ill. In one urban center, one-fifth of HIV-infected patients did not fill their prescriptions. It seems logical that the instability of homelessness would automatically lead to a lack of adherence, but that has not proved to be the case universally. One program had a 70 percent adherence rate in homeless HIV-infected individuals, and the high rate of compliance was attributed to the program's flexible clinic hours, accessible clinic staff, and incentives. Predictors of poor adherence include lack of rapport between clinician and patient, drug/alcohol use, mental illness, lack of patient education, inability of patients to identify their medications, lack of access to medical care or medication, and domestic violence. The individuals most likely to adhere to a drug regimen in a reliable manner are ones who have strong support systems, the ability to adapt to taking medication as a part of their routine, an understanding of the importance of taking all medications, and a comfort level with taking medication when other people are present.

Since patient reporting is not considered a reliable source of adherence information, using aids to measure adherence, such as pill counts, pharmacy records, and smart pill bottles with computer chips that record each opening, is preferred.

Improving adherence to HAART can usually be accomplished via several strategies: setting up a treatment plan that the patient understands and commits to following, providing education on goals of therapy, clarifying reasons for strict adherence, informing family of the importance of adherence, and recruiting supporters to enhance the likelihood of adherence.

According to the *2001 Guidelines for the Use of Antiretroviral Agents in HIV-Infected Adults and Adolescents,* some interventions that appear to improve the adherence of those using drug therapy for HIV are pharmacist counseling, clinic personnel counseling; discussion of adherence at each visit; reminders, alarms, pagers, and pillbox timers; patient education aids (regimen pictures, stickers, calendars); and clinician education aids.

advocacy Action by a patient or an interested party that is designed to enhance the likelihood of having full and ample access to health care options and services. In today's health care system, it is believed by many that delivery of proper care is facilitated and promoted by having an assertive patient advocate. Such efforts for those with HIV/AIDS are many and varied.

affective disorder See MOOD DISORDERS.

affirmations Declarations of specific emotional-health platforms, the repetition of which is meant to soothe tension and heighten resolve. Some patients battling HIV/AIDS repeat affirmations as a means of helping them cope with the emotional aspect of the disease.

African Americans and HIV/AIDS The AIDS epidemic has had a devastating effect on African Americans. By December 2001, the CDC had reports of 315,000 cases of AIDS in African Americans, of an overall figure of 816,000 cases of AIDS. Of 362,827 Americans living with AIDS as of December 2001, 42 percent were African Americans.

Researchers estimate that one in 50 African-American men and one in 160 African-American women are infected with HIV. Sadly, African-American children represented two-thirds (65 percent) of all reported cases of pediatric AIDS.

New HIV infections among African Americans in the United States in 2001 were 54 percent, although they are only 13 percent of the U.S. population. Of new HIV infections in women in the United States in 2001, 64 percent were in African-American women. Of new infections in men in the United States as of December 2001, half were in African-American men.

Health care professionals are acutely aware that the prevention thrust to reach African Americans must take into consideration that in those African Americans with AIDS, men who have sex with men are the largest percentage (37 percent) of reported cases since the start of the AIDS epidemic. In African-American men, the second most frequent exposure is injection drug use (34 percent), followed by heterosexual exposure (8 percent cumulative cases). In African-American women, injection drug use accounts for 42 percent (since the outset of the AIDS epidemic), and 8 percent of cumulative cases stem from heterosexual exposure.

In studying prevention challenges for African Americans, researchers have found that two common ways substance abuse leads to HIV and other STDs are trading sex for drugs and sharing needles. Another arm of the prevention effort has looked at enlisting the help of local leaders in acknowledging the problem and helping to combat HIV/AIDS in their communities.

AIDS   See ACQUIRED IMMUNODEFICIENCY SYNDROME.

AIDS-associated retrovirus (ARV)   The name given in the early '80s to a retrovirus that was isolated in people with AIDS and in people without any symptoms but in AIDS risk groups. In 1985, ARV and two other viruses—human T-lymphotropic virus type III (HTLV-III) and lymphadenopathy-associated virus—were analyzed and determined to be in the same retroviral family. In 1986, these viruses were renamed the human immunodeficiency virus (HIV).

See also HUMAN IMMUNODEFICIENCY VIRUS.

AIDS Clinical Trials Group   The AIDS Clinical Trials Group is a nationwide network of multicenter clinical trials that focus on testing HIV drugs and treatments. These drugs are used for treating HIV and opportunistic infections and tumors and stimulating the immune system. It is notable that these trials have spawned most of the information available today on treatments for HIV patients. Also known as AIDS Clinical Trial Units, these make up a consortium of ACTUs called ACTG, which is funded federally through the National Institutes of Health. The ACTG is the largest clinical trials group for HIV in the world, boasting the most researchers, the largest number of participants, and the biggest budget.

AIDS Coalition to Unleash Power (ACT UP)   The AIDS activist group that is the best known, the AIDS Coalition to Unleash Power—a group that sought to get HIV/AIDS issues out on the table in order to enhance proper treatment of those who suffer from the disease—was launched in 1987 in New York. This group has influenced public health policy through action-oriented development of political clout, intended to reduce bias and ensure equal treatment.

AIDS denialists   Those who do not believe that HIV is the cause of AIDS are termed AIDS denialists, because, in essence, they are denying what the scientific community worldwide acknowledges as truth—that HIV does cause AIDS. Not surprisingly, these people are the bane of the existence of those who have spent decades promoting safe sex, HIV testing, and HIV/AIDS treatment.

The term *AIDS denialists* applies to members of a movement called Homosexuals Intransigent and others who believe that attributing causation of AIDS to the human immunodeficiency virus is a government plot to sabotage homosexuals. Their contention is that homophobic politicians want to "scare people out of homosexuality." The denialists call Centers for Disease Control and Prevention data fraudulent and claim that it is very suspicious that AIDS has been redefined at least three times—undoubtedly, in order to encompass a greater number of indicator diseases and, thus, inflate the numbers of those infected. Another tenet of their argument is that it makes no sense for a sexually transmitted disease to be distributed unevenly in the United States; in other words, more than half of new AIDS cases in 1998 were among people living in New York, Florida, New Jersey, California, and Texas. The writer of the article "Everything Government Says about AIDS Is False" also claims that there have "always been far more heterosexuals than homosexuals with AIDS from the very start," and that "the patterns of AIDS are not consistent with a viral disease spread by sex and blood." These AIDS dissidents believe that AIDS is a chemical injury that results from using recreational drugs and from having toxic "treatments" for HIV, especially AZT—and that the government and media have collaborated to hide the truth of the true origin of AIDS from the American public. The denialists further urge gay men to avoid HIV tests and anti-HIV therapies, and they protest that AIDS is not infectious—that it occurs independently. For more on their theories, see http://www.virusmyth.com.

On the same note, the retrovirologist Peter Duesberg has been a very vocal critic of the causal association made between HIV and the immune suppression that leads to an AIDS-indicative illness. His assertion is that drug use is a major cause of AIDS-associated immune suppression. To respond to this claim, a study was designed wherein cohorts of homosexual and heterosexual men were compared; when subjects were matched for use of marijuana, cocaine, or amphetamines, it was found there was no link between development of AIDS and use of drugs. The homosexual cohort did use more nitrites than did the heterosexual one, but the development of AIDS was related to presence of infection (HIV) and not to drug use. (Nitrite inhalants, originally used to treat certain heart conditions, have sometimes been used as sex stimulants by gays.)

Duesberg also asserted that promiscuity is a cause of AIDS, a theory that history disproves, in that promiscuous behavior has been around for centuries. Cases would have been seen in prostitutes before 1978 if promiscuity were behind AIDS. Duesberg noted, "In America, only promiscuity aided by aphrodisiac and psychoactive drugs, practiced mostly by 20- to 40-year-old male homosexuals and some heterosexuals, seems to correlate with AIDS diseases."

If he were correct, why did AIDS not appear sooner? It has been documented in studies that many homosexuals had multiple sex partners in the pre-AIDS period. In a 1969 survey, more than 40 percent of white homosexual men and one-third of black homosexual men reported that they had had at least 500 partners over their lifetime, and one-fourth more reported 100 to 500 partners. Furthermore, most of them said that more than half of the partners had been strangers. There were also numerous cases of rectal gonorrhea and anal herpes simplex virus infection among men in the years before the onset of the AIDS epidemic.

Although it is almost impossible to fulfill strictly Koch's postulates for HIV and AIDS because there is not an animal model in which HIV causes immune suppression, scientists and others of the HIV-causes-AIDS camp point to cases associated with blood transfusions, congenital infection, and sexual transmission, which are as close to Koch's postulates as is possible in humans. Physician and bacteriologist Robert Koch, (1843–1910) set up criteria (postulates) that were to be used to judge whether a certain bacterium was the cause of a given disease.

Nevertheless, there are still those in the scientific community and AIDS activists who remain unconvinced that HIV causes AIDS. Some critics' doubts are based on the circumstances under which the HIV/AIDS hypothesis was advanced. In 1984, Secretary of Health and Welfare Margaret Heckler told the media that an American discovery of the (probable) viral cause of AIDS had been made even though not a single peer-reviewed article on HIV had appeared. The press soon dropped the qualifier *probable* in their reporting of the announcement, and all scientific monies for AIDS research were directed to HIV studies. Others point to dealings that they deemed suspect between the U.S. government and Burroughs Wellcome, leading to approval and use of AZT.

Most of the doubts of HIV skeptics stem from the scientific evidence for the HIV/AIDS hypothesis, which they consider slim to nonexistent. Critics underscore that HIV and HIV antibodies are undetectable in a large percentage of AIDS cases—estimated to be 2 to 10 percent. Also, Duesberg and others say that AIDS-defining diseases are disorders that occur in many people who are never defined as having AIDS because they are HIV-negative. So, they think if both AIDS and AIDS-defining illness do occur without HIV, HIV is not the sole cause of AIDS but possibly one of many contributing causes in those who are HIV-positive.

They also argue that most who have AIDS have been exposed to many immunosuppressive risks besides HIV, even if most have also been exposed to HIV. Just as prevalent as HIV in AIDS patients are hepatitis viruses, herpesviruses, including cytomegalovirus, *Treponema pallidum* (the cause of syphilis), Epstein-Barr virus, and mycobacteria. The critics think that AIDS immunosuppression results from the cumulative effect or synergistic interactions of these pathogens.

Other elements that are thought possibly to result in autoimmunities similar to those in AIDS are exposure to large amounts of foreign antigenic tissue (blood products or semen) and exposure to drugs with immunosuppressive effects: opiates, nitrites, cocaine, high-dosage antibiotics (chronically), and chemotherapeutic agents.

Listing their doubts related to existing data (immunological and virological), skeptics say that the rate at which HIV infects T cells is so low that even if it killed every cell infected, the human body would be able to replenish them. However, retroviruses have never been shown to kill host cells consistently.

Responding to skeptics' objections concerning rates of T cell infection, HIV scientists propose a pathogenesis of AIDS in HIV-triggered autoimmunities caused by the similarity of HIV surface proteins to those of immune system cells. Even so, CD4 homologies by which HIV is said to cause malfunction of the immune system also exist for other pathogens and foreign tissue, including many pathogens that are commonly found in AIDS patients. In addition, the long latency period from infection to AIDS development is not like that of other viruses, a finding that is inconsistent with established retrovirological principles.

AIDS drug assistance programs The most accessed AIDS programs in the United States, AIDS drug assistance programs (ADAPs) were begun in 1987 in order to dispense free drugs to those without insurance who contracted AIDS. States administer their own programs, and thus eligibility requirements and drugs covered have differed from one place to another. In the face of today's changing health care system and the high costs of HIV/AIDS drug therapies, the ADAPs are having difficulty meeting the demands.

AIDS Education and Training Centers Program
Begun in 1987, the National AIDS Education and Training Center Program was created to promote education and prevention efforts and increase the field of health care providers well versed in diagnosis and treatment of HIV. Regional programs exist in all U.S. states.

AIDS orphans Children whose parents, grandparents, caregivers, or foster or adoptive parents have died of AIDS. Some are in shelters and foster care facilities; others live with relatives. In some cases, these children have HIV.

AIDS prodrome A term used early in the AIDS epidemic referring to signs or symptoms that are precursors of AIDS. AIDS prodrome is synonymous with the term *AIDS-related complex.*

AIDS-related complex A group of symptoms such as weight loss, fever, and lymphadenopathy associated with the presence of antibodies to HIV and often progressing to AIDS. This term is used less often now than in the early days of the AIDS epidemic, and is synonymous with the term *AIDS prodrome.*

AIDS service organization A community group whose goal is to provide ongoing assistance to those with HIV/AIDS. Some of the services are support groups, counseling, testing, food banks, housing information, and legal services. Staffers are usually volunteers.

alcohol Ethyl alcohol, or ethanol, which is in alcoholic drinks, when taken into the body depresses central nervous system activity. In those who drink excessive amounts of alcohol problems such as cirrhosis of the liver, gastritis, cardiomyopathy, and peripheral neuritis can develop. Alcoholism is an addiction to alcoholic beverages and is considered a disease.

Alcohol can definitely play a role in contracting STDs in that an intoxicated person may have impaired judgment. That can lead to lax or deficient safe-sex practices, as well as the possibility of lowered standards, facilitating high-risk behaviors and risky sex partners.

alpha-interferon Under investigation as a possible way to treat AIDS symptoms, alpha-interferon is a natural protein secreted by the body's immune cells in response to viral infection. It is thought to have immunomodulatory actions and may affect virus multiplication and spread. Different versions are manufactured for treating hepatitis B and C and Kaposi's sarcoma. There is also a form for injection into refractory external genital warts.

American Foundation for AIDS Research (amfAR)   This group is the country's leading nonprofit group supporting HIV/AIDS research, prevention, education, and advocacy. The organization is known for its instrumental role in accelerating the pace of HIV/AIDS research. Funded by individuals' donations and contributions from corporations and foundations, amfAR has invested about $207 million in support of its mission and funded grants to 1,960 research teams worldwide, from 1985 to 2003. In the early days of the AIDS epidemic in the United States, Mathilde Krim, Ph.D., who was then a researcher at New York's Memorial Sloan-Kettering Cancer Center, joined with some of her colleagues in demanding research efforts and public information campaigns. At the time, theirs were among the few voices willing to speak out on behalf of those with HIV and AIDS and insist on federal funding of research and prevention. In April 1983, the AIDS Medical Foundation was founded in New York to address these ends, and in September 1985, amfAR was formed through the unifying of the AIDS Medical Foundation with the National AIDS Research Foundation (a group begun in California). Today, one of amfAR's most important thrusts is funding an AIDS prevention program aimed at reaching drug users by providing needle exchange, whereby drug users can exchange used needles and syringes for sterile ones. The goal of this program is to reduce the spread of HIV transmission via contaminated drug paraphernalia. As in the past, amfAR continues to go where needed in its efforts to respond to emerging needs and invest in cutting-edge science.

Americans with Disabilities Act   An important equal opportunity law, as well as one designed to prevent discrimination, the Americans with Disabilities Act (1990) protects those with disabilities, a term that includes people who have asymptomatic HIV to full-blown AIDS. Its protection against discrimination is so far-ranging that it even covers those individuals who could be perceived as being carriers of HIV, such as caretakers, volunteers, and family members.

amfAR   See AMERICAN FOUNDATION FOR AIDS RESEARCH.

anabolic steroids   Steroid hormones sometimes abused by athletes seeking to increase muscle mass. These can have serious harmful effects. Synthetic steroid hormones have also been used to treat men with AIDS who are experiencing low testicular function or testosterone deficiency due to HIV. As a treatment for AIDS-related wasting, however, anabolic steroids have not yet been proved effective in studies.

analgesic   An agent that relieves pain. Examples are acetaminophen (Tylenol) and aspirin.

anal intercourse   Sexual intercourse, with insertion of one person's penis into the other partner's anus. Without the use of a condom, this is considered high-risk sexual activity. Small tears in rectal tissue that can result from anal intercourse are facilitators for sexually transmitted diseases. Although either partner can become infected with HIV during anal sex, the one receiving semen is at greater risk (the lining of the rectum is thin and can allow the virus entry during anal sex). The person inserting his penis into an infected partner can become infected with HIV through the urethra or through penis cuts, abrasions, or sores. Also important to note: condoms break more often during anal sex than they do during vaginal sex. A water-based lubricant is recommended, in addition to a condom, to reduce the likelihood of breakage.

anal-oral sex   Sexual contact between one partner's mouth and the other's anus (also termed analingus). This is sometimes called "rimming."

anatomy, female   Normal female pelvic anatomical components include the vulva—the outside parts, including labia, clitoris, and vaginal opening. The labia encompass the labia majora (outer lips) and the labia minora (inner lips); the clitoris sits at the top of the vulva and is a site of extreme sensitivity in sexual arousal and pleasure (analogous to the male's glans of the penis). The urethra serves to convey urine from the bladder to the outside of the body. Skene's glands on each side are suppliers of sexual lubricants. The two fallopian tubes are located between the wider part of the uterus and the ovaries—key female anatomical components in their role in transporting the egg from the ovaries to the uterus, where it can implant after fertilization. The two ovaries sit at the ends of the fallopian tubes. Ovaries are egg containers and producers of estrogen and progesterone.

anatomy, male   The major male organ is the three-tissue-tubed penis, whereby a man urinates and makes semen. The glans, or head, at the end of the penis, contains more nerve endings than any other part of this organ. The glans is analogous to the woman's clitoris. Foreskin, often clipped at birth via circumcision, covers the head of the penis. In many men, the head of the penis hosts a group of shiny bumps, which are sometimes mistaken for genital warts. The scrotum is the bag of skin beneath the penis that holds the testicles, epididymis, vas deferens, and blood vessels. The two testicles inside the scrotum produce sperm and testosterone. Above the testicles are the epididymis (sperm storage), vas deferens (carrier of sperm when the male ejaculates), and blood vessels. The male also has the urethra, a hollow tube that carries urine outside the body when the bladder empties, and the prostate, which is the gland at the base of the bladder that secretes fluids that help make up the semen.

anemia   A deficiency in the normal red blood cell mass within the body that is characterized by fatigue and pallor. In HIV patients, anemia can result from HIV infection or opportunistic infection, or it can be a side effect of drug therapy.

anogenital wart   A raised, bumpy growth in the anal or genital area resulting from human papillomavirus infection.

anonymous testing   Generally speaking, this refers to testing for HIV that is done anonymously. Many cities host testing centers that perform anonymous testing, which keeps track of patients via a numbering system. This method ensures that the agency itself does not have information on the person's identity.

anorexia   The loss of appetite that accompanies some diseases. Anorexia is common in those with HIV and should not be confused with anorexia nervosa, an eating disorder in which the person suppresses appetite.

antibody   A specific kind of blood protein synthesized in lymphoid tissue, after stimulation by an antigen, which acts specifically to attack and render harmless the antigen in an immune response. Whereas B lymphocytes take about two weeks to produce antibodies to most antigens, they may take months to produce antibodies to HIV, and even then they are not able to prevent the HIV infection from progressing.

antibody-dependent cell-mediated cytotoxicity   Via lymphocyte-mediated cytotoxicity, an effector cell kills a target cell coated in antibodies. T cells are the critical effector cells of the adaptive immune response.

antidepressant   Affecting neurotransmitters in the brain, an antidepressant is a medication used to relieve depression and other mood disorders.

antigen   Any substance that the body interprets as foreign, and, as such, foreign material that causes an immune response with production of an antibody. Antigens are proteins, toxins, or microorganisms that the body's immune system sees as foreign and thus tries to destroy. The immune system manufactures antibodies in response.

antioxidant therapy   Antioxidants are substances that are believed to reduce the damage that is caused by oxidants in the blood. Free radicals damage the immune system, so those living with a compromised immune system often seek to reduce the ravaging by augmenting their system with antioxidant therapy, which includes vitamins E and C, beta-carotene, and selenium, as well as foods that are rich in antioxidants: yams, squash, tomatoes, apricots, broccoli, spinach, pumpkin, and carrots.

antiretroviral   A drug with an antiretroviral effect, that is, activity against retroviruses. Antiretroviral drugs are known for reducing the replication rate of retroviruses such as HIV. As a way to treat asymptomatic patients with HIV in its intermediate stage, these drugs have a dramatic effect in that they often serve to increase the length of time before development of opportunistic infections or death. The therapy is determined for the individual patient; it usually features a combination of three drugs.

Over time, the effectiveness of highly active antiretroviral therapy (HAART) wanes in some patients, probably as a result of the emergence of drug-resistant strains of HIV. HIV/AIDS health care specialists conjecture that using combination therapy will increase the time that is needed for resistant virus strains to develop. Some researchers predict that drug-resistant HIV strains will cause 42 percent of all HIV infections in San Francisco by the year 2005.

anxiety   An extreme uneasiness or apprehension that can be based on real or perceived fears. In respect to sexually transmitted diseases, anxiety often goes hand in hand with such a diagnosis, particularly in the cases of those that are not curable: genital herpes and HIV.

ARC   See AIDS-RELATED COMPLEX.

ARDS   See ACUTE RESPIRATORY DISTRESS SYNDROME.

artificial insemination   The introduction of semen with viable sperm into the vagina or uterus in order to induce pregnancy. In the context of sexually transmitted diseases, it is important to note that donors for sperm banks are asked to test for HIV at the time of donation. The sample is frozen

and quarantined. Then the donor is required to be retested six months later. When the results of both HIV tests prove negative, the sperm is thawed for possible use. Thus, it is important for a woman who is interested in artificial insemination to investigate the procedures used by the particular sperm bank facility. If they are not scrupulous in their testing, a woman could be inseminated with HIV-positive semen that puts her, as well as her infant, at risk of infection.

ASCUS Pap smears   *ASCUS* is the acronym for "atypical squamous cells of undetermined significance"—a classification of an abnormal Pap smear finding. This indicates that there were cellular abnormalities seen under a microscope. It is usually further qualified as to whether it appears to indicate a reactive process (related to an infection) or a premalignant process. In the realm of sexually transmitted diseases, women who have had HPV infection should be especially vigilant about getting their Pap smears done. Via the Bethesda system developed in 1988, HPV status was taken into consideration, and cytologic abnormalities are classified as low- or high-grade squamous intraepithelial lesions—LSILs and HSILs. LSILs include normal cells with koilocytosis and mild dysplasia; HSILs encompass moderate to severe dysplasia and carcinoma in situ. For those atypical cells that remain unclassified, *ASCUS* is the label—meaning atypical squamous cells of undetermined significance. Your health care provider will discuss with you whether you need a repeat Pap smear or a colposcopy, in which your cervix is viewed with a microscope.

aspergillosis   An opportunistic fungal infection that, in AIDS patients, usually affects the lungs, resulting in a thick-walled cavitary disease of the upper lobes, diffuse unilateral or bilateral infiltrates, ulcerative tracheobronchial disease, or obstructive bronchitis. Second most likely organ for involvement is the brain. The *Aspergillus* species exist as molds that grow on decaying vegetation and soil all over the world. Transmission is via airborne spores. A person with pulmonary (lung) involvement can have shortness of breath, fever, cough, and chest pain. Extrapulmonary aspergillosis usually causes abscesses and aneurysms. Central nervous system involvement also is manifested in focal neurologic deficits and other problems stemming from an intracranial mass lesion.

asymptomatic infection   An infection that is symptom-free and does not cause an individual to feel ill. This is a problem with early stages of some sexually transmitted diseases: the carrier does not have symptoms and is thus unaware of infection, although the disease can still be spread to other people.

atrophy   Decreased size or wasting away of a body part or tissue. Facial atrophy is part of the lipodystrophy that can occur in people taking highly active antiretroviral therapy (HAART). This can have a negative effect psychologically because the person looks ill. At the AIDS 2002 XIV International AIDS Conference, a Brazilian study was presented that showed the successful use of PMMA (polymethylmethacrylate) facial implants to correct lipodystrophy. These patients reported an improvement in their quality of life.

autoantibodies   These antibodies are produced by or associated with various autoimmune diseases.

autoimmune disease   An illness caused by inflammation and destruction of tissue by a person's own antibodies. In essence, an individual with an autoimmune disease has an immune response to his or her own tissues or cells.

autovaccination   A patient can be vaccinated with vaccine that is made of organisms taken from his or her own tissues. The goal is to stimulate the body's immune response to the disease.

azidothymidine (AZT)   A synthetic thymidine (one of the components of DNA), azidothymidine is the primary antiviral drug used to combat HIV. Although AZT does not prolong the life of the HIV-infected individual on a long-term basis, it does slow the decline in CD4 counts and delay the development of opportunistic infections in patients who have asymptomatic HIV. It is also appropriate for patients with symptomatic HIV. Studies have shown that AZT is vulnerable to emergence of mutations that produce resistance. At almost every stage of infection, there are large numbers of HIV-containing cells and thus ongoing production of new HIV particles (some of these contain mutations that confer AZT resistance). Common side effects of azidothymidine are insomnia, headaches, and gastrointestinal distress.

Because this was the first drug used to fight HIV, it is still called AZT, even though the correct name is now *zidovudine* (ZDV). Serving to inhibit the growth and proliferation of the virus, AZT is approved for treating adults who have CD4 counts below 500 cells/mm3 and children who are at least three months old. Prevention of maternal–fetal HIV transmission is another approved use.

AZT monotherapy   Drug therapy for an HIV patient that includes only zidovudine (AZT), versus the more common administration of a combination of drugs in highly active antiretroviral therapy (HAART). Monotherapy has limited application because HIV shows resistance to the drug as time passes.

AZT resistance   When a person has HIV and his or her body shows resistance to the antiviral effect of AZT, this response may be indicative of more rapid progression of the disease.

bacterial STDs Types of sexually transmitted diseases caused by bacteria include syphilis, gonorrhea, chancroid, chlamydia, and granuloma inguinale.

bacterial vaginosis (BV) The belief that bacterial vaginosis is sexually transmitted is supported by its association with multiple partners, rare occurrence in virgins, and lack of prevalence in couples who are monogamous—but the final word is that BV should be viewed as a "sexually associated infection." Once referred to as nonspecific vaginitis, or *Gardnerella*-associated vaginitis, this is the most common vaginal infection in women who are of childbearing age.

Causes

Although not classified as a sexually transmitted disease, BV is so prevalent in sexually active women that researchers believe this prevalence suggests a link with sexual activity. Virgins, however, also can have this infection. What triggers the overgrowth of bacteria that sets up this problem is unknown, although it does appear that douching can disturb the ecosystem of the vagina. Epidemiological studies suggest that risk factors include nonwhite race, a history of trichomoniasis or other sexually transmitted disease, early sexual experience, multiple sex partners, and use of an IUD.

Bacterial vaginosis is a condition resulting from an imbalance in the normal bacteria in the vagina. A normal vagina has high amounts of helpful lactobacilli bacteria, which play an important role in maintaining a healthy vaginal ecosystem. When a woman has bacterial vaginosis, for some unknown reason, lactobacilli decrease, and there is an overgrowth of other bacteria, which are normally present in the vagina in lesser numbers.

The exact origin has not been determined, but researchers have established that BV is associated with activities that can change vaginal pH: douching, having an STD, and changing sexual partners. What occurs is that, instead of the usual prevalence of *Lactobacillus* species bacteria, the vagina of a woman with BV has an overgrowth of *Gardnerella vaginalis, Bacteroides* species, *Mycoplasma hominis,* and *Mobiluncus* species.

The common gynecologic disorder vaginitis is seen in three forms: yeast, usually caused by *Candida albicans;* trichomoniasis (caused by *Trichomonas vaginalis*); and bacterial vaginosis, caused by anaerobic pathogens. BV results from an imbalance of the vagina's microorganisms rather than infection by a single microorganism.

Symptoms

Half of women who have BV have no symptoms or disease that is clinically apparent, and many women who do have symptoms treat themselves inappropriately with over-the-counter yeast-infection remedies. However, women with BV often have an abnormal white or gray vaginal discharge that can be thin in nature and has an unpleasant smell. Some women report a fishlike odor that is especially strong after intercourse. Burning during urination and itching on the outside of the vagina are other signs.

Sometimes accompanied by discharge, odor, pain, itching, or burning, BV has as its main symptom an odd, odorous vaginal discharge, but it is also not a good idea for physicians to diagnose vaginitis exclusively on the basis of color, consistency of discharge, and description, because a complex exam is necessary for women who have vaginal discharge, odor, itching, or irritation. At the same time, further confusing diagnosis is the fact that about half of women who have BV do not have symptoms.

For the diagnosis, a woman must have a minimum of three of these symptoms: fishy odor of vaginal secretions on whiff test, homogeneous vaginal discharge, vaginal pH greater than 4.5, and clue cells.

Testing

To diagnose BV, a doctor does a physical exam to look for signs and obtains a sample of vaginal discharge to evaluate. A wet-mount preparation, which consists of vaginal discharge diluted with saline solution on a slide, is viewed under a microscope to check for clue cells that are indicative of bacterial vaginosis. Other testing may include pH evaluation and a whiff test.

Treatment

Bacterial vaginosis sometimes clears up spontaneously, but a woman with BV should be treated in order to make sure she is not subject to complications such as pelvic inflammatory disease. In nonpregnant women, the Centers for Disease Control and Prevention recommends that physicians treat bacterial vaginosis with topical formulations of metronidazole (MetroGel) and clindamycin (Cleocin) or oral metronidazole (Flagyl). A doctor prescribes antimicrobial medicines, such as metronidazole or clindamycin, and the patient must use all of the medicine prescribed. Metronidazole can be used by pregnant women after the first trimester.

Any pregnant woman who has ever had a premature delivery or low-birth-weight infant should be examined for BV and treated if she does, indeed, have it. In most cases, male partners of women with BV do not need to be treated. Female sex partners, conversely, can spread the disease between them.

Recommended treatment of bacterial vaginosis is to screen to reduce infectious complications before abortion or hysterectomy (pelvic inflammatory disease is a risk) and to treat with antibiotics: metronidazole or clindamycin. The common "remedy" of eating yogurt has shown no benefits.

Complications

When a woman is pregnant, she is more likely to have complications if she has bacterial vaginosis.

Pregnant women with BV are five times more likely to have postpartum endometritis than uninfected women, and BV patients who have positive culture results for both *Bacteroides* species and *Mycoplasma hominis* are the women most likely to have a preterm delivery of a baby with low birth weight.

BV bacteria also may infect the uterus and fallopian tubes. Such infection constitutes pelvic inflammatory disease, a potentially serious infection that can result in damage of the tubes that sometimes leads to a risk of ectopic pregnancy and infertility.

BV can heighten one's susceptibility to HIV infection on exposure to the disease. Also, an HIV-positive woman is more likely to pass HIV to her sex partner if she also has BV. In addition, having BV increases a woman's susceptibility to other STDs.

New evidence points to lack of vaginal *Lactobacillus* species and presence of BV as factors increasing the risk of acquiring HIV infection. Of special concern are several studies that point to a link between BV and HIV seropositivity. In a look at 144 women in one study and 4,718 in another study, researchers found that HIV may promote growth of abnormal vaginal flora or that bacterial vaginosis may increase an individual's susceptibility to HIV via sexual transmission. The researchers concluded that it appears that treating women with BV to restore normal vaginal flora may effectively lessen their likelihood of acquiring HIV.

The association of bacterial vaginosis with pelvic inflammatory disease, endometritis, preterm birth, cervical intraepithelial neoplasia, low-birth-weight infants, and acquisition of HIV makes careful diagnosis and treatment important. Since bacterial vaginosis is often asymptomatic (in up to 50 percent of women), an accurate diagnosis based on clinical indicators (most patients self-diagnose and treat themselves for yeast infection) is critical.

Transmission

BV has a cause that is not well understood, and its transmission is equally foggy. Most likely to contract bacterial vaginosis is a woman who has a new sex partner or who has had multiple partners. It is rare to see BV in virgins. Women do not, however, get BV from bedding, toilet seats, swimming pools, or objects they touch. This is a common malady in young women of reproductive age, and in the United States, up to 16 percent of pregnant women have BV. The highest prevalence is in African Americans and the lowest is in Asian Americans.

Prevention

The Centers for Disease Control and Prevention suggests that sexually active people use condoms when they have sex, limit the number of sex partners, and avoid douching. Guidelines from the Centers for Disease Control, however, do not recommend treatment for sexual partners of a person with BV.

balanitis An inflammation of the head of the penis, often associated with tight foreskin; in other cases this problem may develop as a result of failure to clean under the foreskin regularly. Redness, smelly discharge, and swelling are characteristics of an acute attack. A patient is treated with antibiotics and encouraged to wash off smegma—white "cheese" made by the glands at the head and neck of the penis. To ward off future bouts of balanitis, a man may choose to have his penis circumcised. Balanitis also can be caused by *Candida albicans* or by bacteria. An individual should not have sexual intercourse until the infection is gone. Sex makes the infection worse.

bareback sex A common term bandied about as a reference to the act by HIV-positive men of intentionally having unprotected sex with other men who are HIV-positive. Along with the AIDS denialists movement, bareback sex appears to be compelling testimony to a strange new wave of thinking that began with the new millennium and continues to be pervasive and a contributing factor in rising rates of HIV infection in gay men. It seems clear that improved treatments for HIV ushered in the alarming new trend of complacency among homosexual men, and thus unsafe sex reemerged as a major problem. Many experts believe that bareback sex puts an HIV-positive man at risk in terms of reinfection with other HIV strains, which then make him more difficult to treat successfully with drug therapy.

Bartholin's abscess A Bartholin's abscess sometimes forms when the duct to one of the two Bartholin's glands on each side of the vaginal orifice get blocked. The secretions in the glands can become infected with one of many bacteria, including chlamydia and gonorrhea. These are usually treated with incision and drainage of the abscess. Sometimes, antibiotics are also prescribed. The Bartholin's glands produce a lubricant for intercourse.

bathhouse Serving as the sexual extravaganza centers of the 1970s, bathhouses offered gay men an assortment of plentiful partners and extreme emphasis on sexuality. With promiscuity the norm, these places became breeding grounds for HIV infection, and soon a frightening connotation was attached to the bathhouse phenomenon. Eventually, the havens became extremely controversial, even though some owners saw fit to disseminate information on safe sex as the AIDS epidemic gained impetus and the dangers of risky sex became common knowledge.

bedsore A skin sore that results from ulceration of tissue arising from inadequate blood supply via the prolonged pressure of bed confinement. In the realm of sexually transmitted diseases, those most likely to suffer bedsores are emaciated patients with HIV/AIDS. Rendered immobile, they develop bedsores in skin that covers bony prominences.

For prevention/treatment information, see Appendix III.

behavioral risk factors See RISK FACTORS.

behavioral surveillance data monitoring To develop interventions that will effectively decrease the spread of STDs, it is important to collect and analyze behavioral surveillance data concerning high-risk behavior and reasons that people neglect to pursue treatment or delay treatment. It is believed that the upshot could be a level of undetectable prevalence of STDs many years sooner than could occur without such a system in place. The savings would be billions of dollars.

A behavioral surveillance network is designed to estimate the sizes of populations at risk for STDs, monitor knowledge of STDs and attitudes toward STDs and sexuality, monitor people's ability to recognize STD symptoms and thus face the need for medical treatment, link behavioral and biomedical disease indicators, and evaluate the effectiveness of education programs.

In the case of community surveillance, the focus is aimed at the ways the populace accesses health care, their health surveys, and monitoring of sentinel sites. The course of an epidemic can thus be traced by using data on behavior, by checking for changes that occur on the heels of prevention campaigns, by estimating health care coverage of STDs, by determining the extent to which private providers are involved, and by tracking links between risk behavior and prevention efforts.

benefit Many types of government benefits are available to those with HIV/AIDS; these include Social Security, welfare, Medicaid, Medicare, food stamps, social services, and medications. By the same token, the indigent, disabled, and elderly are eligible for similar benefits. The downside of federal programs is that the applicant must endure the cumbersome aspects of extensive red tape, varying standards, and services that are often non-user-friendly.

benign Does not threaten life; not malignant (as in tumors).

bestiality Sexual gratification achieved via sexual contact with animals.

beta-2-microglobulin test Beta-2-microglobulin is released into the blood when a cell dies. Elevated levels of B2M are indicative of disease. The test is used to monitor immune status of an individual with HIV, because a correlation exists between high levels of beta-2-microglobulin and disease progression.

beta-carotene A carotene isomer that is found in dark green and dark yellow vegetables and fruits and converts to vitamin A in the body. Beta-carotene is an antioxidant that destroys free radicals.

bisexual The orientation of a person who can achieve arousal and/or gratification through sexual contact with both men and women.

biting In documented cases of HIV transmission, biting has not been considered a threat unless the bite draws blood or breaks skin, in which case the transmission becomes a blood issue. According to records kept by the Centers for Disease Control and Prevention, no cases of HIV transmission have been attributed exclusively to saliva or a bite.

bleach Ordinary chlorine bleach, available in grocery stores, is a preparation used to bleach fabric and household surfaces, and one that also is used to kill HIV and other viruses and microbes existing in stool, blood, and saliva. Typically, bleach is diluted 1:10 (in other words, one part bleach to 10 parts water). This solution is commonly used with great effectiveness on household surfaces and in washing of clothing and bedding.

blindness Lack of the ability to see. A person can become blind in the late stages of AIDS, and blindness also has multiple other causes, including glaucoma, cataracts, and macular degeneration.

blood bank A facility where blood is taken, processed, and stored for future use. The safety of blood used for transfusions has been an enormous issue since the AIDS epidemic raised worries and increased precautions. Because of cases of AIDS diagnosed in hemophiliacs who had had blood transfusions, blood banks began to exclude donors who indulged in high-risk sex practices and instigated tests to screen for AIDS/HIV. At the same time, the use of autologous transfusions became increasingly popular and encouraged in health facilities.

Use of HIV antibody tests became standard practice in the 1980s; however, the problem is that a person who has just contracted HIV does not immediately have a detectable antibody response. On the contrary, the length of time that passes before HIV becomes evident varies. Usually, it is no more than a few months. Clearly, it is possible for a donor's blood test to have a negative finding during this brief period before emergence of sufficient antibody response to produce a positive test result. Thus, the existing situation at blood banks is this: most facilities can boast greatly improved safety of the blood supply but there is no guarantee that HIV will not be transmitted via transfusion.

blood components The composition of blood includes plasma, red blood cells, white blood cells, platelets, fat globules, chemical substances, and gases.

blood screening The process of testing blood that has been donated to ascertain whether it contains disease. The blood that is infected is subsequently destroyed.

blood supply safety See BLOOD BANK.

blood test A lab analysis of a blood sample that is performed to determine its characteristics. Blood tests are effective in diagnosis of various conditions and progression of disease.

blood transfusion The process of using whole blood or blood products to replace blood in a person's body.

body fluids The human body contains a number of fluids, including blood, urine, saliva, sweat, tears, breast milk, cervical secretions, semen, and sputum; the only ones that are known to transmit HIV are vaginal secretions, blood, breast milk, and semen.

bone marrow suppression A condition characterized by the bone marrow's decreased ability to produce white blood cells, red blood cells, and platelets. This may result in anemia, bacterial infections, and bleeding that is excessive and/or spontaneous. Some drugs used to treat HIV have the side effect of causing bone marrow suppression.

bone marrow transplantation Often used in treating some cancers, bone marrow transplantation is the removal of healthy bone marrow from a donor and its transfusion into an ill patient who needs it. This restores stem cells that have been destroyed by chemotherapy and/or radiation therapy. Thus, when the person with lymphoma, for example, has bone marrow transplantation, usually he or she becomes better able to battle infections. The types of marrow transplantation are autologous, using the patient's own marrow, which was harvested before chemotherapy, cryopreserved, and then reinfused; allogeneic, using marrow from a parent, sibling, or compatible unrelated donor; and syngeneic, using marrow from an identical twin. Marrow transplantation differs from organ transplantation in that the removed stem cells are replaced spontaneously within a short period (in the person from whom they were harvested). For this procedure to help the patient, he or she must be at a relatively early stage of disease and have the capacity to respond to treatment.

booting An activity that involves a drug user's withdrawing blood in a drug-filled syringe before injecting the contents. Health care professionals believe that this practice constitutes high risk for HIV transmission because of the increased blood–syringe contact.

branched DNA assay An HIV test that employs a light-detecting system to measure the amount of HIV in blood plasma. The brightness of the test's luminescent signal varies depending on the amount of viral RNA present. This test is used to evaluate the effectiveness of the current drug treatment an individual is undergoing and the degree of HIV progression.

breast-feeding A method of giving nourishment to a child by glands in the breasts that secrete milk. Cytomegalovirus and HIV can reach an infant via breast-feeding when the mother has one of these diseases.

buddy In many communities all over the United States, the term *buddy* took on a whole new meaning with the advent of the AIDS epidemic. This label was attached to the volunteer caregivers who help individuals with HIV or AIDS. After training, the buddy can be responsible for duties ranging from running errands to providing hands-on care. There are numerous AIDS organizations that organize buddy system programs so that those who have AIDS and have no relatives to care for them or lend support can receive the help of a volunteer.

Burkitt's lymphoma   A malignant tumor of the lymphatic system. Epstein-Barr virus plays a role in the origin and growth of this fast-growing tumor.

buyers' clubs   Known mainly for making "unapproved" drugs available to people with HIV and AIDS, these groups are regarded as underground systems. Not surprisingly, the U.S. Food and Drug Administration offers caveats concerning these clubs: remember that one does not have a physician supervising each individual patient's regimen; the products are of uncertain origin and purity; and there is no proof of effectiveness of offerings sold.

BV   See BACTERIAL VAGINOSIS.

Candida albicans The fungus that causes candidiasis.

candidiasis ("yeast infection") A superficial infection with a fungus of the genus *Candida* that can affect various locations including the vagina.

Causes

More than 95 percent of candidal vaginal infections are caused by *Candida albicans*. Causes of the others are usually *Candida glabrata* and *Candida tropicalis*.

Symptoms

People with candidiasis can have beefy red plaques in the groin area, spreading to scrotum or labia; satellite lesions extending onto thighs; and curdy white patches on inflamed vaginal mucosa. The classical symptoms of recurrent candidal vaginitis are itching and a curdlike, cheesy discharge. A man may have pain with urination and/or red, itchy skin with peripheral pustules.

Candidiasis is more common in diabetics and in people who are taking or have recently taken antibiotics. In immunosuppressed women severe and treatment-resistant vaginal yeast infections that consist of milky white discharge and white patches develop. One report indicated that 37 percent of those who started out with recurrent yeast infections eventually were receiving care for HIV. Conditions that occur so often in HIV that they have become considered signs of the disease include herpes zoster, oral candidiasis (thrush), and oral hairy leukoplakia.

Testing

Diagnosis is usually made through clinical findings and by microscopic examination of candidal vaginal infection's vaginal discharge. A potassium hydroxide (KOH) preparation involves applying a 10 percent KOH solution to a microscope slide with vaginal secretions on it.

If there is no sign of *Candida* species in testing, a patient may be screened for bacterial vaginosis, chlamydia, human papillomavirus, *Trichomonas* species, and gonorrhea. An individual who has frequent candidal infections should consider the possibility of other risk factors: frequent antibiotic or steroid use, pregnancy, diabetes, immunosuppression, HIV infection, poor perianal hygiene, or wearing of tight clothing or underpants of silk or nylon.

Treatment

The primary goal of treatment is alleviation of symptoms. In most patients, over-the-counter antifungal topical agents can be used to treat an acute case effectively but should be used only by women who have been previously diagnosed with vaginal candidiasis and are experiencing similar symptoms again. If symptoms are not relieved or if symptoms recur, then the patient needs to be reevaluated by her doctor. An oral medication called fluconazole (Diflucan) is another option for treatment but is only available by prescription. Using antifungal agents cuts down the number of vaginal organisms to a level that is undetectable by culture; however, this does not get rid of the organism in the vagina completely. In women who are healthy and whose immune systems are functioning well, infection of mucosal surfaces by *Candida* species is readily treated and usually does not recur.

If a person has recurrent candidal infection, the physician usually wants to test further for diabetes or immunosuppression. Note: some of the creams used to treat candidiasis render condoms ineffective because they destroy the latex.

Prevention

In women who seem to be hypersensitive, it appears that the best treatment is to prevent growth of *Candida* species by using antifungal agents aggressively and oral antihistamines for symptom relief. In cases of recurrent infections, it may well be that the best therapy is hyposensitizing the patient to *Candida* species.

Psychosocial Issues

In a study reported in *Sexually Transmitted Infections* (October 1998), researchers sought to identify the psychological factors that accompanied chronic recurrent vaginal candidiasis. A group of 28 women with recurring candidiasis were compared with 16 women with no history of this disease. Although the groups were similar in demographic characteristics and most sexual health issues, the ones with recurrent disease were much more likely to suffer clinical depression and stress, to have low self-esteem, and to report decreased life satisfaction. They also believed that their candidiasis interfered greatly with their relationships, both sexual and emotional. Thus, the study underscored the need for psychological treatment for such patients.

Research

New research suggests that the common medical practice of using heparin in intravascular catheters to discourage blockages by blood clots may accidentally trigger events that change a benign fungal infection into a deadly incident in some patients. *Candida albicans* is the leading cause of invasive fungal disease in premature babies and others with weakened immune systems, such as those with HIV, postsurgical patients, and cancer or bone marrow transplantation patients. Findings reported in the *Journal of the American Medical Association* (November 28, 2001) suggest the link between use of heparin in intravascular catheters and its role in setting off events that lead to a toxic shock–like reaction.

CBC   See COMPLETE BLOOD COUNT.

CD4 cell count   A person's CD4 lymphocytes, or T helper cells, are important in the immune system. At the outset of HIV infection, the number of CD4 cells declines as a result of the large amount of virus in the person's system. Then, in many cases, the immune system goes into action and suppresses the virus, often for years. But when the virus finally overcomes the body's immune system, the person becomes more susceptible to malignancies and opportunistic infections. This is the point when a patient officially has AIDS.

CD8 cell count   A type of immune cell, or T suppressor cell, this can be measured, and many who treat HIV/AIDS monitor the progression of the infection by studying the ratio of CD4 to CD8 cells. When researchers have studied the lack of infection in an HIV-exposed person, they have seen an association with a strong CD8+ cell noncytotoxic anti-HIV response. The population of people who despite repeated exposures to HIV remain uninfected is a source of much interest to researchers in that those individuals have either natural or acquired resistance to the virus. In a study documented in the *Proceedings of the National Academy of Sciences of the United States of America* (February 2, 1999), researchers investigated four exposed and uninfected cohorts, representing 60 people, to see whether protective immunity could be occurring. What was observed was CD8+ cell noncytotoxic inhibition of HIV replication in acutely infected CD4+ cells in most of those most recently exposed to the virus, and the levels of this response were sufficient to inhibit the in vitro infection of these people's peripheral blood mononuclear cells. Thus, this strong noncytotoxic CD8+ cell anti-HIV response may be an antiviral immune activity that seems to offer protection from infection to these individuals.

CDC   See CENTERS FOR DISEASE CONTROL AND PREVENTION.

CDC Global AIDS Program   Since 1999, the CDC has set up Global AIDS Programs in India and 14 countries in Africa. In 2001, the CDC supported programs in Asia and more nations in

Africa and sought to address the problem of the HIV/AIDS epidemic in the Caribbean and Latin America. The Caribbean's rates of HIV are the highest in the world outside Africa, and as of 2002, heterosexual intercourse the was main mode of transmissions. The CDC is working with the Caribbean Epidemiology Center to promote HIV prevention efforts. Sir George Alleyne, then director of the Pan American Health Organization, noted in 2002 that in the Region of the Americas, one of every 200 people between 15 and 49 was HIV infected, and in the Caribbean, one in every 50 people. Worldwide, there are 2,784,317 cases of AIDS documented in the 2002 Pan American Health Organization report. Globally, about 40 million are living with HIV/AIDS. AIDS deaths in the world in 2001 were about 3 million. As of June 2002, a total of 1,202,147 AIDS cases were reported in the Americas, and 653,825 AIDS deaths have occurred since 1986, based on preliminary figures for 2000–2001.

For the fiscal year 2001, the CDC appropriated more than $104 million for its Global HIV/AIDS Programs. In the same fiscal year, the National Institutes of Health spent more than $130 million on AIDS research conducted in international settings. The NIH also spent about $282 million on HIV vaccine research in fiscal year 2001. The Health Resources and Service Administration, working through the U.S./Mexico Border Health Initiative, helps with cross-border HIV/AIDS issues and targets $13 million over five years in grant funds for those with HIV and AIDS who live in the United States along the 2,000-mile area of the U.S.–Mexican border.

The World Health Organization and the Joint United Nations Programme on HIV/AIDS estimate that about 42 million people worldwide have been infected since the pandemic's beginning—and about 16,000 more are infected daily. The CDC is aware of the drawbacks of health care in developing nations, which lack sufficient research capacity, public health infrastructure, and resources (financial and human).

In collaborations with the governments of Cote d'Ivoire, Thailand, and Uganda, plus other places, the CDC supports field stations for research on HIV/AIDS and participates in studies that seek increased understanding of the epidemiological features of HIV-1 and HIV-2 infections. The following activities are occurring in research facilities:

- Attempting to reduce vertical transmission of HIV in developing countries (1,600 babies are born with HIV or infected through breast-feeding each day in these countries). Continuing research the CDC conducted in collaboration with the Thai Ministry of Public Health and Mahidol University had a promising outcome—the findings that a short course of zidovudine given to an HIV-infected mother late in pregnancy and during delivery reduced the rate of vertical HIV transmission by half (if there was no breast-feeding) and that this treatment is safe for use in the developing countries. The CDC has worked with host countries and public health agencies to implement the AZT regimen widely and examine single-dose treatment with nevirapine.

- Instituting programs for high-risk populations in Thailand and Cote d'Ivoire. HIV prevention interventions are targeting IV drug users, female sex workers, and others at risk.

- Pinpointing factors that may confer HIV immunity. Researchers from the CDC and the ministries of health (Thai and Ivorian) are studying groups of female sex workers who have repeatedly been exposed to HIV yet have remained uninfected. They have looked at genetic traits that may convey immunity, and researchers hope that this research will help in the development of an HIV vaccine.

- Using a treatment regimen that can effectively reduce the HIV/AIDS impact in developing countries. A joint study unveiled information that a drug regimen of trimethoprim-sulfamethoxazole greatly reduced the rate of death of HIV-infected TB patients in Africa.

- Doing genetic analyses and collecting data on genetic variations and drug resistance of HIV strains in host countries. Researchers believe that because of the increased spread of HIV subtypes across international borders, the data can help them develop vaccines and facilitate detection and treatment of different HIV strains worldwide.

- Gathering data on HIV/AIDS trends among sentinel groups (female sex workers, pregnant women, STD patients, injection drug users, and children) that can be used in establishing new interventions.
- Improving modes of care and survival for HIV patients.
- Investigating the diseases that are related to HIV, such as other STDs and TB. The goals here are to ascertain whether there are links between illnesses and to develop prevention/treatment strategies for populations around the world.
- Studying factors associated with HIV transmission that occurs heterosexually. Around the world, no kind of exposure has infected more people than heterosexual contact. In the United States, this form of transmission is responsible for a growing percentage of HIV infections and AIDS cases. It is imperative that researchers discover the biomedical and behavioral aspects of heterosexual transmission in order to squelch the spread of HIV worldwide.
- Supporting a vaccine trial in Thailand. The CDC helped Thai health officials identify subjects for the vaccine study, measure the level of new infections in Thailand, and work with the community to implement the trial. The CDC also worked with Thai authorities and the U.S. manufacturer VaxGen, Inc., to ensure that the trial participants were given risk-reduction counseling and gained a full understanding of the trial mechanisms, potential risks and benefits of taking part in the study, and need for maintaining behavioral risk reduction during the span of the trial. The CDC also provided support for a similar VaxGen-sponsored trial in the United States.
- Working with developing countries on setting up programs for HIV testing and counseling. The CDC has aided in evaluating rapid HIV tests, assisted with piloting of the testing algorithm chosen, collaborated on setup of counseling protocols and guidelines for same-day HIV test results, and assisted in developing HIV counselor materials and courses.

Center for Infectious Diseases   A center under the auspices of the federal Centers for Disease Control and Prevention.

Centers for Disease Control and Prevention Widely known as the CDC, the Centers for Disease Control and Prevention is a federal public health agency whose activities include tracking the epidemiological characteristics of sexually transmitted diseases and doing proactive work to prevent and control the spread of these and many other diseases.

cervical cancer   A malignant growth of the cervix. A woman's risk of cervical cancer is increased by having first sexual intercourse at an early age, having multiple sex partners, having five or more pregnancies, and having a history of sexually transmitted diseases. Important diagnostic tests are the Pap smear and colposcopy. It is recommended that a woman have an annual Pap smear starting at age 18 or sooner if she has had intercourse. Because many women avoid having yearly Pap smears done, cervical cancer is usually present for many years before it is finally diagnosed, when the woman experiences abnormal bleeding.

cervical cancer screening   The gold standard for cervical cancer screening is the Papanicolaou (Pap) smear, which sexually active women should have on a regular basis, according to the recommendations of gynecologists.

cervicitis   This inflammation of the cervix can have several symptoms: vaginal discharge that is white or yellow–green, low back pain, burning during urination, and a cervix that looks red and friable. In most cases, cervicitis is due to a sexually transmitted disease—chlamydia, gonorrhea, or trichomonas.

cesarean section   A surgical procedure by which a physician delivers a baby by making an incision in the abdomen and uterus and using it as the route of removal.

chancre   The primary lesion of syphilis. It is usually painless and solitary, with a raised border; however, chancres can vary in appearance. After an average incubation period of three weeks, the lesion begins as a red bump that ulcerates and then heals within several weeks.

chancroid   A sexually transmitted disease that is characterized by a papule that turns into a pustule that ulcerates and becomes painful.

Cause

It is an ulcerative lesion, caused by *Haemophilus ducreyi,* which can affect the vulva, vagina, cervix, urethra, penis, or anus. Chancroid is an endemic disease in Korea and Vietnam and is highly prevalent in Africa. This disease has decreased in the United States, the peak number of cases since World War II, 5,199 for the entire United States in 1989, was followed in 1990 by 3,099 and in 1991 by 2,358. Chancroid is a genital ulcerative disease once common in the United States and considered one of the five classic sexually transmitted diseases that became infrequent until the 1980s, when it became epidemic in a number of U.S. cities and Canada; it was believed to be spread primarily by prostitutes. The end of epidemics in North American cities coincided with the widespread use of the antibiotic ceftriaxone for gonococcal treatment. If that is the reason for the demise of the epidemic, it points to the many people who are effective spreaders of microorganisms who may be incubating chancroid or who may have lesions and are not seeking medical care, according to *USTD 2001.*

Symptoms

Often multiple (one to three) lesions occur; they are of four types: transient, phagedenic, giant, and serpiginous. These usually are painful red ulcers, with ragged borders and yellow–gray exudates at the base. Incubation period is three to five days. Inguinal lymphadenopathy (enlarged, tender lymph nodes in the groin area) can be present. Half of sufferers complain of fever, headaches, and malaise. This can be distinguished from syphilis in that the ulcers of chancroid are painful.

Complications

Since chancroid is an ulcerating disease, it predisposes the patient to HIV infection. Male to female ratio is high in chancroid, and this ratio leads one to infer that prostitutes are involved in transmission. Both men and women are symptomatic, but often female prostitutes with ulcers do not seek medical treatment. These lesions are believed to be a major risk factor for the heterosexual spread of HIV. Male genital secretions containing HIV can enter through genital chancroids.

Diagnosis/Testing

A Gram stain of an ulcer that reveals gram-negative rods in chains ("schools of fish") suggests the diagnosis of chancroid. Culture on enriched chocolate agar with vancomycin may yield a positive result, and a biopsy specimen is diagnostic. Chancroid should be differentiated from genital herpes and syphilis. A blood test should be done to rule out the diagnosis of syphilis, which is curable.

Treatment

For patients without HIV, four drug regimens can be used effectively for chancroid: azithromycin, ceftriaxone, ciprofloxacin, or erythromycin, the last two of which have had, worldwide, several isolates reported to have intermediate resistance to them. The ulcers and lymph nodes usually take approximately 10 days to heal. However, sometimes the lymph nodes become fluctuant and have to be drained.

children with HIV/AIDS   In the early years when U.S. children became infected with HIV, they died early. But now many of those who have been infected by vertically transmitted HIV are being treated aggressively, and their lives are thus lengthened. Nevertheless, the fact remains that AIDS has become the leading cause of death in children and young adults in some parts of the United States.

A child can contract HIV if he or she has an open sore or cut that is exposed to HIV-contaminated body fluids or blood. A baby can contract HIV from his or her mother during pregnancy, labor, delivery, or breast-feeding.

It is important to note that HIV-positive children cannot spread the disease by hugging, holding hands, sharing bathrooms and swimming pools, and having other forms of casual contact. It is unlikely for HIV to be spread in a child care facility from one child to another. However, a parent of an HIV-infected child should inform the center director of the child's HIV status.

In children, early symptoms of HIV include failure to thrive (grow and gain weight), chronic diarrhea, enlarged spleen and liver, swollen lymph glands, chronic yeast infections, skin infections, pneumonia, and other infections that healthy children rarely get. A physician should monitor an HIV-positive child carefully. When a daycare facility has an outbreak of an infectious disease, it is important to remove the HIV-infected child from the facility until the other youngsters are healthy again.

Caveats for reducing the risk of HIV spread in childcare settings are an emphasis on frequent, thorough handwashing and very careful hygiene measures. Caregivers should use gloves when changing diapers and when cleaning up blood and body fluids, and they should quickly wash with soap and water when breast milk is spilled onto skin. Children should not be allowed to share toothbrushes. Caregivers should disinfect surfaces that are splashed with blood or body fluids, cover any open wounds, and ensure that special measures are followed if someone is accidentally exposed to HIV.

Chlamydia trachomatis   Chlamydia is the most common of all bacterial STDs: 4 to 8 million new cases occur each year, according to the *Journal of the American Medical Association* Women's Health Sexually Transmitted Disease Information Center.

Cause

The bacterium *Chlamydia trachomatis* causes chlamydia infection, and it is transmitted during vaginal, oral, and anal sex with an infected partner. Tropical climes have seen a strain of *C. trachomatis* that causes the STD lymphogranuloma venereum, characterized by swelling and inflammation of the lymph nodes in the groin, but this is a rare infection in the United States.

Symptoms

Often men and women have no symptoms for weeks or months after they contract chlamydia. In women, symptoms that do appear are likely to take the form of an unusual yellowish vaginal discharge from the cervix. In fact, in both sexes, chlamydial infection may cause an abnormal genital discharge and painful burning with urination.

It is believed that about half of infected males and 75 percent of infected females do not suspect a problem even though they have chlamydia, because they are symptom-free. The natural outcome of this silent stage is that the disease may not be diagnosed and treated until there are complications, so, meanwhile, the disease is unwittingly spread to new partners. A physician suspects that a woman has chlamydia if she has a typical cervical discharge and if her cervix appears red and swollen and seems to bleed easily.

Testing

The U.S. Centers for Disease Control and Prevention recommends chlamydia testing at least once a year for all sexually active women up to age 19, and annual testing for any woman 20 or older who is at risk (does not use condoms and has had a new sex partner or multiple partners). Only about a third of doctors routinely screen their young female patients for chlamydia.

A sample of secretions from the patient's genital area is submitted to a lab to test for the *Chlamydia* organism. The inexpensive, quick test for this infection uses a dye to detect bacterial proteins. This can be done during a routine checkup. A process called DNA amplification detects the genes of the organisms in genital secretions.

The FDA has approved this process for detection of *C. trachomatis* in urine—a major move because it does not require an invasive sample and can be used in settings where a pelvic exam is not feasible (health fairs, for example). In 24 hours, the patient gets the results of the test. In the future, it is likely that testing for chlamydia by using a urine sample will become commonplace. This will facilitate screening, making it simpler than in the past.

Women who should be tested for chlamydia include those with mucopurulent cervicitis; sexually active women 20 years old or younger; and women 20–24 who meet one of these criteria—inconsistent use of barrier contraception or new or more than one sex partner during the last three months, and women 24 and older who meet both criteria.

Complications

Left untreated, chlamydia in women can lead to pelvic inflammatory disease, a common culprit in future ectopic pregnancy and infertility in women. Since statistics show that the highest rates of chlamydial infection are seen in adolescents who are 15 to 19 (regardless of location or demographic characteristics), chlamydia is one reason that pelvic inflammatory disease (PID)—a serious complication of chlamydia—has emerged as a major cause of infertility.

Aggressive treatment of chlamydia is imperative and should be considered if there is any evidence whatsoever of uterine spread. If the infection is allowed to reach the fallopian tubes, the woman is at risk for scarring, tubal obstruction, ectopic pregnancy, and infertility. Thus, the longer the infection lingers untreated, the greater the risk of permanent damage. It is estimated that in about 40 percent of women whose chlamydia is untreated pelvic inflammatory disease will develop; of that group, about 20 percent become infertile. Furthermore, of those 40 percent, about 18 percent have chronic pelvic pain and 9 percent have a tubal pregnancy.

A woman who has chlamydia has a greatly heightened chance of contracting HIV if she is exposed, and some research shows a link between chlamydia and cervical cancer. About 60 percent of babies who are exposed to chlamydia infection at birth have pneumonia or chlamydial eye infections.

In rare instances in men, chlamydial infections lead to pain or swelling in the scrotal area—a sign of epididymitis, an inflammation of a part of the male reproductive system that is near the testicles. Infertility can result if the man is not treated. Chlamydia can also cause proctitis (inflamed rectum), conjunctivitis (inflammation of the lining of the eye), and trachoma—the most common preventable cause of blindness worldwide.

Women should be made aware of the complications associated with chlamydia, and it is important to note that when a woman has chlamydia infections time after time, these repeated episodes increase the likelihood of permanent damage to her reproductive organs.

Concerned about the high rate of this disease, researchers recommended that all sexually active women below age 25 be tested for chlamydia twice a year, in an article in the journal *Sexually Transmitted Diseases* (February 2001). Researchers report that about 4 million cases are diagnosed in the United States every year. Therefore, chlamydia is the most frequently reported infectious disease in the nation and the most common bacteria-caused STD. Furthermore, the reported figures are undoubtedly lower than the actual figures, because not everyone knows he or she has chlamydia, and some do not seek treatment.

Treatment

Once an individual receives a diagnosis of chlamydia, an antibiotic is prescribed. This could be a one-day course of azithromycin or seven days of doxycycline. Other effective options are erythromycin and ofloxacin.

If a woman is pregnant, the doctor usually prescribes azithromycin, erythromycin, or amoxicillin. Penicillin does not eradicate chlamydial infections.

If the problem is not resolved a week after completing the medicine, the patient should return to the doctor for follow-up evaluation.

All sex partners should be evaluated and treated to prevent reinfection. Furthermore, the person with chlamydia and all of her sex partners should have follow-up exams about five or six days after treatment to be sure the problem is eradicated. Intercourse should be avoided until follow-up testing confirms that the disease is cured; the infected person's partner(s) should use the same precaution.

Prevention

It is common for people to infect sexual partners, because chlamydial infection often is present in the absence of symptoms. Those who have multiple sex partners, especially women 25 or younger, should have regular chlamydia testing. People who are sexually active and use condoms or diaphragms during intercourse may reduce the likelihood of transmission of chlamydia.

Researchers are studying topical microbicides and a vaccine as modes of preventing infection. An urgent research priority, too, is the development of a simple, inexpensive test for diagnosis of chlamydial infection.

Psychosocial Issues

A woman who is diagnosed with chlamydia often is very concerned about her ability to have children—a situation the woman must live with because treating the disease may not prevent its causing infertility. Thus, doctors cannot reassure women about their future reproductive ability.

Researchers report that when women find out they have chlamydia, they have several reactions: they are shocked to discover they have a sexually transmitted disease, they feel anxiety about their future fertility, and they often experience difficulty in disclosing the infection to partners. Women report feelings ranging from self-disgust to distress.

A group of UK women who were surveyed said that they felt isolated, reluctant to confide in friends, and disturbed because they had previously believed that STDs primarily affected only women who were promiscuous or "deviant."

Research

In the article "Chlamydia Toxin and Chronic Illness," in *JAMA,* December 19, 2001, Brian Vastag noted that scientists have finally found a gene in *Chlamydia trachomatis* that produces a toxin responsible for an array of chronic illnesses. This discovery also helps explain why only some strains of *C. trachomatis* turn out to be harmful. Chronic inflammation is at the root of the diseases, differing by site, but even decades ago, researchers suspected a toxin caused the inflammation. It was the sequencing of the organism's entire genome that provided answers. At the National Institute of Allergy and Infectious Diseases' Rocky Mountain Laboratories in Hamilton, Montana, Harlan Caldwell, Ph.D., and Robert Belland, Ph.D., found that *C. trachomatis* makes a toxin that collapses protein scaffolding inside cells; that finding explains how toxin B wreaks havoc. The hope is that this finding will lead the way to antitoxin vaccines (*Proceedings of the National Academy of Sciences,* early edition online, November 13, 2001).

chronically infected cells   T cells that carry HIV blueprints and make new HIV.

circumcision   The surgical procedure that removes the end of the prepuce, or foreskin, of the penis. Usually performed on newborn infants, circumcision has an element of preventive maintenance, and, in some cultures, this relates to religious customs. Some researchers conjecture that absence of circumcision makes a man more likely to contract sexually transmitted diseases. More uncircumcised than circumcised men have STDs.

There is growing evidence from sub-Saharan Africa that male circumcision is effective in reducing the risk of acquiring HIV. Researchers concluded that there was ample reason to look at issues of safety, acceptability, feasibility, and cost-effectiveness of promoting male circumcision in African populations as a means of controlling the spread of HIV infection and other sexually transmitted diseases running rampant.

cirrhosis   A condition in which the liver is scarred. Causes of cirrhosis include hepatitis, alcoholism, autoimmune diseases, chronic heart failure, and chronic obstruction of the bile duct. There is no cure for cirrhosis, but its progress can be curtailed. About 30 percent of those with hepatitis C ultimately have cirrhosis of the liver. Of those people in whom cirrhosis develops, about 20 percent experience eventual liver failure.

civil liberties   In the context of sexually transmitted diseases, bias against those with HIV/AIDS is a problem because this has carried over into various forms of discrimination that hamper the individual's civil liberties. Examples are job harassment and firing, housing discrimination, and public accommodation discrimination. Hotly debated in this arena are many topics: disclosure of HIV status, mandatory testing of pregnant women, shared activities or sports that could be conduits of transmission, pros and cons of prevention and educational efforts as means of promoting behavior that is sexually "deviant" or promiscuous, universally required testing, and employers' rights to hire and fire.

clap   See GONORRHEA.

clinical trial Scientific study that is used to test an experimental medicine in human beings in order to gauge its safety and effectiveness for the purpose(s) cited. In respect to sexually transmitted diseases, there are trials set up by research centers, such as those being done by the AIDS Clinical Trials Units, under the auspices of the National Institute of Allergy and Infectious Diseases.

CMV See CYTOMEGALOVIRUS.

cofactor A factor that exists in addition to the main cause of a disease and speeds up disease progression. Cofactors can also be the presence of other factors (stress, environment), proteins, microbes, hormones, genetic resistance or predisposition, and age.

cohort studies Scientific studies that follow groups made up of similar individuals over a period in attempts to find out why some people contract a disease and others do not and to examine factors contributing to the outcomes. In medical research, cohort studies involve people who share a demographic or a specific trait that is the focus of the study. Via cohort studies, researchers are able to glean information on the epidemiological characteristics of diseases.

colitis An inflammatory disease of the colon, colitis has symptoms of diarrhea, abdominal pain, and bloody stools. HIV-infected individuals often suffer from colitis that results from cytomegalovirus. Some patients with colitis have a colon that is diffusely inflamed and thus bleeds readily during colonoscopy.

combination therapy Two or more therapies used in combination in order to treat a disease more effectively. This is done with alternate or simultaneous administration of the drugs. In the case of HIV treatment, researchers and physicians have found that combination therapy works better than monotherapy (the use of one drug alone). It appears clear that drugs work together to fight progression of HIV for many people as well as to stifle the evolution of drug-therapy-resistant strains.

community outreach Operating on the premise that information and knowledge serve to limit or decrease the spread of sexually transmitted diseases, administrators of public health and private prevention programs nationwide are seeking to stem the trend toward increasing proliferation of STDs among those who are sexually active and, in some cases, promote the idea of abstinence as the only surefire way to prevent contracting a sexually transmitted disease.

Community Programs for Clinical Research on AIDS Sponsored by the National Institute of Allergy and Infectious Diseases of the National Institutes of Health, the Community Programs for Clinical Research on AIDS (CPCRA) focus on the patients of community physicians in studies for clinical research pertaining to HIV.

complacency In the late 1990s, the Global Commission on AIDS identified complacency—relaxing safe-sex measures and taking more risks by sexually active people—as a huge issue in that longer lives and improved quality of living for those with HIV/AIDS have given people with high-risk lifestyles a false sense of security. This complacency manifests itself in relaxed attitudes toward condom use, multiple partners and a general lack of vigilance about prevention of sexually transmitted diseases. Some pundits argue that many Americans are also convinced that a cure for AIDS is just around the corner, and others cite the view that highly active antiretroviral therapy (HAART), often resulting in increased longevity, makes a dire health threat look much less ominous. A multistate study of 1,976 HIV-negative or untested people who were at risk for HIV infection showed that, because of the availability of HAART, 31 percent were "less concerned" about becoming infected, and 17 percent were "less safe" about sex or drug use because of the HIV treatments that lengthen lives.

The findings came by way of the HIV testing survey HITS, a seven-state study that used anonymous interviews done from July 1998 to February 1999. Subjects were 693 gay and bisexual men recruited at gay bars, 600 street-recruited injection drug users, and 683 heterosexuals recruited at sexually transmitted disease clinics. The results of the study definitely confirmed fears that HIV therapies have made some high-risk individuals more complacent. Prevention programs must address this matter by disseminating the information that the long-term efficacy of HAART is uncertain and that these treatments also have limitations.

complete blood count Referred to as a CBC, this blood test measures the blood's chief cellular components, including the total white blood cell count, counts of specific kinds of white blood cells, red blood cell count, hemoglobin level, and platelet count.

Comprehensive AIDS Resource Emergency Act of 1990 See RYAN WHITE COMPREHENSIVE AIDS RESOURCE EMERGENCY ACT OF 1990.

Concorde Study This important study weighed the effects of zidovudine (AZT) therapy on asymptomatic HIV patients. Conducted in Great Britain, France, and Ireland as a project of the British Medical Research Council and the French National AIDS Research Agency, Concorde sought to find out whether early treatment with AZT did indeed prolong the lives of those who were HIV-infected but showing no symptoms. The researchers did not know which participants received a placebo and which had AZT, nor did the approximately 1,800 participating in the study. Launched in 1988, Concorde researchers followed subjects for an average of three years and reported that they saw no significant difference in survival rate or disease progression in the two groups. They did find that CD4 levels showed a statistically significant difference, but critics would point to a flaw in the study: there had been a divergence from the original protocol in 1989, when the study was modified on ethical grounds, allowing participants who had a CD4 count below 500 cells/mm3 to start taking AZT. They, and those who began AZT because they had begun to experience symptoms, were included in the preliminary analysis, a fact that was pointed to as having skewed the results.

The authors drew a conclusion that was hotly criticized: in HIV-infected people who were symptom-free, they saw no significant benefit of the immediate use of AZT, compared with deferred therapy, in terms of improved survival rate or reduced disease progression, irrespective of initial CD4 count. Another criticism was that the researchers had not used the optimal dose of AZT, thus rendering the results invalid insofar as predicting potential benefit of the drug. Further, this study looked exclusively at AZT monotherapy, rather than the more beneficial route of combination therapy. The upshot was that Concorde appeared to shoot down the gains that had been made in AIDS research and raised many disturbing questions about the direction that future AIDS research should take.

condom A latex sheath that fits over the penis and is used to prevent pregnancy and STDs, although it cannot be considered 100 percent safe in either case. Health organizations worldwide endorse and promote the use of condoms, but high-risk practices remain common, as 13 percent of men and 5 percent of women in U.S. metropolitan areas report heterosexual activity with two or more partners in the previous 12 months without consistent condom use.

With sexually transmitted diseases wreaking havoc all over the world, most of those who are sexually active know that they should use condoms (also known as rubbers and prophylactics) to prevent unwanted pregnancies and to help reduce the spread of sexually transmitted diseases. It is no secret that genital, anal, and oral sex can be ways of contracting HIV, chlamydia, genital warts, herpes, gonorrhea, hepatitis B, and syphilis.

Of course, it is also well known that many men dislike condoms and that condoms are not 100 percent effective in preventing transmission of sexually transmitted diseases. Thus, the only way a person can make sure he or she is never put at risk is to forgo sex altogether and be abstinent.

An individual can reduce risk by limiting sexual activity to only one partner (monogamy), but this is not 100 percent safe, either, unless the person can be 100 percent sure that the partner is totally monogamous, too. But, even then, one still does not know about the partner's past partners.

One fact a sexually active person can count on is that condom use reduces the risk of contracting an STD. Consider the fact that about two-thirds of those with AIDS in the United States contracted HIV during sexual intercourse with an infected partner—a misfortune that health experts contend probably could have been prevented had the partners used condoms.

Latex condoms offer some protection against genital warts, genital herpes, and hepatitis B virus. They provide good protection against HIV, chancroid, syphilis, chlamydia, gonorrhea, pelvic inflammatory disease, and vaginitis caused by infections such as trichomoniasis and vaginitis caused by changes in pH due to exposure to semen. In this context, it is important to note that condoms made of plastic and those of animal tissue are not recommended for protection against sexually transmitted diseases.

An option for women who are sexually active and want to prevent pregnancy and STDs is the female condom, which fits inside the vagina as a diaphragm does and also covers the vulva. This is not as effective as a man using a condom.

Many couples do use condoms for birth control or reduction of risk of disease, but some people make the mistake of thinking that they are protected from STDs by using other types of birth control, including the IUD, levonorgestrel (Norplant), medroxyprogesterone acetate (Depo-Provera), vasectomy, tubal sterilization, diaphragm, and oral contraceptive pills. These in no way provide protection against contracting STDs. Those who rely on birth-control methods other than condoms still need to use condoms in order to protect against disease.

A sexually active pregnant woman must be especially vigilant about using condoms because she is protecting her fetus as well as herself. Sexually transmitted diseases contracted before pregnancy can cause a tubal pregnancy, which can result in the death of the mother and most certainly results in the death of the unborn infant. STDs can also cause damage to a baby born to an infected woman.

So these are the facts: the "rumor" that condoms are not totally reliable is true, but when used properly, they reduce the likelihood of contracting a sexually transmitted disease, including HIV.

Condoms and Adolescents

As of 2003, rates of many STDs are highest among adolescents; chlamydia and gonorrhea rates are highest among females who are 15 to 19 years old, yet studies show that teens use condoms only occasionally—approximately half the time. Adolescents generally view themselves as bullet-proof, and attempts at HIV education have not been as successful as intended. A 1998 Harris Poll done for the American Foundation for AIDS Research and reported in *Patient Care* (October 1999) noted that 46 percent of participants ages 18 to 24 claimed they had no chance of contracting AIDS, but the foundation also offers statistics that show about half of all new HIV infections in the United States occur in people younger than 24.

Countering Partner Objections

A difficult aspect of condom use is countering partner objections, since there remain many people who are adamantly opposed to using them during sexual activity. Thus, anyone who is sexually active needs to be ready with good responses to such objections. Here are some common objections and appropriate responses that can be used to shoot down these arguments:

"If we plan sex, that detracts from the passion."

Your answer: "We are not actors in the movies; we can get HIV." Suggest that communication and honesty are great foundations for the kind of relationship you would like to have. If no basic intimacy is established, why would you have sex with that person?

"Just trust me."

Your answer: "I will trust you if you agree that safe sex is right for us, until we are both tested and can be sure we're not transmitting any STD." Being naive and assuming that your new partner is telling you the truth is risking your future ability to have children, and you could also be risking your life.

"My religion doesn't allow the use of condoms."

This is true of some religious beliefs, but they probably also do not advocate premarital sex. It can be consider a taboo subject for a woman to initiate, or a man may regard using a condom as a matter of deficient masculinity.

"Don't you think I'm worth taking a chance over?"

No one is worth risking your life over—and hearing someone say this should send up the red flag of selfishness. Basically this person is saying to you, "I'm so cool that, to my mind, my giving you an STD is no problem because you'll think it was worth it, because the sex was so good." Ask yourself whether that logic holds true: will you have fond memories of hot sex when you are sitting in the sexually transmitted disease clinic trying to figure out a way to get rid of a very unsexy case of genital warts?

"I hate condoms—that's like wearing a raincoat."

Many men persuade women to abandon the safe-sex idea because they claim their satisfaction will be severely compromised. This can make a woman feel very fearful: if I do not do it the way he wants, he will turn to another girl. Again, remember that no one is worth risking your life for or suffering the complications of a sexually transmitted disease for.

"I don't have a condom with me."

Whether male or female, a sexually active person should carry a condom. For women, it is a mistake to assume that a man will come prepared, and it is important to take responsibility for one's own health by having condoms on hand when sex is planned. Being prepared is not synonymous with being promiscuous; it is synonymous with being proactive and smart.

How to Handle Condoms

Handling condoms gently and storing them properly (in a cool, dry place) are important. Those using condoms should also apply a drop or two of lubricant (unless using the kind that are prelubricated). It is important to bear in mind that oil-based lubricants can damage latex; these, which are to be avoided, include petroleum jelly (Vaseline), butter, cold cream, and mineral and vegetable oils. Storing condoms in a glove compartment, wallet, or pocket can damage them, thus rendering them ineffective.

When a user opens a condom package, he or she should take care not to tear it, and in instances when a condom seems brittle or sticky, do not consider it safe for use.

A drop of lubricant should be put inside if the condom is unlubricated. To put a condom on, an uncircumcised user should pull back his foreskin before rolling it on. For the circumcised, this is not a consideration. The man should place the rolled condom over the tip of the hard penis, with a half-inch left at the tip for semen collecting. With one hand, he should pinch the air out of the tip (most condom breaks are caused by friction against air bubbles). He should use his other hand to unroll it over the penis, rolling it all the way down the base. Next step: he smoothes out air bubbles and lubricates the outside. As far as proper placement, a condom should be put on before the penis touches the vulva because males leak fluids before and after ejaculation that can carry sperm and germs that might cause STDs. A condom is good for one use only. Also, the expiration date on the package should be checked.

After a condom has been used, correct removal is also important; the man should pull out of the vagina before the penis softens, and the condom should be held against the base of the penis to prevent semen spillage. After disposing of the condom, the man should wash his penis with soap and water before reinitiating contact or cuddling.

condyloma acuminata This is the scientific name for genital warts. These are sexually transmitted warty growths that usually project outward and that appear on the external genitalia, vagina, cervix, or anus. Sometimes, though, the warts are flat or even require the application of acetic acid solution by a physician in order to see the lesions. The person who has genital warts is infected with the human papillomavirus.

condyloma lata In the secondary stage of the sexually transmitted disease syphilis, condyloma lata, which are genital lesions, appear. These are highly infectious.

confidentiality In medical records terminology, information concerning a patient that is confidential cannot be released without written authorization by the patient. In the case of HIV testing, the information takes on added gravity in that the individual who was tested does not want to be identified as having HIV or even as having been tested for HIV. This restricts the medical facility's disclosure of the information, but the negative or positive test result still remains in the medical file of the individual tested, within the records section of the medical facility. Some believe that having this information as a part of one's permanent medical file is unwise in that it presents a clear and present danger that even confidential results could be leaked without the patient's permission.

congenital syphilis Syphilis that is transmitted to a baby by intrauterine infection from a mother who has the infection. When this is untreated, about 40 percent of congenital infections result in the death of the children. Those children who contract syphilis and are untreated sometimes suffer neurological impairment, seizures, deafness, and/or tooth and bone deformities.

More often than in the past, in the United States syphilis is detected in pregnant women, and they are treated. A woman usually needs a single dose of penicillin, which is considered safe for her and the infant in utero.

As a result of the Centers for Disease Control and Prevention's national initiative on syphilis elimination, launched in 1998, doctors saw (as of 2001) a remarkable drop in rates of syphilis in infants. In the year 2000, 529 congenital syphilis cases were reported to the CDC: about 13 of every 100,000 live births. Of these, 434 occurred because the mother had no or poor syphilis treatment. In 123 of the cases, the mothers had no prenatal care. From 1997 to 2000, congenital syphilis rates have dropped 51 percent.

Rates of congenital syphilis are highest in the South. African Americans posted the highest rate, which was 49.3 per 100,000 births; Hispanics and Latin Americans had a rate of 22.6; whites' rate was 1.5. A large part of the overall decline in syphilis in infants and women was a result of the CDC's prevention program, in cooperation with local and state agencies.

One problem that still exists is that health care providers must be able to do screenings for syphilis in order to treat pregnant women who have syphilis. According to a survey conducted in 1998, only 85 percent of obstetricians in the United States screen pregnant women routinely for syphilis.

The current CDC recommendation is that women be tested for syphilis during early pregnancy. In areas of high prevalence of syphilis, providers are asked to test patients early in pregnancy and twice in the third trimester, including once at delivery. It is also recommended that syphilis screening be offered in jails, emergency rooms, and other settings that sometimes take care of pregnant women who are in high-risk STD categories.

contact tracing A treatment-and-prevention practice that involves tracing sexual partners of those with sexually transmitted diseases—in particular, HIV and AIDS—in order to spur those individuals to seek medical testing. In some cases, the name of the infected individual is given to the contact; in other cases, there is no identification of the person who has the disease.

contraceptives Methods of preventing unwanted pregnancy, none of which is 100 percent effective. Most of the contraceptives commonly used are good methods, each of which has pros and cons. The first concern in choosing a contraceptive should be reliability and safety. Methods of birth control that have a rate of only about two or fewer pregnancies per 100 couples per year in scientific studies, when instructions were followed carefully, include birth control pills, IUDs, diaphragms, latex condoms (spermicidal), medroxyprogesterone acetate (Depo-Provera) injections, and sterilization. Some couples whose religious beliefs forbid use of hormonal or mechanical methods of contraception use the rhythm method, which limits sexual intercourse to those days of the month in the menstrual cycle that are deemed most unlikely to result in conception.

Those who deal in dispensing contraceptives always do so with the caveat that the effectiveness of a method of contraception is dependent on how carefully and consistently partners use it. According to reports from pregnant women and from studies, there are times when couples are least likely to take precautions and use contraceptives; these include the beginning of a new relationship, the end of a relationship, times of emotional turmoil, after a pregnancy scare or abortion, and after diagnosis or treatment of a sexually transmitted disease. Methods of contraception that have a low rate of effectiveness include withdrawal, suppositories, gels, sponges, foams, and creams.

In the context of the study of STDs, it is important to remember that a contraceptive does not automatically convey protection against a sexually transmitted disease. Latex condoms do, however, provide some protection.

Clinical prevention guidelines for patients in STD clinics include: avoid sexual intercourse with an infected partner until that person has been adequately treated; if you are with a new partner, use a new condom with each act; be aware that vaginal spermicides reduce infections but do not protect against transmission of HIV; know that using nonbarrier contraceptives offers no protection. Preexposure vaccination for hepatitis A and B is also recommended.

copayment   The amount of money paid by an insured person when he or she sees a doctor for medical treatment. It is usually a small fixed amount and is separate from what is paid by the individual's insurance.

correctional facilities   The umbrella term for facilities that house and confine criminals who have been convicted in the American court system and sentenced to various periods in jail. This term is significant in regard to sexually transmitted diseases because prisoners need to be in the loop of prevention information, particularly concerning HIV transmission, but also including all types of sexually transmitted diseases.

counseling   The act of health care providers' offering guidance and support for patients. In the realm of sexually transmitted diseases, counseling is necessary to get the individual through the ini-

tial shock, particularly in respect to HIV/AIDS and genital herpes. Learning to live with a lifelong disease or infection takes strong support from family and friends, and a qualified counselor can certainly be an important part of the treatment team.

Counseling describes the meeting between a patient and a health care professional to discuss issues and concerns during periods of crisis, anxiety, or confusion or simply to understand herself or himself better and make wiser choices. In respect to sexually transmitted diseases, counseling services are critical, especially for those diseases that have lifelong implications, such as genital herpes and HIV. With these diseases, the infected individual faces psychological and social problems that are extremely complex and often devastating. Counseling can help a person make his or her way through the maze of shock, fear, anger, and confusion that typically surrounds these STDs.

cryosurgery   See CRYOTHERAPY.

cryotherapy   The use of liquid nitrogen to produce extremely cold temperatures in order to freeze and destroy particular tissues, such as cancer tissue. Cryotherapy is used to treat problems such as Kaposi's sarcoma and abnormal cells on the cervix.

cryptococcal meningitis   The fungus *Cryptococcus neoformans* is the cause of the infection cryptococcosis, which is generally very severe in those who have HIV infection, often leading to meningitis. Headaches, fever, seizures, and vision difficulties are common symptoms. Typically, doctors diagnose this form of meningitis by blood analysis and a spinal tap (a lumbar puncture). After the patient is treated, this disease often recurs.

cryptococcosis   The infection that is caused by *Cryptococcus neoformans*. Immunosuppression predisposes a person to cryptococcal infection. Infection of the lung occurs after inhalation of dust containing *C. neoformans*. Central nervous system involvement is the most common manifestation of cryptococcosis.

cultural barriers   In certain ethnic groups, condom use is still viewed as a less macho approach to sexuality, and this belief becomes a barrier to commonsense use of methods for prevention of sexually transmitted disease. Thus, one of the goals of community education efforts is to erase the misconception that protecting oneself against sexually transmitted diseases makes a man less masculine.

cytomegalovirus (CMV)   Cytomegalovirus is a common virus of the herpes family that infects about half of all young adults in the United States. Though it usually does not have dire consequences, and, in fact, most adult CMV infections are asymptomatic, it also affects AIDS patients, who often have serious cases of CMV because of their compromised immune system. Such infections can occur in the eyes, lungs, liver, gastrointestinal tract, brain, or bone marrow. One of the worst spinoffs of this disease is retinitis; CMV eye infection can lead to blindness.

The virus can be found in saliva, urine, and other body fluids. Also found in cervical secretions and semen, CMV can be spread by sexual contact. Even kissing can spread it. Evidence indicates that most CMV infections are acquired via close personal contact or sexual transmission. An incurable virus, CMV stays with a person for life, though usually in a dormant state, as does genital herpes, and both can reactivate occasionally.

Doctors use the ELISA test to diagnose CMV. Treatment for CMV involves the use of the antiviral drugs foscarnet and ganciclovir when the sufferer has AIDS-associated CMV retinitis. Currently in testing are new antiviral drugs for use in CMV infections.

One serious complication is that CMV can infect a baby in the uterus of a mother who becomes infected with CMV or has a recurrence during pregnancy. In the United States, almost 1 percent of newborns are infected. For an infant, congenital CMV can have serious complications: mental retardation, deafness, or epilepsy.

Prevention is difficult, but there is evidence that male condoms may reduce the likelihood of transmission of CMV by oral, vaginal, and anal intercourse. Handwashing and proper handling of diapers of infected infants are important, because CMV is shed in saliva and urine.

dating   After the 1980s, the concept of dating was radically altered by HIV, which put a considerable pall on the freewheeling sexual activity of previous decades. Suddenly, sex took on a whole new character, as people who had never before even considered the idea of condom use had to face the reality that HIV could be the result of engaging in sexual activity with an infected person.

delta hepatitis   Also known as HEPATITIS D.

dental dam   A latex device made for use in dentistry, but often used as a barrier when a person is involved in sex acts—oral and anal. A dental dam is usually a small six-inch square of latex. Sometimes people also use unlubricated condoms that have been cut open. Dental dams are believed to prevent the transfer of vaginal secretions, blood, and fecal matter. Some health care professionals recommend that a dental dam not be reused.

depression   A mental state characterized by sad mood, hopelessness, and general despondency. Symptoms vary from mild depression's sadness and tearful episodes to major depression's sleep and appetite disturbances; withdrawal; dysfunction in work, school, or home; loss of energy; lack of focus; and, in some cases, suicidal thoughts. In people with sexually transmitted diseases, periods of "the blues" are not unusual, especially immediately after initial diagnosis. In those with HIV, a clinical diagnosis of major depression is sometimes made more difficult by the fact that many symptoms of depression can be caused by HIV infection, related conditions, even the drugs used for therapy.

digital-anal sex   A sex act in which one partner uses a finger to stimulate the other's anus. This is pertinent in respect to sexually transmitted diseases in that genital secretions can be a means of transmitting HIV, so the partners involved in digital-anal sex need to be cognizant of this fact and use safe-sex measures.

digital transmission   The transmission of a sexually transmitted disease by one partner's fingers touching the other partner's genitals.

dildo   A sex toy that is used in sex play to mimic the feel of an erect penis. In prevention of sexually transmitted diseases, the dildo must be considered a possible means of transmission when it has genital secretions on it.

disability   An illness, injury or other state that impairs an individual physically or mentally.

disclosure   The revelation of one's health status regarding HIV or another disease has long been a hotly debated issue. In *Child Care Health Development* (January 2000), C. Thorne, M. L. Newell, and C. S. Peckham looked at the aspect of disclosure of infection status in families affected by HIV and planning for the social care of children of infected parents. This information was collected as part of a large survey on clinical and psychosocial service use of these families, including parents and other caregivers for HIV-affected children, in follow-up in 10 pediatric centers from seven European countries. Of 182 surveys returned, most were filled out by parents (73 percent), of whom 92 percent were HIV-infected. Of the 226 children cared for by respondents, 62 percent were HIV-infected. The researchers reported that the child's and parent's infection statues were rarely disclosed, and this lack of communication was associated with the child's age in both cases. Also, it was seen that infected children who lived with their parents were less likely to know their own diagnosis than were those who lived in alternative care. Uninfected parents and caregivers were more likely to need professional guidance in disclosing the information to an infected child than were infected parents. Of infected parents, half had made plans for the care of their children in the event that they became unable to care for them. As a result of improved management of pediatric HIV, greater numbers of vertically infected children are reaching adolescence.

discrimination *Discrimination* was one word that took on new layers of meaning when the 1980s ushered in bias against those with HIV/AIDS, as the epidemic's frightening proportions caused many people to focus unprecedented scrutiny on the homosexual male segment of the population. An HIV diagnosis was such a stigma that many people with HIV experienced conflict in their feelings about disclosure. It soon became clear that some people were discriminating against those with HIV/AIDS. People lost jobs, and the firings were attributed to loosely worded "nonperformance" causes. Mortgages and leases were refused those with HIV or AIDS. Some insurance companies dropped coverage when they discovered that certain clients were HIV-positive. Although matters have improved somewhat now that highly active antiretroviral therapy has allowed HIV-infected individuals to live longer, symptom-free, many people with this diagnosis still choose not to tell coworkers because they do not want to be treated as pariahs.

For those with HIV/AIDS who do face discrimination, there are attorneys well versed in legal rights and obligations. A good source of information on lawyers is the state bar association, a local AIDS-advocacy agency, or a civil rights commission.

It is not hard to find a professional who will handle complaints about discrimination. In this context, it is important to note that people with AIDS are protected against discrimination on grounds of disability (Section 504 of the Rehabilitation Act of 1973). The Americans with Disabilities Act of 1990 prohibits discrimination against people with HIV infection, even if they do not show signs of infection, and the law applies even to service providers and groups that do not receive federal funding. Federal law also protects HIV-infected people from discrimination in recruitment, hiring, assignment of job, sick leave, and other benefits. Health care rights encompass treatment without discrimination by hospitals, nursing homes, hospices, and other health care providers. Social services—welfare, Medicaid, Medicare, and other programs—must also be administered without discrimination because a person has HIV/AIDS.

Those whose rights are violated can report a violation to the Office for Civil Rights, U.S. Department of Health and Human Services, 200 Independence Avenue, SW, Washington, DC 20201, or can submit the complaint directly to a regional office instead of having it forwarded by the federal bureau. The complaint must be filed within 180 days of the alleged infraction; must include name, phone number, and signature; must cite the company, service provider, or organization filing against; must indicate the complaint and the date it occurred; and must include an explanation of attempts to resolve the problem.

DNR An indication on a patient's medical chart that is an order to those providing health care that the person does not want to be revived by means of CPR if he or she is near death—as in cardiac or pulmonary arrest. The order means "do not resuscitate." In the case of advanced AIDS, patients sometimes do not want to continue being treated and kept alive. DNR does not apply to offering or giving other forms of treatment. Some physicians discuss DNR orders with a patient who has a serious condition. A patient can also broach the subject. Some patients choose to deal with this decision before the disease has debilitated them by assigning a durable power of attorney for health care and by making a living will.

do not resuscitate   See DNR.

donovanosis   A very rare sexually transmitted disease. Donovanosis is most common in New Guinea, Africa, India, the Caribbean, and Australia. In the same way that genital ulcers are most commonly caused by herpes in the United States, in other countries donovanosis is the most common cause.

Cause
Donovanosis is caused by the bacterium *Calymmatobacterium granulomatis.*

Symptoms
Also called granuloma inguinale, donovanosis is characterized by ulcers. Symptoms show up about 80 days after exposure, and people usually see ulcers in the genital or anal area and sometimes in the mouth. These are dark red and large, starting as nodules and ulcerating. The ulcer(s) slowly enlarges, causing tissue destruction. The tissue can bleed easily.

Testing
A biopsy of the infected skin is required. Sometimes, this infection is also detected when a woman has a Pap smear.

Treatment
Antibiotics should be taken for a minimum of 21 days as directed by a physician. Treatment with antibiotics is also important because studies suggest that the person with donovanosis has a greater risk of getting HIV if exposed to the virus.

A person who is infected must be sure to complete the course of the antibiotics because treatment is effective only with a full course of antibiotics. Various medications have been used successfully, including doxycycline and trimethoprim-sulfamethoxazole (TMP-SMX) (Bactrim). A person with HIV may need to take the medications for a longer period to achieve successful eradication.

Permanent scarring is possible in areas such as the urethra. If this obstructs the drainage of lymphatic fluid, it can cause genital tissue swelling and result in a condition called genital elephantiasis.

Prevention
Since it is known that transmission can occur through sexual contact with an infected partner, condoms are recommended. Also, all sex partners of a person with donovanosis should take the antibiotics even if they have no symptoms. Anyone who has had sexual contact within a 60-day period before the donovanosis symptoms developed should receive antibiotic treatment.

double-blind study   A clinical study that can claim total objectivity in that it does not allow the researchers or the subjects information as to which treatment has been applied to which group of subjects. Used in drug trials to prevent tainting of results because of bias or preconceived expectations or notions, the study gives an experimental drug to one group and a placebo to the other.

drug abuse   A person's attempts to self-medicate, often with drugs that are illegal, but also with ones that have been prescribed but are used in a manner other than the way that they were intended. The correlation between drug abuse and STDs is multifaceted. In respect to HIV/AIDS, disease is often transmitted when drug users share drug injection paraphernalia. Furthermore, drugs can lessen the likelihood of using safe-sex measures when their mood-altering aspect hazes the judgment of sexually active individuals. Another problem arises when some drug users turn to drug sales and/or prostitution in order to provide money for their drug habits; this puts them at high risk for STDs in yet another way.

It is also believed by many researchers that the immune system can be damaged by use of alcohol, cocaine, amphetamines, and other drugs. Thus, users have heightened risk for contracting HIV and other sexually transmitted diseases.

Drug abuse can also put the drug abuser's children at risk. Consider the fact that most pediatric AIDS cases in the United States have resulted from prenatal transmission when a parent used IV drugs.

drug-associated HIV transmission   One of the biggest problems with the spread of HIV, despite the fact that many people in the United States are aware of this mode of HIV transmission—via sharing of needles or other drug paraphernalia. Nevertheless, the U.S. government budgets a great deal of money every year for information and prevention programs that seek to inform intravenous drug users not to share equipment and to encourage them to seek help from needle exchange programs nationwide as well as from drug rehabilitation programs.

drug cocktail   A combination of drugs used to treat a disease. In the case of HIV, the combination of drugs known as highly active antiretroviral therapy (HAART) is called a drug cocktail. This has proved very effective at lengthening the lives of many people with HIV.

drug interaction   The interaction—positive or negative—between or among drugs that are used in conjunction with one another. It is important for a doctor to supervise a drug regimen because some drug interactions can prove fatal. In the case of HIV, monitoring of the combinations of drugs used in HAART is important to foster good results and to prevent unpleasant side effects and reduced effectiveness caused by some drug interactions.

drug-resistant gonorrhea   Strains of gonorrhea that have developed a resistance to the traditional antibiotics used to treat this disease.

See also GONORRHEA.

drug user   A person who self-medicates using illegal drugs or legal drugs to the point of overuse. In the context of sexually transmitted diseases, it is important to note two points: intravenous drug use is one of the main risks of contracting HIV, and persons who use drugs sometimes do not demonstrate good judgment in practicing safe sex via condom use. Thus, they put themselves at greater risk of contracting STDs. Health care experts caution that the use of mood-altering drugs often results in unsafe sexual activity—in some cases, even with strangers. Yet another offshoot of vulnerability of the drug user is in respect to suppression of the immune system, which leaves a person more vulnerable to HIV if exposed.

duty to warn   A person diagnosed with HIV has an ethical obligation to inform current and past partners they may have been exposed to the virus, and in some places, the HIV-infected individual also has a legal obligation. Usually, this means informing any partner with whom he or she had a sexual relationship during the past two years. Also, it is wise to encourage those people to be tested for HIV. It may take several tests to confirm that they have not contracted the disease, because the blood test usually takes about three months to show positive results. Most states have laws that make notifying past partners a legal requirement. More controversial is the physician's role in notification: the American Medical Association has advised physicians that they should inform partners if the patient refuses to inform them. Beyond partners, though, a person who has HIV has no obligation to inform anyone else, and in many cases, attorneys advise clients not to do so.

Tarasoff v. Regents of the University of California established a precedent in this arena: a psychologist knew a patient wanted to kill a young woman and, clinging to the issue of a patient's right to confidentiality, took no steps to protect the proposed victim, who subsequently was killed. Thus, the Supreme Court went on to establish the "duty to warn" standard, which later became a California statute. Later *Tarasoff* was defined more broadly by other state courts, requiring physicians to warn others of the danger a patient may pose if the risk of disease transmission is foreseeable.

Persons who have been infected with HIV must tell all sex partners they have had within the last year or two, and anyone with whom they have shared needles and syringes, so they become aware they may have been exposed to the virus. People diagnosed with HIV who do not want to contact partners can ask the health department to help in this matter of notification.

Beyond the HIV realm, there is also the duty to warn of other sexually transmitted diseases, some of which doctors are required to report to the Centers for Disease Control and Prevention. (As of 2003, syphilis, chlamydia, and AIDS are reportable diseases in every state. HIV and chancroid are reportable in many states. Requirements for reporting other STDs differ by state.)

dysphagia A condition in which the act of swallowing is difficult. Sometimes dysphagia causes the sensation of having something stuck in the throat. Causes can be conditions of the mouth or throat, pharynx or esophagus obstruction, or muscular activity abnormalities of the esophagus.

early detection In all sexually transmitted diseases, knowledge of having the disease is desirable because treatment modalities are usually more effective when applied early on. Furthermore, early detection prevents the spread of the sexually transmitted disease—ideally when the individual realizes that there is an infection and discontinues sexual activity until the disease is cleared—or in the case of HIV, continues to use protection indefinitely. Also in HIV patients, early detection allows treatment with drug therapy before the disease has ravaged the immune system and thus can serve to lengthen life and improve quality of life as well.

ear piercing The insertion of a needle into the earlobe in order to create a hole to accommodate an earring; also, a possible means of becoming infected with HIV in that the needle used in piercing has contact with blood. If a needle used on an HIV-infected person is reused on another client of the ear piercer—without being cleaned and sterilized—HIV may be spread via the needle. However, it is usually standard practice for the personnel of piercing salons to clean their equipment before each piercing, so the likelihood of contracting HIV in this manner is very remote. However, inquiring about salon practices in regard to reuse of equipment is still a good idea.

ectopic pregnancy The development of an embryo at a site other than the uterus. This can occur if the fertilized egg remains in the ovary or the fallopian tube or if it lodges in the abdominal cavity. A tubal pregnancy is the most common type of ectopic pregnancy; it can occur in fallopian tubes that become blocked or have been inflamed. When the fetus grows, the tube may rupture and bleed. Typically, the fetus dies within three months of conception and is absorbed into the woman's body. In the realm of sexually transmitted diseases, a past history of pelvic inflammatory disease (due to infection with chlamydia or gonorrhea) is a risk factor for ectopic pregnancy.

education In respect to all types of sexually transmitted diseases, health care professionals are in agreement that education is a key part of prevention, and public health agencies go to great lengths in order to facilitate the dissemination of educational materials and programs. The goals are to make sexually active people aware of the importance of practicing safe sex and to enhance their awareness of the kinds of diseases that can be communicated when individuals indulge in risky practices and have sexual activity with high-risk partners.

ejaculation The discharge of semen from the penis at the time of orgasm (climax) in a male. The elements of semen are released in the following sequence: the secretion of Cowper's glands, followed by sperm and the secretion of the prostate gland, and, finally, that of the seminal vesicles.

ELISA test The ELISA—enzyme-linked immunosorbent assay—is a blood test commonly done to detect antibodies in the blood—particularly applicable to HIV disease. Because this test can produce false positive results in testing for HIV, there is a second test that is done for confirmation—the Western blot, which is 99 percent accurate. Many community health clinics offer these tests free. The person being tested can choose to have the test anonymously (he or she is not identified) or confidentially (he or she is listed in clinic records by name, and the information is regarded as private).

emaciation   Wasting of the body caused by conditions, diseases, or lack of nutrition. This term is sometimes associated with the final stage of AIDS, in which some people become very thin.

e-mail HIV prevention news updates   An online source of information on HIV is the CDC National Prevention Information Network at http://www.cdcnpin.org/services/listserve.htm. Submit your e-mail address and you will receive regular news updates on HIV.

emotional problems   For many people, the diagnosis of a sexually transmitted disease can result in a great deal of emotional turmoil, which can turn out to be a significant aspect of the disease. This is especially true in the case of the life-threatening disease HIV and the lifelong disease genital herpes. With each of these, the individual must adapt to living with a disease that not only has tremendous physical ramifications, but also can cause social ostracism and depression. Helping the sufferer of one of these diseases to adjust and cope should be considered an important part of treatment.

employee benefits   Usually health and life insurance and retirement savings, the "perks" received by a worker in addition to salary.

employment discrimination   The 1993 movie *Philadelphia* was a hallmark film effort that gave graphic clarity and poignancy to the issue of employer discrimination against employees with HIV/AIDS. In the early days of the AIDS epidemic, there were many cases in which people reportedly lost jobs because they had AIDS, and the workplace was wrought with fears and misconceptions concerning how HIV could be spread. As people became better educated about HIV and the courts made decisions based on their interpretation of the Americans with Disabilities Act, the reaction subsided somewhat.

encephalitis   An inflammation of the brain that may be caused by a viral or bacterial infection or may be a part of an allergic reaction to a systemic viral illness or vaccination. This infection manifests itself in headaches, fever, seizures, and other neurological problems—symptoms that, when combined with the results of a CT scan, MRI, lumbar puncture, or EEG, confirm the diagnosis. People who are HIV-positive may have encephalitis caused by infection with HIV, CMV, *Toxoplasma* species, or herpesvirus.

endemic   A disease that is indigenous to a certain region; the constant presence of a disease or an infectious agent in a specific geographic area.

enteritis   With the primary symptom of diarrhea, enteritis is an inflammation of the small intestine. Viruses and bacteria can cause infective enteritis. X rays and radioactive isotopes can cause radiation enteritis. The causes of enteritis in a person with HIV are typically *Cryptosporidium* and *Microsporidium* species, CMV, and *Mycobacterium avium* complex.

enzyme-linked immunosorbent assay   See ELISA TEST.

eosinophilic folliculitis   Occurring in advanced HIV disease, eosinophilic folliculitis features itchy papules signaling an inflammatory reaction around the hair follicles. In most patients, there are hundreds of lesions. Eosinophilic folliculitis is chronic, with spontaneous exacerbations and remissions.

epidemic   A disease that is affecting many people at the same time in a given area, when this prevalence is in excess of what may be expected on the basis of past statistics for that population. The word *epidemic* also refers to the unarrested spread of a disease—AIDS, for example.

epidemiology   The science that focuses on studying a disease and its links to various factors that may affect the likelihood of increased or decreased incidence in a certain environment.

epididymitis   An inflammation of the epididymis, a tube that connects the testis to the vas deferens in a man. In men younger than 35 years old, epididymitis is usually sexually transmitted and is most commonly caused by chlamydia or gonorrhea. In men 35 and older, it is usually caused by bacterial prostatitis, underlying structural urologic problems, or recent manipulation (such as catheterization) of the genitourinary tract. Different bacteria result in epididymitis in these cases. Pain, swelling, and redness of the scrotum occur over one to two days. Initially, tenderness is limited to the epididymis; it then spreads to the testis. Treatment includes antibiotics and scrotal elevation.

Epstein-Barr virus (EBV)   Epstein-Barr virus is the causative agent of infectious mononucleosis and is also associated with Burkitt's lymphoma and nasopharyngeal carcinoma. The virus is spread from person to person by exchange of saliva and close contact. Nasopharyngeal carcinoma is most common in China. Historically, Burkitt's lymphoma has been most common in Africa. However, more recently, there has been an increasing incidence in nonendemic countries of Burkitt's lymphoma in AIDS patients. There are also B cell lymphomas—which are distinct from Burkitt's lymphoma but also associated with EBV—that occur in immunocompromised patients, such as those who have AIDS. Hairy leukoplakia of the tongue is another EBV-associated disease.

erythropoietin   A hormone secreted by certain cells in the kidney that stimulates red blood cell production. For HIV-associated anemia, there is a genetically engineered version of erythropoietin that has lessened the need for transfusion and thus allowed HIV patients to continue antiviral therapy even when the drugs induce anemia.

esophagitis   An inflammation of the esophagus. In reflux esophagitis, caused by regurgitation of stomach acid, the symptoms are heartburn, difficulty in swallowing, and regurgitation of bitter fluid. A very serious form of this inflammation is corrosive esophagitis, caused by ingestion of caustic acids or alkali. Infective esophagitis often results from a fungus (*Candida* species) infection in debilitated patients, especially those being treated with certain drugs; it also can occur in people with viruses, such as cytomegalovirus and herpesvirus. Chiefly characterized by painful swallowing, esophagitis often occurs with AIDS.

exercise   Exerting oneself in a regimen of exercise or workouts is a way to enhance health and overall lifestyle. The fitness enthusiast often benefits psychologically as well as gaining physical and health advantages, in that a sense of well-being accompanies frequent and regular exercise. In tandem with proper nutrition, an exercise regimen can help people heal and recover more readily.

experimental drug   A drug that has not been approved for use as a treatment. In sexually transmitted diseases, the term *experimental drug* commonly refers to the assortment of medication options under review for HIV and AIDS.

exposure   Contact with a sexually transmitted disease that is incidental or that results from high-risk behavior and its frequency. In such cases, there is a window of opportunity for the infectious disease to infect a sex partner. In many cases, though, one exposure is sufficient to produce infection with a sexually transmitted disease.

facilitated DNA inoculation The thrust of this process is the input of noninfectious HIV genes into a person's blood via injection; this occurs in concert with administration of an agent meant to promote uptake of the genes into host cells. The HIV-fighting premise is based on an effort to cause an individual's own cells to produce HIV proteins and to stimulate the individual's immune system to produce antibodies and killer T cells.

facts on STDs The National Institute of Allergy and Infectious Diseases, a division of the National Institutes of Health, has published the following information on sexually transmitted diseases in the United States:

- STDs affect the entire population, people in all walks of life. Most STD sufferers are teens and young adults. Almost two-thirds of all STDs occur in people younger than 25.
- The higher incidence of STDs in the American public is partly attributable to a growing tendency for earlier sexual activity combined with later marriages. Also, divorce is common, sending people back into the dating realm. The net result is that those who are sexually active are now more likely to have multiple sex partners and, thus, put themselves at risk for contracting STDs.
- It is important to remember that some STDs do not produce symptoms, particularly in women. Also, when there are symptoms, they are easily confused with the symptoms of diseases that are not transmitted via sexual contact.
- Even when an STD does not cause symptoms, the infected individual may be able to pass on the disease to a sex partner. That is why periodic

testing is advisable for those who have multiple sex partners.

- Women generally experience more severe and more frequent health consequences from STDs. This is partly because the upshot of having an asymptomatic infection is that many people delay seeking medical care until they have serious problems. Examples are STDs that spread into the uterus and fallopian tubes, causing pelvic inflammatory disease (PID), which can result in infertility and ectopic pregnancy. Human papillomavirus can lead to cervical and other genital cancers, although this is rare. There is also a problem of vertical transmission, mother to baby, of STDs. Some infections can be cured; others may cause death or disability to the infant.
- Diagnosed and treated early in their course, most STDs are treatable. The most serious STD is acquired immunodeficiency syndrome (AIDS), a fatal viral infection of the immune system. Health experts agree that contracting STDs other than AIDS increases one's risk of acquiring the AIDS virus.

Fair Housing Act The Fair Housing Act (1968) specifies the tenets of governmental protection against housing discrimination in sales and rentals.

Fair Housing Amendments Act When the Fair Housing Act was amended in 1988, it enlarged the Fair Housing Act of 1968, which had undergone several amendments in the 1970s and 1980s. The point was to ban housing discrimination that was disability-based (in this case, in relation to HIV). It prohibits landlords from ostracizing those with HIV; they cannot evict these people, legally harm them, or refuse to rent or renew a lease.

Specifically, the Fair Housing Act prohibits housing discrimination based on race, color, religion, sex, disability, familial status, and national origin. Its coverage includes private housing, housing that receives federal financial assistance, and state and local government housing. This law makes it illegal to discriminate in any aspect of selling or renting housing or to deny a dwelling to a buyer, renter, or individual who intends to live in the residence. Also covered are financing, zoning practices, new construction design, and advertising. Further, the act requires housing facility owners to make reasonable exceptions to afford those with disabilities equal housing opportunities. (A landlord who has a no-pet policy can be required to grant an exception to this rule to allow a blind person with a guide dog to live in the residence.)

The act also requires that landlords allow disabled tenants to make reasonable access-related modifications to their private living space, as well as to common-use spaces, although the landlord does not have to pay for such changes. Also, new multi-family housing with four or more units must be designed and built to allow access for individuals with disabilities. This includes accessible common-use areas, doors wide enough for wheelchairs, kitchens and bathrooms that allow a wheelchair-bound person to maneuver, and other adaptable features within units.

A *handicap* is defined as a physical or mental impairment that substantially limits major life activities, as in the instance of persons living with AIDS. Protection extends to those who are perceived as having a handicap, even if they do not. The definition was gleaned from the Rehabilitation Act of 1973, which courts interpreted as encompassing HIV/AIDS.

false-negative A blood test result that is inaccurate in that the individual being tested has a negative result when in fact he or she has contracted a disease. The reason for a false-negative result typically is that too few antibodies or antigens are currently present to produce a positive result.

false-positive A positive test result that is inaccurate. The blood test incorrectly indicates that the person tested has a specific infection.

family law In respect to issues of divorce, custody, and so on, the American Bar Association prohibits revelation of a party's HIV status as leverage in a divorce or custody case or as an indication of a party's sexual orientation. Some states bar same-sex couples from becoming foster parents. It is important to check state laws and consult an attorney to resolve issues that involve family law.

fatigue A feeling of tiredness is a nonspecific symptom that can result from a basic cause such as sleep deprivation, common sources such as anemia or hypothyroidism, or more serious illnesses.

FDA See FOOD AND DRUG ADMINISTRATION.

female condom Designed as a vaginal barrier to help prevent HIV transmission, this contraceptive and disease-prevention barrier prevents the entry of semen and other fluids. Rated as safe and effective as condoms for males, this lubricated sheath of polyurethane fits into the vagina and is anchored behind the pubic bone. A woman does the insertion in much the same manner as putting a diaphragm in place. Lubricants (water-based) can be used to make insertion easier. No prescription is required. Female condoms are available in medical clinics and drugstores. As for male condoms, correct use is key to providing protection, and the device is not 100 percent effective in preventing STDs and pregnancy. The CDC's *Sexually Transmitted Diseases Treatment Guidelines 2002* call the female condom Reality "an effective mechanical barrier to viruses including HIV." With the exception of one study on trichomoniasis, no clinical studies have been completed to evaluate the effectiveness of female condoms as protection from STDs. It is believed that the use of female condoms does reduce the risk for STDs.

feminine hygiene products Items such as vaginal douches, many of which are not usually recommended by doctors.

Fitz-Hugh–Curtis syndrome Named for the doctors who reported this condition (Fitz-Hugh and Curtis), a condition marked by "violin-string" adhesions between the liver and the diaphragm—usually as a result of infection with chlamydia or gonorrhea. Bacteria travel to the right side of the abdomen and collect in fluid above the liver, causing pain in this area.

flagellation The act of striking or beating with hands or devices (whips, paddles, etc.). Sometimes used as a means of achieving sexual gratification, flagellation can be an element of sadomasochistic sexual activity and is of concern in relation to HIV in that skin can be broken, thus allowing a potential route of entry for blood contaminated with HIV.

follicular dendritic cell Characterized by thready tentacles, this cell is found in lymphoid follicles and is investigated for its role in HIV's stalwart endurance after the immune system has rallied to battle disease. The virus's continued infectiousness on follicular dendritic cells astounds researchers in that these are covered with antibodies and other protective proteins, which should serve to neutralize the virus. Unfortunately, that is not the case, and infection in secondary lymphoid tissue stealthily continues wreaking havoc by destroying tissue, although causing few symptoms.

follow-up Return to a clinic as directed by a physician after diagnosis of a sexually transmitted disease and/or initiation of treatment. A patient may need to be monitored for response to therapy, possible side effects of medications, and other conditions.

Food and Drug Administration Based in Rockville, Maryland, this well-known U.S. agency has the overall responsibility for protecting the public against health hazards. Thus, it regulates new medical devices and the testing, sale, and promotion of pharmaceutical drugs and food products and additives. This agency became the focus of AIDS activists in the 1980s as they sought to speed the approval of medications that might offer appropriate therapy for those with HIV/AIDS in the epidemic sweeping the United States. Drugs are not sold in the United States until they receive FDA approval, which is dependent on the results of drug trials that are used to confirm a medication's safeness and effectiveness or lack thereof. Its regulators classify some drugs as over-the-counter, others as prescription-only, and others as controlled substances.

French kiss Also known as a deep kiss and a wet kiss, this mode of sexual foreplay and/or affection involving the tongue is important in the realm of STDs for its exchange of saliva, believed by some people to be a possible mode of HIV infection. In actuality, though, no cases of saliva transmission in which the saliva did not contain HIV-infected blood have been documented. The CDC has found no cases of saliva transmission of HIV infection.

FTA-ABS test The fluorescent treponemal antibody-absorption (FTA-ABS) test is used to detect antibodies to *Treponema pallidum,* which is the organism that causes syphilis.

fungal infection Fungi include yeasts and molds; some species cause infections in human beings, ranging from a minor vaginal yeast infection to a more serious illness such as cryptococcal meningitis in an immunocompromised patient.

gallbladder disease Occasionally the first sign of AIDS, gallbladder disease can occur in the form of enlarged or obstructed bile ducts that block the flow of bile and thus result in jaundice and pain. Sometimes AIDS patients are found incidentally by ultrasound to have nonspecific gallbladder wall thickening. Symptoms of gallbladder disease include upper right abdominal pain, fever, vomiting, jaundice, and diarrhea.

gay bowel syndrome A phrase that encompasses the intestinal diseases proctitis, proctocolitis, and enteritis, the syndrome is thought to result from infection with parasites and other organisms in the intestinal tract, most likely as a result of anal or oral–anal intercourse. Because these forms of sexual activity are prevalent among gay partners, it is assumed that gay men have increased risk of exposure to fecal matter that can lead to intestinal disease.

Gay Men's Health Crisis A prevention and care organization created to promote services for those with AIDS. Begun in New York City in 1981, the Gay Men's Health Crisis spawned numerous similar organizations nationwide, all of which focus on preventing isolation and ostracism of people who have HIV/AIDS.

General Medical Assistance Those programs that provide health care to the indigent who are not covered by Medicaid. General Medical Assistance has a state and local scope.

gene therapy A means of delivery of new, functional genes to patients who have genetic diseases.

genital herpes Herpes simplex virus (HSV) type 2, because it primarily affects the genital area, is referred to as genital herpes and should be differentiated from the very common HSV type 1, associated with fever blisters on the mouth or face (oral herpes). However, both types of HSV can cause genital herpes. HSV-1 usually causes lip sores (fever blisters, cold sores), but it can cause genital infections, too. HSV-2 causes genital sores most of the time, but it also can infect the mouth.

It is important to note, in the context of genital herpes, that the immune system cannot completely rid the body of herpes. Always, a small colony of the virus lives on, evading the immune system by traveling nerve pathways and hiding in nerve roots. A latent phase, during which it hides and causes no problems or symptoms, may last weeks or years, but it can be reactivated at any time. Certain triggers cause the virus to reproduce and set out on the nerve pathways once again, reaching the skin in large enough quantities to be contracted by a sex partner. When it is active, however, herpes does not always manifest itself in visible signs, and therein lies one of the largest problems.

Genital herpes is extremely common in the United States, affecting about 50 million people 12 and older—or one in five of the total adolescent and adult population, according to the Centers for Disease Control and Prevention. More women (one in four) contract HSV-2; in men, the frequency is one in five, probably attributable to the fact that it is easier for a male to transmit the disease to a female than vice versa. More blacks than whites have herpes. The group in which herpes is proliferating most quickly is young white teens; in those who are age 12 to 19, HSV-2 was five times more prevalent at the start of the new millennium than it was two decades earlier.

About 89 percent of those with genital herpes are unaware of their disease because they have no symptoms—ever—or do not recognize the symptoms. One of the most startling facts about genital herpes is that most people who are HSV-2-infected have never actually received a diagnosis. Lacking any awareness that they have genital herpes, these individuals often spread it unknowingly. This obviously poses an enormous health risk for those who are sexually active and underscores the importance of STD testing before initiation of a sexual relationship with a partner. This disease has major health consequences because the virus stays in the body in certain nerve cells, periodically causing lifelong symptoms in some but not all individuals. Stress, illness, poor nutrition, excessive activity, and sunlight have all been known to trigger bouts of herpes in herpes sufferers, even when the disease has lain dormant for a long time. These triggers set the virus in motion, causing it to travel along nerve pathways to the site of outbreak.

Cause

Caused by the herpes simplex virus (HSV), genital herpes is a sexually transmitted disease. Medical experts report that approximately four of five people do not know they have it; therefore, it is important to be well informed about the ways in which this disease is transmitted. Of this recurrent, incurable disease's two serotypes—HSV-1 and HSV-2—the latter causes most cases of genital herpes.

Symptoms

The primary episode of genital herpes varies greatly, and as a result, many of those infected are unaware of the infection. Those who do have pronounced symptoms usually have lesions within two weeks of transmission. Flulike symptoms, including fever and swollen glands, are not unusual. First episodes last two to three weeks. Other early symptoms are sensations of itching or burning; pain in the legs, genital area, or buttocks; vaginal discharge; and abdominal region pressure.

The site of the infection hosts the first sores (lesions), but these also can occur inside the vagina and on the cervix in women or in the urinary passage of either sex. Small red bumps morph into blisters, finally turning into painful open sores. They crust over a period of a few days and then heal. Some people with genital herpes experience headache, fever, muscle aches, painful urination, vaginal discharge, and swollen glands in the groin.

The primary episode of genital herpes is usually the worst and is often followed by four to five more symptomatic periods the first year. However, many who have HSV-2 experience no symptoms, and in some people, the symptoms are mild, but this disease can also cause painful genital ulcers that recur frequently.

What sometimes makes herpes hard to detect is that it manifests itself in different forms. Some are easily missed; others are overt and dramatic. Obvious signs are painful blisterlike sores, which eventually crust over in a scab before they heal. Herpes causes ulcers, sores, and crusted lesions in various places: anus, buttocks, upper thigh, vagina, labia, scrotum, and penis. It also can infect the urethra and cause burning. Subtle signs of genital herpes are skin redness, tiny pimplelike sores, small skin slits, and irritation around the anus that is sometimes confused with hemorrhoids.

Herpes symptoms in some women resemble yeast infection. Small sores in the urethra can cause painful urination. Aching or itching during the menstrual period is another symptom. Some women mistakenly think they are having a skin irritation caused by sexual activity when it is actually caused by herpes. Men who contract herpes may initially believe that they have acne, irritation caused by sexual activity, or jock itch.

Testing

Lab testing is important because herpes can resemble an ingrown hair, a pimple, or a rash. If a person has multiple typical-appearing lesions, a presumptive diagnosis of herpes is often made by a physician while test results are pending. Physicians diagnose genital herpes by visual examination, test of a sample from the sore, and blood tests that can detect herpes even when no symptoms are present. Anyone who thinks he or she may have been exposed or who has genital symptoms of herpes should see a physician for testing and assessment.

Early detection is easier than late detection because there are amounts of virus large enough to provide a good sample.

Lab tests for those with sores (lesions) are viral culture and blood tests. Blood tests can be performed when people have no symptoms, too. The antigen test—less often used—can also detect virus in a lesion.

Most available is the viral culture, considered the gold standard of herpes detection. Viral culture is also viewed as the most accurate method; a new sore is swabbed or scraped, and the sample is placed in a lab culture medium that contains healthy cells. The lab technician who examines the cells one to two days later sees changes that indicate growth of the herpesvirus when there is a positive diagnosis of genital herpes. In a serologic (blood) test, the important aspect is to have a *type-specific* assay, to distinguish HSV-2 from HSV-1 antibodies.

A newer diagnostic technique is faster but a bit less accurate. Swabs of a lesion are examined to detect viral protein components, but this kind of test should be done when sores first appear to ensure reliable results. This virus is hard to find. And because it is true that tests often do not detect the virus in an active sore, a negative test result is not a certain indication that the individual does not have genital herpes.

Blood tests cannot determine the existence of active genital herpes infection, but they can detect antibodies to the virus that show that the person has been infected with HSV at some prior time and thus antibodies to it have developed. (A person's immune system produces antibodies to fight infections.) Unfortunately, in the case of antibodies to herpes, they only partially protect the person against another infection with a different strain or type of herpesvirus, and reactivation of the latent virus is not usually prevented, either. Furthermore, standard blood tests can reveal only whether a patient has had a herpes infection—not whether it was oral or genital. Blood tests that can distinguish whether the prior infection was type 1 or type 2 or both can help determine a person's prognosis because, for example, recurrences are less frequent for genital HSV-1 infection than for genital HSV-2 infection.

When an individual goes to a health care provider for diagnosis of a possible STD, the first step is to provide details about medical history, listing any symptoms that have aroused concern and giving a sexual history, including number of partners and use of condoms. This is information that helps the doctor make a correct diagnosis, not an attempt to judge the patient's personal habits.

A doctor performs an examination, including a visual study of the genital area. In men, this means closely examining the penis, scrotum, and rectum in an effort to spot blisters and lesions indicative of herpes. The area may be swabbed for a lab test. In the case of a woman, the doctor performs a pelvic exam with speculum to inspect the cervix and vagina. He or she may take swabs for lab evaluation. In both sexes, lymph nodes are inspected. Also, those being tested should know that usually antibodies do not show up in the blood until a few weeks after herpes exposure.

Viral culture rarely gives a false-positive result, but it is not unusual to miss herpes even when it is present. If lesions are present but lack sufficient active virus, a false negative finding may result. This suggests to the health care provider that no herpes exists even when the individual does have herpes. Recurrent episodes have a high rate of producing false-negative results. The upshot is that an individual may require repeated doctor visits to confirm diagnosis.

In contrast, a blood test detects herpes with or without symptoms. However, weeks may pass before the antibodies that a blood test detects develop, and some blood tests cannot distinguish the two types of herpes. The individual who has never had symptoms but wants to be tested must have a type-specific blood test. This approach is a good idea for an individual whose partner has herpes—or a person who has had numerous sex partners and wants to be tested for common STDs.

The best type-specific blood test is the Western blot. A patient can simply ask the doctor whether this is being used. Several research labs perform such type-specific tests; call 1-888-ADVICE8, the Herpes Advice Center, to find one. Physicians can request the Western blot from the University of Washington's virology lab.

The FDA-approved finger-prick test for herpes is called the POCkit HSV-2 Rapid Test. Done widely in medical clinic settings, this test offers results in five minutes. This can be used 12 days after exposure and gives accurate results. Antigen tests provide quicker results than culture but also require a better sample and may not distinguish HSV-1 from HSV-2.

Because the active phases can be hard to identify, herpes is frequently spread during times when those infected do not know that the virus is active. Also, it is important to realize that an individual can get herpes without even recognizing the first episode because of the possibility of "silent" transmission.

When genital herpes is in the active stage, there may or may not be visible lesions. Several laboratory tests may be required to differentiate herpes sores from those of other infections. Some first episodes, on the other hand, are so severe that they require hospitalization of the person affected.

Complications

A herpes-infected woman who sheds herpesvirus at the time of childbirth can cause potentially fatal infection in her infant. Thus, since having a first episode during pregnancy presents a much greater risk of transmission to the newborn and a greater risk of intrauterine infection of the fetus, it is important that pregnant women prevent contraction of herpes.

The woman who has active genital herpes at the time of delivery usually requires a cesarean section. However, in women with genital herpes, infection of an infant is rare. Though very rare, herpes infections in newborns are life-threatening. Herpes can be transmitted to infants during delivery if the baby in passing through the birth canal is in direct contact with herpes.

For the woman who had herpes before becoming pregnant, the risk of transmitting infection to her baby during childbirth is very low—unless she has active herpes signs or symptoms in or near the birth canal at the time of delivery. A normal vaginal birth can be expected if the woman begins labor with no symptoms of herpes. During pregnancy, a longtime herpes sufferer transmits protective antibodies to her fetus. These help protect the baby from infection, even if some virus exists in the birth canal.

Most likely to transmit virus to a baby is the woman who gets herpes for the first time while she is pregnant, because the rate of viral shedding in the first six months after acquiring this infection is especially high. Furthermore, her own immune response to herpes, including antibodies to be transmitted to the fetus in the uterus, will not have developed. Also, she may run the risk of premature delivery and considerable problems for her baby. Half of babies infected with herpes die or suffer neurological damage; a baby who is born with herpes can experience encephalitis (brain inflammation), severe rashes, and eye problems.

Acyclovir can improve the outcome of babies with neonatal herpes if they are treated immediately. Serious complications can be ameliorated with early treatment.

The pregnant woman who does not have herpes but has a partner with herpes should use condoms throughout the nine months of gestation. During the last trimester, refraining from intercourse is wise.

The woman who contracts herpes for the first time during her second trimester will undoubtedly have an abdominal delivery (cesarean section) whether or not she has signs of active herpes, because a mother having her first outbreak of herpes simplex virus near or at the time of the baby's birth passes on to her child a one-in-three risk of infection. In cases of recurrence of this disease, the risk is lower—only about one in 30.

A physician who detects herpes lesions in or near the birth canal during labor performs a cesarean section to ward off danger of infection to the baby.

A woman nearing the last months of her pregnancy should be careful to avoid unprotected oral and genital sex with a partner whose infection status is unknown or one who has oral or genital HSV. When labor is beginning, it is important to ask the doctor to check carefully for signs of genital herpes. Vaginal delivery is acceptable for women with herpes who have no prodromal signs or symptoms of genital herpes. Even with a cesarean section, the infant is not 100 percent safe from risk of HSV infection.

Those who have suppressed immune systems often experience herpes simplex virus episodes that are very severe and long-lasting. It is important to note that many health experts believe that HSV-2 may play a major role in the heterosexual spread of HIV in that the virus that causes herpes can make people more susceptible to HIV infection. It is also believed that genital herpes provides an accessible point of entry for HIV. Before there was effective therapy for AIDS, people with HIV had severe herpes outbreaks, which may have helped transmit both herpes and HIV infections to others.

An HIV report from the Johns Hopkins AIDS Service on the Internet in 2002 reported new observations on interactions between STDs and HIV. In the Enders Lecture, Dr. L. Corey of the University of Washington presented data showing a large and perhaps growing role of HSV-2 in facilitating sexual transmission of HIV.

Both HSV 1 and 2 can produce sores around the vaginal area, on the penis, around the anus, and on buttocks and thighs. It is also possible for broken skin on other body parts such as fingers to come in contact with HSV, which generates lesions in that new location.

Prodrome

The signal of a new recurrence of herpes is called a prodrome, which feels like itching or tingling in the genital area, a backache, leg pains, or another type of sensation. These are referred to as prodromal symptoms, and some people find them the most painful part of recurrent episodes.

A prodrome is often a precursor of skin lesions soon to appear—although that is not always what happens. What it does mean invariably is that herpes is in its active phase. Symptoms of recurrent episodes tend to be milder than those of the first episode and last about a week.

Prevention

Before and during an outbreak, herpes is contagious. It is most contagious when the virus is replicating externally before an outbreak and during an outbreak when the sufferer has fluid-filled blisters. Contact with a toilet seat or hot tub rarely, if ever, spreads the virus.

Direct contact spreads the herpesvirus. An easy target is the soft skin of the genitals, vagina, anus, and mouth. The individual who has sexual contact or kisses a partner who has herpes in that location in the contagious stage is likely to contract herpes.

A person who has early signs of a herpes outbreak or has visible sores should avoid sexual contact until sores are healed completely and would probably be prudent to wait at least a few days after that. Condoms should be used between outbreaks for partial protection. The herpes patient who uses chronic suppressive antiviral therapy probably reduces the chance of transmission to a partner.

No precaution listed here absolutely guarantees that a partner will be protected from contracting genital herpes. Although few statistics exist, it appears that in monogamous couples, the likelihood of transmission is extremely low when couples do not have intercourse during outbreaks. Typically, average transmission rate is about 10 percent. Uninfected men are three times less likely than uninfected women to acquire the disease. The risk of contracting herpes type 2 is higher in those who do not have herpes type 1.

Herpes can even reactivate without producing visible sores, although the virus may still be shedding around the original infection site, in genital secretions, or from lesions that are barely noticeable. Although this shedding may last only a day and may not cause any discomfort, the infected individual can infect a sex partner.

Once an individual is infected with HSV, that person is infected for life. Both types are transmitted through direct contact: kissing and sexual contact (oral, vaginal, anal, or skin-to-skin contact). It is extremely important for sexually active individuals to understand that genital herpes can be transmitted even if the infected partner has no sores or symptoms. It should be emphasized that people with oral herpes can transmit the infection to the genital area of a partner during oral–genital sex. A third route of transmission is through a herpes-infected individual who transmits the disease with no concern for his or her victims. A study of 66 women *(Update in Sexually Transmitted Diseases, 2001)* revealed that 62 percent were unaware of the fact that they had genital herpes at the time of transmission; 71 percent were asymptomatic or did not attribute their symptoms to genital herpes at the time of transmission. During an active herpes episode, people with genital herpes should take steps to speed healing and to prevent spread of the infection to other parts of the body or to other people with whom they have contact.

Using latex condoms consistently is the best protection, but no one should count on these to provide 100 percent protection because viral shedding, and thus exposure, can occur when a herpes lesion (sometimes invisible to the naked eye) is not totally covered by the condom. If your partner has genital herpes, abstain from sex when symptoms are present and use latex condoms between outbreaks.

An individual with herpes sores on the lips can spread herpes to the lips of another person through kisses. Oral sex can spread the infection from lips to genitals. For that reason, many cases of genital herpes are caused by herpes type 1. When there are herpes sores on the genitals, vagina, or other unprotected areas, sexual activity is a means of spreading the virus.

Treatment

For herpes, there is no quick fix, nor is there a cure. Medications called antiviral drugs can, however, attack the virus and give those afflicted with this disease some relief, helping to reduce the duration and severity of symptoms. Many herpes sufferers take small doses of antiviral medications daily to prevent symptoms. Plus, these individuals can take the drugs in larger doses when they do experience symptoms. Research shows that daily use of antiviral therapy dramatically lessens the rate of asymptomatic viral shedding, as well as reduces outbreak frequency. Controlling outbreaks and minimizing discomfort are two goals of antiviral agent use. The severity of a first episode of genital herpes can be dramatically minimized by the use of an initial 10-day course of medication that helps sores to heal faster, reduces swollen glands, and curbs viral shedding.

Recommended for those who have severe or prolonged recurrences and prodromes is episodic therapy, taking medication at the first warning sign of an outbreak; this serves to shorten dura-

tion of symptoms and speed sore healing. The patient who takes the drug before lesions appear makes more significant gains, and, in some cases, early preventive medication forestalls formation of lesions altogether.

A third kind of treatment regimen is suppressive therapy, intended to reduce the likelihood of recurrences or to extinguish them. The patient takes a small dose of antiviral medication daily for long periods. Typically, those on suppressive therapy dramatically reduce their symptom recurrence, and in about one-fourth, there are no recurrences at all. Often, the physician treating the herpes sufferer stops suppressive therapy once a year to assess the need for the medication.

Recent research suggests yet another advantage of suppressive therapy—a 95 percent reduction in days per year of viral shedding and risk of transmission. It has not been shown, however, that transmission can be completely prevented by use of suppressive therapy.

The most commonly used medications for herpes are acyclovir (Zovirax) and valacyclovir (Valtrex), which disrupt the replication process of the virus and thus its spread. A patient who takes either drug can reduce the duration and severity of symptoms during a first episode and speed healing during recurrences and prodrome (when there are warning signs and symptoms). They work especially well when initiated within 24 hours of onset of symptoms.

Many experts think that this therapy also may reduce the risk of transmission to sexual partners. Acyclovir is taken at different doses either three or five times a day for a first episode and usually 400 mg is taken three times a day for treatment of recurrences. This drug is used worldwide and is only rarely associated with any serious adverse effects. The Acyclovir in Pregnancy Registry has shown no rise in birth defects or other problems in more than 10 years. Similar safety is reported in the newer entries on the market—valacyclovir (Valtrex) and famciclovir (Famvir). Valtrex has acyclovir as its active ingredient but has the advantage of being better absorbed by a person's body. For episodic therapy, the dosage is only twice daily for three days. For chronic suppression, Valtrex is taken once daily. Famciclovir (Famvir) lasts longer in the body than acyclovir, and the herpes patient takes only twice-daily doses.

Recurrences

It has been seen that people having six or more episodes of herpes a year can reduce the rate of recurrences by 75 percent by availing themselves of daily suppressive therapy. Furthermore, daily use of acyclovir has been shown to be safe and effective for patients who have taken it for as long as six years.

It has been noted that in immunocompetent patients, doctors have not seen incidences of clinically significant acyclovir resistance with suppressive therapy.

Herpes sufferers who use suppressive medication should be aware that these drugs do not eliminate asymptomatic viral shedding. The extent to which this kind of therapy reduces the likelihood of HSV transmission is still undetermined.

It is important to note that in the population of women of childbearing age in the United States, one in three has genital herpes—yet herpes infection in newborns is extremely rare—less than one in every 2,000 births.

In a CDC-sponsored study of neonatal herpes, 140 mothers were evaluated; 77 percent had no known history of genital herpes, had no lesions during pregnancy, and did not have genital ulcerations at delivery. The crux of the neonatal herpes problem involves women who lack immunity to HSV-2 and are experiencing their first episode of genital herpes in a later stage of pregnancy. The women are asymptomatic, are shedding virus at delivery, but lack immunity that they could pass on to the infant. The women tend to be young and unmarried and to have had a history of an STD.

Using systemic acyclovir and valacyclovir during pregnancy has not been proved safe. However, a registry that is maintained by the firm Glaxo-Wellcome, Inc., in collaboration with the CDC, reports that its findings on women who are using these drugs do not show a higher incidence of major birth defects than that in the general population. Because this registry keeps tabs on the effects of using these medications during pregnancy, women who take acyclovir or valacyclovir while pregnant should be reported to the registry (800-722-9292, extension 38465).

Oral acyclovir may be taken by a woman who has her first episode of genital herpes during pregnancy. Basically, though, the routine use of acyclovir during the pregnancy of a woman with recurrent infections is not recommended.

The neonatal HSV transmission rate (with rate of transmission dependent on clinical characteristics of maternal disease) is as follows: for mothers in a symptomatic first episode, 50 percent; in an asymptomatic first episode, 33 percent; in a symptomatic recurrence, 4 percent; in an asymptomatic recurrence, 0.04 percent. As for risk of recurrence of HSV at delivery, it is 30 percent for women having their first episode of HSV during pregnancy; 15 percent for women with long-standing recurrent disease; and 3 percent for those who have asymptomatic shedding.

The 1999 American College of Obstetricians and Gynecologists recommendations follow: primary HSV during pregnancy should be treated with antiviral therapy; cesarean delivery should be done with active first-episode HSV genital lesions at delivery; antiviral therapy should be considered at approximately 36 weeks' gestation after a first episode of HSV during the current pregnancy; cesarean delivery should be performed with recurrent HSV infection for people who have active genital lesions or prodromal symptoms at delivery; expectant management of preterm labor or preterm premature rupture of membranes and active HSV may be warranted; for women at or beyond 36 weeks of gestation at risk for recurrent HSV, antiviral therapy also may be considered, although such therapy may not reduce the likelihood of cesarean delivery; when there are no active lesions or prodromal symptoms during labor, cesarean delivery should not be performed on the basis of a history of recurrent disease.

If a baby is exposed to herpes during delivery, careful follow-up is necessary. Cultures of mucosal surfaces may be taken to detect HSV even before clinical signs develop. When mothers contract herpes near the time of delivery, it may be necessary to give the baby acyclovir.

It is important to note that some people with compromised immune systems (those on chemotherapy or AIDS patients) may have drug-resistant strains of herpes. Abnormal strains seem more likely to flourish in these individuals. By the same token, no increase in drug-resistant strains of herpes in the general population has been observed since the advent of acyclovir use.

As of 2003, the recommended regimens for genital herpes in non-HIV-infected people are:

For episodic recurrent infection:

Acyclovir: 400 mg orally three times a day for five days, or
Acyclovir: 200 mg orally five times a day for five days, or
Famciclovir: 125 mg orally twice a day for five days, or
Valacyclovir: 500 mg orally twice a day for three days

Regimens for daily suppressive therapy:

Acyclovir: 400 mg orally twice a day, or
Famciclovir: 250 mg orally twice a day, or
Valacyclovir: 500 mg orally once a day, or
Valacyclovir: 1,000 mg orally once a day

The dosing of these antiviral medications varies slightly in a person with HIV.

Studies suggest that valacyclovir and famciclovir are much like acyclovir in effect but are easier to use on a long-term basis. In patients who experience very severe bouts of herpes or complications that make hospitalization necessary (hepatitis, pneumonitis, disseminated infection, etc.), it is important to provide IV antiviral therapy.

There are also prescription topical medications available for herpes labialis (cold sores) that can shorten the duration of pain by about one day. The available creams are penciclovir (Denavir) and acyclovir cream. For severe herpes labialis, the oral medications such as acyclovir can be used.

Without a prescription, biooxidative creams are available. These creams combine an antiviral agent with infused oxygen to kill the herpesvirus because viruses cannot live in an elevated-oxygen environment. When cellular oxygen levels are increased, diseases such as genital warts, herpes, flu, and measles cannot proliferate.

A second aspect of treating herpes is counseling. Understanding the circuitous route that herpes often takes is key to coming to grips with having a disease for which there is no cure.

Psychosocial Issues

Psychological distress among those infected is an enormously devastating result of herpes. In personal relationships, having herpes can feel like having leprosy, and, unfortunately, once it is contracted, there is little one can do other than try to suppress the symptoms and frequency of bouts and take an honest approach with prospective sexual partners.

Decreased sense of self-worth is a huge problem with herpes, in that many people, after recovering from the initial feeling of betrayal and shock when they realize they have contracted the disease, move into a state of malaise and inaction. During this time, a redefinition of self can take place, as the individual assigns herself or himself the stigma of being "undesirable." Withdrawal and depression are not unusual, and this is a time in which the loved ones of the infected person should be vigilant to provide support and monitor behavior for declining interest in life.

A belief that repeated rejections will occur because of this diagnosis can prove to be an immense burden for a person to carry during youth. Emotional difficulties can cause mood swings and destructive thoughts, as the herpes sufferer experiences relationship rebuffs over months and years after the disease is contracted. When the sex partner who passed on the disease is relegated to a distant memory, resentment remains as the person rehashes the unfairness of being harnessed lifelong with this distressing and often relentless disease.

To combat the feeling of helplessness that often accompanies this disease, the person with herpes needs to be fortified with knowledge. Knowing how this is spread and how it can be treated can go a long way toward easing the load of self-recrimination and low self-image. Some have a supportive confidante who helps soothe them during bluesy periods; others are comforted by fellow sufferers in support groups.

One of the major difficulties occurs in learning how to broach the subject of herpes with a new sex partner, and some should be encouraged to seek counseling with a mental health professional on how to address this subject. In many people with herpes, the fear of rejection as a result of disclosure of herpes is mixed with chagrin and anxiety. At the same time, herpes sufferers learn, sometimes the hard way, that establishment of an intimate and satisfying relationship must be based on honesty at the appropriate time. Of course, no one should feel compelled to reveal personal health issues to someone with whom he or she is not sexually intimate and probably never will be. It is important to remember that those rejections that follow on the heels of disclosure of herpes status should be chalked up as "screening," in that partners who showed little promise for a mutually beneficial, loving long-term relationship are eliminated.

Counseling, family support, and preventive measures can help patients cope successfully with this disease. Those who have distress and no confidante should be encouraged to seek help via hotlines that answer questions and assuage concerns.

A person who has contracted herpes needs to understand that this disease does recur, and that episodes can vary in severity. In some individuals, episodes tend to become less severe after a year or so; in others, herpes is treacherous to handle indefinitely. Because this disease has asymptomatic shedding, it is extremely important for the infected person to understand that sexual transmission can occur at times when he or she is not aware that the disease is resurfacing. During counseling, a doctor is likely to caution that it is imperative to refrain from sexual intercourse during times when there are prodromal symptoms or lesions. Consistent use of condoms during sexual activity with new or uninfected partners should be a rule of thumb for those with genital herpes. People who have HSV-2 infections are more likely than those with HSV-1 to have viral shedding minus symptoms.

Another key fact that should be shared in counseling is the risk of neonatal infection. Some women are reluctant to disclose that they have herpes when their doctors ask for their gynecologic history, and it is very important that the doctor who is delivering the baby be aware of the herpes.

To alleviate the anxiety of a person who is newly diagnosed with this lifelong disease, doctors usually point out that episodic antiviral therapy can help to shorten the duration of lesions and that suppressive antiviral therapy can help prevent recurrent outbreaks of herpes or render them less frequent and less severe. The first year after initial infection is marked by the most frequent outbreaks of herpes. In succeeding years, most people experience fewer outbreaks. However, some people have outbreaks that are frequent and severe for many years.

Self-Care

Attention to peace of mind is important for those dealing with the lifelong stress generated by having herpes. Only those who have herpes can fully understand the burden of dealing with recurrences of genital herpes, which are distressing, bothersome, and painful. There usually are ongoing concern and worry about transmitting the disease to a partner and about the necessity to have no sexual activity during active periods of the sores. Thus, it is important, emotionally, to find ways to soothe oneself via meditation, affirmations, exercise regimens, or hobbies.

Also as means of self-care, *JAMA* Women's Health STD Information Center recommends these measures:

- Keep the infected area clean and dry to prevent development of secondary infections.

- Try to avoid touching the sores you have, and wash your hands after you do have contact with the sores.

- Avoid sexual contact from the time when you first have symptoms until complete healing has occurred. This can be defined as the time when the scab has fallen off and new skin covers the lesion spot.

Periods of latency and activity vary with the individual, but it remains unclear what causes the virus to activate. Some research suggests that friction to the genitals can trigger herpes. Stress, fatigue, sunlight exposure, and menstruation are also cited as causes. Often recurrences are not predictable.

When treatment is started within the prodrome period or within a day after the appearance of lesions, many people with recurrent herpes do well with episodic therapy. Thus, it is important to have the medication on hand so that it can be started as soon as lesions or signs of prodrome are detected.

Research

Areas of investigation are focusing on causes of reactivation, better treatments to prevent transmission and recurrence, and development of a safe and effective vaccine, as well as safe and effective topical microbicides.

For more information, call the National Herpes Hotline, (919) 361-8488.

genital intercourse　A form of sexual intercourse that involves insertion of a man's penis into a woman's vagina. Also called vaginal intercourse.

genital secretion　In respect to sexually transmitted diseases, genital fluids and secretions are important in that HIV and other STDs can be contracted by contact with an infected person's genital secretions.

genital ulcer　Superficial skin ulcerations in the genital area can be a manifestation of different STDs such as herpes, chancroid, syphilis, granuloma inguinale, and lymphogranuloma venereum. In the United States, genital ulcers are most commonly associated with genital herpes.

genital warts　Although sexually transmitted human papillomavirus—the cause of genital warts—is not a disease that doctors must report to the Centers for Disease Control and Prevention, it is believed, on the basis of epidemiological studies, that there are about 500,000 to 1 million new cases every year. More than 100 types of human papillomavirus (HPV) have been identified in humans, and researchers expect the final number to be around 200.

Causes

External genital warts (EGWs) are most often caused by human papillomavirus type 6 (HPV-6) and sometimes by HPV-11, both of which researchers rate as low-risk in that these are not the types that typically lead to cervical cancer. Skin-to-skin contact with productive lesions that are shedding HPV DNA is the number-one means of transmission of HPV. Thus, genital sexual contact is the cause of HPV. Condoms give some protection, but their overall efficacy in curbing transmission rates is dubious. HPV can be contracted from parts of the penis and groin that are not covered by condoms. Furthermore, HPV transmission appears to take place even when there are no visible lesions: human papillomavirus DNA has been detected during asymptomatic infection stages.

Genital warts (condylomata acuminata or venereal warts) are caused by certain types of HPV, whereas other HPV infections tend to cause warts on the hands and soles of the feet but not genital warts. It is rare (but possible) for genital warts to be transmitted by fomites (any nonliving material such as surgical gloves) and by infected mothers to newborns.

Incubation period for EGWs is about one month to two years, and in most cases, the infected individual has warts within a few months of exposure to HPV. Left untreated, these can regress, remain the same, or get larger. In people with clinical HPV infection that manifests itself in external genital warts, about 20 percent of lesions actually resolve spontaneously—typically, within the year that they first became apparent. It has been observed that HIV/AIDS patients, transplant recipients, and others with suppressed immune systems experience florid warts and have high rates of recurrences after treatment, suggesting that a key player in containment of HPV is cell-mediated immunity. HPVs, members of the papovavirus family, can live in a human being dormantly for months or years and then, if the person's immune system becomes weak, respond by activating and replicating.

Anogenital HPV has far-reaching effects: 24 to 40 million people are affected in the United States, and each year, about 1 million more new cases are diagnosed. Of all people in the United States who are sexually active, about 2 percent have genital warts that are clinically visible. Many more show signs of infection that is subclinical.

As illustration of the prevalence of HPV, a 1999 study of 608 college women in New Jersey showed a startup prevalence of 26 percent, which was followed by a cumulative 36-month incidence of 43 percent. This translates to a high incidence in these young women of being infected with HPV at some point during the three years. Similarly high percentages are seen in other studies of college women. In a 1991 University of California at Berkeley study, 33 percent of 467 subjects had cervical HPV infections, and HPV was detected in vulvar or cervical swab specimens of 46 percent of subjects.

Research has also shown that HPV-16 incidence is at least twofold higher in women than in men. Of people with one lifetime sex partner, only 7 percent had HPV-16, whereas 20.1 percent of those who had had 50 or more lifetime sex partners had HPV-16.

About 15 percent of U.S. men and women between the ages 15 and 49 have genital warts that can shed HPV DNA, according to statistics in *Family Practice Recertification* (August 1999). It is believed that another 60 percent in the same age group probably have antibodies to genital HPV as a result of previous HPV infection.

According to the *Update in Sexually Transmitted Diseases 2001,* human papillomavirus is the most common viral STD and probably the most common STD. There has been a dramatic rise in visits to doctors for clinical HPVs since the 1960s. There are more than 100 known types, varying in affinity for the genital tract (about 35 types), clinical expression, and potential for causing cancer. HPV risk factors are lifetime number of sexual partners, sexual activity, low socioeconomic status, cigarette smoking, and immunosuppression.

HPV infections can cause genital warts and benign or malignant neoplasms, or they can be totally symptom-free. Sites where genital warts occur are on the external genitalia or perianal area, and warts can be seen in the vagina, on the cervix, and inside the urethra and anus.

According to *Update in Sexually Transmitted Diseases 2001,* HPV types include the following:

- Those with low malignancy potential—types 6 and 11—which produce warty lesions, rarely progress to high-grade neoplasia, and have a high regression rate.

- Types with high malignant potential—types 16, 18, 31, 33, 35, and others—which are usually subclinical, are occasionally found in genital warts, and are strongly associated with lower genital tract neoplasia (dysplasia, invasive squamous cell carcinoma, and adenocarcinoma of the cervix).

Infection with multiple types of HPV is common, and doctors are vigilant for signs of lower genital tract neoplasia.

As far as duration, most HPV infections are transient, with an average period of about eight months. It is not known whether regression equates with eradication. The prevalence of HPV decreases with the age of the population.

Of the many types of HPV scientists have identified, one-third are spread via sexual activity and live only in genital tissue. The most recognizable sign of genital HPV is the genital wart, but this disease usually causes a silent infection, free of visible symptoms. In fact, one study sponsored by the National Institute of Allergy and Infectious Diseases reported that almost half of HPV-infected women had no symptoms that were obvious. This silent aspect causes enormous problems because many individuals remain unaware of their infection and the potential risk of transmission to others. Genital warts are highly contagious.

The human papillomavirus has proliferated to epidemic proportions, creating high levels of anxiety among people who are confronted with this problem and know little about it. Concerns about future cancer risk, fertility, and changes in sexuality are often at the forefront of the mind of a newly diagnosed patient. Fear about transmitting the disease is yet another worry. A reluctance to accept the inevitable makes some patients refuse treatment, as if denying that they have genital warts will make them go away.

Symptoms

Condyloma acuminata (warts in the genital or anal area) are the least common manifestation of HPV. These are discrete verrucose or papillary growths, which can be flat or on stalks. They can occur on the cervix, vagina, vulva, urethra, perianal area, or intraanal region. Genital warts can occur as a single lesion or multiple lesions and can be flesh-colored or hyperpigmented.

Subclinical infection is much more common than condylomata. Frequently, the infection is first suggested by an abnormal Pap smear result, which shows cellular changes typical of an HPV infection.

In latent infection, there are no cytologic or histologic changes apparent. It is hard to define the prevalence—20 to 40 percent probably. Natural history is unknown, and latent infection probably accounts for recurrences of infection.

In women, the warts usually occur on the outside and inside of the vagina, on the cervix, and/or around the anus. Genital warts in men are less common, but if they are present, they are usually on the tip of the penis. Others sites in males are on the shaft of the penis, on the scrotum, and around the anus. In rare instances, genital warts develop in the mouth or throat of someone who has had oral sex with an infected person.

Genital warts can appear in clusters; they can be tiny or spread into large masses. Sometimes, even when untreated, these warts disappear. In other cases, they eventually develop into a fleshy raised growth that is cauliflowerlike. Because it is impossible to predict whether genital warts will grow or disappear, it is important for those who suspect they have them to seek a physician's evaluation and, if necessary, treatment. A doctor will need to confirm the diagnosis and evaluate for any related issues, such as an abnormal Pap smear result, which would indicate a need for further monitoring and/or treatment. Also, a woman should be diligent about having regular Pap smears after a diagnosis of genital warts even though high-grade dysplasia or cancer rarely develops in women with HPV.

Physicians report that one of the first questions a patient asks is when she or he contracted it and from whom. No exact answer is available, because HPV, though sexually transmitted, can be an infection that has been present in that person for some time.

Transmission

Skin-to-skin contact with productive lesions that are shedding HPV DNA is the main way genital HPV is transmitted. It enters a person's tissue through inflamed and macerated skin or through microscopic abrasions during sexual intercourse. It appears likely that transmission can occur even when there are no lesions because tests have detected HPV DNA during asymptomatic infection periods.

HPV transmission, according to *2001 Update in STDs*, occurs via sexual contact in the majority of adults; little is known about the mechanics of inoculation; two-thirds of partners have disease after an average incubation period of two to three months; the role of fomites remains unknown for genital HPV; and autoinoculation from nongenital warts in adults is rare.

Although the EGW incubation period can be one month to two years, typically warts appear about two to four months after exposure to HPV, or the infection remains latent or subclinical. In some experts' belief, latent HPV infection lasts throughout the lifetime of the infected person, remaining in the epithelial cells.

Genital warts that are untreated may regress, remain the same, or increase in size. About one-fifth of those with EGWs see the lesions resolve spontaneously—typically, within a year of their appearance.

Although these are unsightly, most are benign. The strains of HPV most likely to result in cancer usually produce only macular warts that are hard to detect unless viewed colposcopically.

A controversial theory being advanced in some circles is that HPV can be transmitted nonsexually. This could mean that an individual can contract genital warts from fomites or from perinatal or digital transmission (via a person's fingers or hand). If this does turn out to be true, nonsexual transmission would explain some of the infections seen in children that are currently being attributed to sexual abuse.

It seems clear that cell-mediated immunity has a major role in containment of this infection, especially considering the course the infection takes in HIV/AIDS patients and transplant patients, who have a high rate of wart recurrence.

Appearing on the genitals and surrounding areas, EGWs usually can be seen with the naked eye. Describing four kinds of lesions in a 1998 report, the American Medical Association Expert Panel on EGWs lists

1. Condyloma acuminata in cauliflower shapes, usually on moist surfaces
2. Papular warts that are dome-shaped, flesh-colored, smaller than 4 mm, and appear on keratinized skin
3. Keratotic warts with a thick, horny layer, which look like common nongenital warts and occur on fully keratinized skin
4. Flat-topped papules that are macular or slightly raised and are seen on moist partially keratinized or fully keratinized skin

Those patients with EGWs who have symptoms report itching, burning, pain, bleeding, and painful intercourse.

Doctors usually diagnose external warts by direct visual examination, using a bright light and handheld magnifying glass. The colposcope is used for detecting cervical and vaginal warts.

Testing

Typically, an initial visit for EGWs features a physical examination, the relating of medical and sexual history, and tests for common sexually transmitted diseases. The results of a Pap smear—the microscopic examination of cells scraped from the uterine cervix to detect cervical cancer—may also reveal that HPV infection is present. Abnormal Pap smear findings are frequently associated with HPV infection.

In a patient with no visible warts, often the first indication of an HPV infection is an abnormal Pap smear finding with specific cellular changes consistent with HPV infection. Depending on the degree of abnormality of the Pap smear result, the patient either needs a repeat Pap smear in several months or proceeds straight to another test, called a colposcopy. In colposcopy, a physician is essentially looking through an instrument that magnifies the patient's cervix and vagina. He or she can apply acetic acid or iodine solutions to the cervix to highlight any cellular changes caused by the HPV. The physician may then find it necessary to take a small sample of cervical tissue to be examined under a microscope. This procedure, called a biopsy, is usually done in a doctor's office.

Complications

In some rare cases, some infants born to women with genital warts have had throat warts (laryngeal papillomatosis). They can be life-threatening and thus require frequent laser surgery in an effort to keep airways open.

It is important to know that high-risk viruses can cause cervical cancer and are also associated with vulvar cancer, anal cancer, and cancer of the penis. Most HPV infections do not progress to cancer, however.

Treatment

Physicians' philosophy on HPV management has changed in recent years, from the immediate treatment of a patient with a mildly abnormal Pap smear finding to a more conservative, wait-and-see approach. This is beneficial because administration of multiple cervical treatments has potential for affecting future fertility, so postponing treatment can benefit long-term health. The downside are the patient's anxiety over facing abnormal Pap smear findings over time and fear of the disease's progression to cancer.

The patient should request as much information from the doctor as he or she needs to alleviate anxiety. If no additional information is wanted, the patient can simply follow the guidelines for treatment advanced by her physician.

The new self-treatment options for patients with EGWs, combined with some older therapies, present a huge array of treatment options. It is interesting to note that today's therapies do not permit the perfect outcome of treatment—that is, eradication of infection, prevention of all sequelae, and elimination of the possibility of transmission to others or of local spread. The treatment can, however, remove visible warts and eliminate symptoms such as irritation, bleeding, and pruritus. Having the warts debulked and the viral load lessened serves to reduce the likelihood of transmission to sex partners and to other parts of the body.

External genital warts were treated with surgery and heat for many years. Then, in 1942, a New Orleans physician reported his use of podophyllum for condyloma acuminata, a treatment he supposedly learned from local Native Americans. Treatment was effective but had the downsides of toxicity on absorption and high recurrence rate. Later cryosurgery, laser surgery, and electrosurgery provided surgical choices; trichloroacetic and bichloroacetic acid were used for physical dissolving of warts. Also used were interferon and 5-fluorouracil, now in disfavor because of their side effects and cost.

The 1990s saw a rapid expansion of understanding of HPV, with two new medicines that allowed private patient treatment of the malady. These are podofilox (Condylox) 0.5 percent gel, a simpler-to-use version of podofilox solution, and imiquimod (Aldara) 5 percent cream; both of these topical medications are for external genital and perianal warts only. They are not for use in treating intravaginal, cervical, urethral, rectal, or intraanal warts.

Unless the doctor states otherwise, a patient should not continue using topical podofilox and imiquimod beyond the FDA recommendation of four and 16 weeks, respectively. Most treatments result in wart-free periods, and some eliminate the warts with no recurrence. Other possible treatments are 5-fluorouracil cream, which is contraindicated in pregnant women, and trichloroacetic acid (TCA).

Over the years, the approach to treating HPV has changed radically. Since physicians have seen that most low-grade cervical intraepithelial lesions regress spontaneously, doctors no longer treat cervical abnormalities as they did in the early 1990s. Then, women in their teens and early twenties were treated more aggressively after detection of the problem. A conservative approach has been adopted by U.S. physicians, most of whom agree that no invasive procedure is needed unless the patient has a high-grade squamous intraepithelial lesion (HGSIL). However, if the infection persists through several positive Pap smear results, treatment will probably be required.

Intraepithelial lesions that are moderate- to high-grade can be obliterated via any one of several safe treatments: cryotherapy, laser vaporization, loop electrosurgical excision procedure (LEEP), or cold-knife cone biopsy (CKCB). Cryotherapy has the disadvantage of a greater probability of recurrent disease than that of the others. CKCB has some downsides: it can increase future risk of second-trimester abortion, preterm labor, and low birth weight. It is important for those with HPV to understand that eradication of their lesions does not eliminate the need for follow-up Pap smears.

Many doctors prefer to remove genital warts with cryosurgery (freezing), electrocautery (burning), or laser treatment. Large warts that do not respond to treatment may require surgery. Some doctors inject the antiviral drug alpha-interferon into the warts, especially when the warts have recurred after traditional treatment. The drug is expensive and has not been proved to affect rate of recurrence; plus, it has the disadvantage of considerable discomfort for the patient, who must endure shots in the genital area.

Most patients go through a regimen that includes several doctor-administered treatments along with patient-applied options. In many cases, what is required are multiple courses of different treatments to solve the problem. Often, a patient is prescribed one therapy for home use and one that the doctor administers.

A wide variety of approaches to treatment exist because of deficient outcome data and lack of access to modalities such as cryotherapy and surgery. There is increasing agreement that some longtime treatments require too many office visits, and one treatment that was commonly used in the past—podophyllin resin—appears to be ineffective.

The following are some of the factors that affect the treatment selection for EGWs:

- There is a lack of studies in pediatric populations of the safety and efficacy of EGW treatments.
- Pain is associated with treatments.
- Wart size and number, anatomic location, circumcision status in men, and epithelial presentation can determine treatment choice; generally, for

example, topical treatments are not ideal for large areas of warts.

- Warts on moist surfaces and between skinfolds respond better than do warts on dry and open areas to topical treatment.

- Aggressive ablative or surgical therapy should not be performed over the clitoris, glans penis, urinary meatus, prepuce, and preputial cavity in the uncircumcised.

- Patient preference insofar as applying self-treatment versus having the health care provider perform treatment is a factor.

- Patient attitude toward the prospect of pain, cost of treatment, and number of visits affects the selection.

One report concludes that the most cost-effective therapy option is to start patients on imiquimod and then switch them to a provider-administered therapy if it is needed. This achieves the highest overall sustained clearance and does so at the lowest average cost per sustained clearance.

The goal of treatment is to remove symptomatic warts. There is no evidence it eradicates infection and no evidence that it affects the natural history or cancer risk, according to *USTD 2001*. Treatment choice should be patient-guided; the health care provider should not overtreat; and no treatment modality is superior. Treatment selection should be determined by considering wart size, number, sites, and morphological features; patient preference; cost; convenience; adverse effects; and doctor's experience.

For keratinized warts, local destructive methods are used. Possible complications of ablation are cosmetic alterations, such as scarring and hypo- or hyperpigmentation. For HPV combined therapies there is potential for increased complications and no increased efficacy.

For external condyloma treatment

- Patients can apply podofilox 0.5 percent solution or gel or imiquimod 5 percent cream.

Doctors can administer
- Cryotherapy

- Trichloracetic acid (TCA) or bichloracetic acid (BCA)
- Sharp excision
- Electrosurgery
- Cavitron ultrasonic surgical aspirator (CUSA)

Alternative therapies for genital warts include intralesional interferon use and laser surgery.

According to the CDC (1998), in the absence of dysplasia, treatment is not indicated for subclinical HPV diagnosed by any technique. There is a high spontaneous regression rate. Also according to 1998 CDC guidelines, evaluation and treatment of the male partner are not needed to confirm the presence of HPV. There are unproven benefits to the female partner of successful treatment and no proven benefits to the male partner or future partners as far as infectivity.

Specific considerations determine treatment of EGWs during pregnancy. Some treatments cannot be used because they carry risk for the fetus. However, treatment is often needed because EGWs can grow during pregnancy, and obstetrical complications of delivery may occur when the mother has large EGWs. Doctors usually use TCA or BCA, cryotherapy, or surgical removal. Since the FDA has labeled imiquimod a Pregnancy Category B drug, it may be an option for use during pregnancy if the patient is properly briefed. Pregnant women are cautioned not to use podophyllin or podofilox because both are absorbed by the skin and may cause birth defects.

Genital warts can wreak havoc during pregnancy: if they enlarge, they can make urination difficult; if they are on the wall of the vagina, they can make the vagina less elastic and cause delivery obstruction. Usually in women who are pregnant and have HPV, lesions enlarge and then regress spontaneously postpartum, but enlargement of condylomata may obstruct delivery, cause hemorrhage, and serve as a nidus of infection. Treatment of HPV in pregnancy is as follows: there should be a rationale for treating, such as allowing vaginal delivery by removing obstructing warts. There is no evidence that treatment or a cesarean section will decrease perinatal transmission (genital HPV, juvenile laryngeal papillomatosis, conjunctival condylomata). In rare cases, a cesarean section is indicated by the nature, location, and extent of HPV disease.

If condylomata will obstruct delivery, they are best treated at 27 to 32 weeks of gestation with TCA (external, vaginal), three applications a week for three weeks. Other treatment options are cryotherapy, laser, excision, and CUSA. Most patients need a course of treatment, or several treatments, in order to clear EGWs after initial diagnosis.

In a minority of women, HPV is believed to trigger the development of precancer and/or cancer of the cervix and, less often, of the vulva, vagina, and anus. For life, such patients need to have yearly pelvic exams with Pap smears.

Prevention

Many researchers and health care professionals see HPV as so ubiquitous that they believe the only people who remain unexposed to this are those who remain celibate lifelong. A figure of 70 percent is advanced as the lifetime incidence of genital HPV infection.

One cannot expect to prevent HPV transmission by condoms because the disease is spread during foreplay and other forms of sexual contact. Condoms do help, however, but it should be remembered that the virus exists all over the genital area—not just the part covered by a condom. The scrotum can infect the vulva, for instance, even when the person is wearing a condom. A man can get genital warts when vaginal secretions with virus infect the base of the penis.

Other modes of transmission may include tampon insertion and sanitary napkin use, oral–genital sex, and anal intercourse. Women who have HPV or whose male partners have HPV should not participate in receptive anal intercourse. Investigators are studying the possibility of nonsexual transmission of HPV. Some possibilities advanced are that the disease is spread by transmission from fomites or by perinatal or digital transmission. Children who have genital warts are assumed to be victims of sexual abuse, but if the nonsexual transmission theory is proved, that will be another explanation for children's infections. If someone sees warts in the genital area of a partner, he or she should refrain from sexual contact until these are treated. A latex condom during intercourse offers some protection, but it is not 100 percent effective.

Psychosocial Issues

High levels of anxiety are related to this disease. Patients need to be educated about HPV, and their concerns should be answered. On initial diagnosis, a patient may be extremely upset by fears about health and sexual future. Patients usually want to know how they contracted this disease and how likely they are to spread it to a partner. Pain and disfigurement are also worries. The uncertainty makes some patients entertain the idea of rejecting treatment and maintaining denial. Some patients who have genital warts experience sleep problems, irritability, crying jags, anger outbursts, weight swings, and relationship difficulties.

During treatment, new problems can arise from fear of the pain of treatment. Some tried-and-true methods are used when treatment occurs for HPV. Doctors like patient distraction, which may involve the nurse's chatting with the patient while colposcopy is done. One study found that entertaining adolescents with music videos reduced anxiety.

Some estimate that about 30 percent of sexually active young women have HPV in the lower genital tract. Most HPV infections occur through sexual contact, but the virus can be dormant for years, so there is actually no way to pinpoint when and where a person got the infection. Intrapartum transmission from mother to baby, from innocent contact between children and caregivers, between children, and through families possibly occurs, although these are thought to account for a small minority of cases in adults. Most HPV infection is time-limited, although it has been thought that all HPV is forever—a presumption that new evidence calls into question. Risk of serious consequences to the male partner, other than warts, is low. Evidence that treating HPV lesions in males decreases the chance of infecting a new partner is lacking. Also, cigarette smoking appears to increase a woman's susceptibility to the adverse consequences of HPV and interfere with success of treatment.

Self-Care

Two patient-applied treatments are handled as follows. Imiquimod 5 percent cream (Aldara) is applied with freshly washed hands. A thin layer of cream is applied to the warts and rubbed in until it vanishes. The packet is discarded and hands are washed again. Cream is left on for six to 10 hours. After that, the area where the cream was applied is washed with mild soap and water. Cream is applied Monday, Wednesday, and Friday or Tuesday, Thursday, and Saturday for up to 16 weeks. When using podofilox gel, a small amount (half the size of a pea) is squeezed onto a fingertip and dabbed onto warts or areas the doctor has said should be treated. It is applied to the wart area only. If a wart is in a skinfold area, skin is spread apart and the gel is applied to the wart. The gel is allowed to dry before skinfolds are returned to their normal position. Hands are washed well with soap and water before and after using gel. Podofilox gel is applied twice daily—morning and evening—for three days; then four days of no treatment follow. The weekly regimen is repeated for four cycles. Ideally, the patient should refrain from sexual activity during the entire treatment period, but especially during the three days of gel application. The gel should not be used on internal warts or other body areas.

Research

HPV vaccines that are both prophylactic and therapeutic are in clinical trials. One would prevent infection or disease, and the other would be used in treatment of cervical cancers.

Scientists have long known that a cause of cervical cancer is an agent that is sexually transmitted. It was presumed to be herpes, but the development of recombinant DNA technology allowed researchers to zero in on the real culprit—human papillomavirus. A detailed analysis became possible after a German team cloned of the important oncogenic virus HPV-16. But even after that information was disseminated worldwide, researchers resisted the idea that HPV—not herpes—was the etiologic agent.

Studies with Southern blot hybridization or polymerase chain reaction have confirmed an extremely strong causal relation between HPV and cervical intraepithelial neoplasia. In fact, it is considered even stronger than the tobacco–lung cancer link. Bearing up these findings are worldwide epidemiologic data that detect evidence of HPV in about 90 to 95 percent of cervical cancers. Admittedly, there are probably other factors at work, but the virus is deemed a prime mover behind the dysregulation of the cell cycle that underlies malignancy.

At highest risk are women with high viral loads and oncogenic types. Having an oncogenic type makes the woman have a greater chance of persistent infection that leads to viral integration and is a more significant predictor of neoplastic progression than is HPV viral load. About half of cervical cancers contain the oncogenic HPV-16. The other high-risk types are HPV types 18, 45, and 31. The high-risk types that are less prevalent are HPV types 26, 33, 35, 39, 51, 52, 56, 58, 59, 68, 73, and W13b.

The risk of a woman's contracting cervical cancer is increased if her body does not get rid of the virus and it persists over a period of years. Thus, women who have long-term HPV infections should be monitored carefully so that growths of abnormal cells can be removed. An infection is termed *persistent* if it lasts a year or more. Studies have noted, incidentally, that among women in whom cervical cancer developed, earlier Pap smear results showed the same type of HPV. The journey from viral exposure to a cancerous lesion takes about a decade, and that is why women usually are diagnosed with cervical cancer in midlife or later. This explains why, despite the fact that HPV infections are most prevalent in young people in their 20s, these women are not the ones with cervical cancer.

Since a faulty immune system inhibits ridding oneself of HPV, it is not surprising that HPV infection in HIV-infected women is about five times that of the general population. Furthermore, these women experience higher HPV viral loads, more precancerous lesions than HIV-negative women, and more severe infections. Further complicating matters is that HIV-positive women are more likely to be coinfected with multiple HPV types.

genotyping HIV genotyping tries to determine the drugs that a certain HIV strain is likely to be resistant toward. This test employs DNA amplification techniques to identify genetic mutations that have been associated with resistance. Since several mutations typically are required to produce resistance that is clinically significant, and the interaction of immune system and multidrug regimens is hard to predict, the results of a genotype assay are not always accurate in prognosticating response to therapy.

Hundreds of slightly different genotypes are circulating at the same time; that means that assays are likely to miss less common mutants, according to "Living with HIV" by Roger Spitzer, M.D., who considers trying a drug regimen and then checking response via a viral load assay the most accurate test. The genotype assay helps to guide initial drug selection in salvage regimens.

In phenotyping, HIV is grown in a test tube in the presence of various antiretroviral agents to give a more direct measure of susceptibility to various drugs. This test is also subject to sampling errors, says Spitzer.

Since 2002, a new genotyping kit, Trugene (Visible Genetics), which ascertains when a patient's HIV is gaining drug resistance, has been used to detect the mutation of a virus that makes a certain medication fail. It is considered a prime tool for helping doctors in their selection of ingredients (drugs) for an HIV-positive individual's drug cocktail. Before this kit was developed, patients could only monitor their treatment by having tests to determine the amount of AIDS virus in the bloodstream. A spike shows growing resistance to one or more drugs, thus signaling the treating physician to switch the patient to a different medicine. Trugene enables the lab to unravel components of the patient's blood sample, decoding HIV genes and pinpointing mutations. A software program matches mutations to a list of those mutations that have already been identified as resistant to specific drugs. In about three days, a lab tech can give the doctor a report detailing the effectiveness of each AIDS drug based on the viral mutations seen in the blood.

gingivostomatitis   Primary gingivostomatitis, which results from herpes simplex virus infection, produces multiple very painful ulcers inside the mouth. The condition can cause a great deal of discomfort.

global strategies   Today there are numerous global strategies that focus on curbing the spread of the HIV/AIDS pandemic. Some strides have been made, but much work remains. At the third International Conference on Global Strategies for Prevention of Mother-to-Infant HIV Transmission in Uganda in 2001, a dramatic report informed the attendees that worldwide mother-to-infant HIV transmission could be dramatically curtailed with $2.5 million worth of drugs. The event, which 700 experts from 52 countries attended, called on corporations, educational institutions, granting agencies, religious groups, governments, and organizations to unite in an effort to help prevent the needless infection of children by mothers with HIV.

Of babies born to HIV-positive mothers, 30 percent get the virus, which is often transmitted in breast milk as well as in the uterus. Most of the infections occur during the infant's passage through the birth canal.

The cost figure was arrived at by estimating the number of HIV-positive pregnant women worldwide and then taking an average transmission rate of 20 percent and an estimated discounted price of nevirapine of 80 cents. For the Republic of Congo and Senegal, German pharmaceutical company Boehringer Ingelheim offered to provide nevirapine free for five years.

golden shower   A sexual act in which one partner urinates on the other, as a means of achieving sexual gratification.

gonorrhea   Also called "the clap" or "drip," gonorrhea is an STD so ancient that it is mentioned in the Bible.

Cause

The cause of gonorrhea is the bacterium *Neisseria gonorrhoeae,* which grows and multiplies in moist, warm areas of the body, including the reproductive tract, oral cavity, and rectum. Sexual intercourse—vaginal, anal, oral—is the means of spread of this disease. Those who indulge in anal intercourse can have gonorrhea of the rectum, and it also occurs there in women when the infection has spread from the vaginal area. Gonorrhea is sometimes passed from an infected woman to her newborn during delivery, producing eye infection. When a doctor sees gonorrhea infection in a child's genital tract, mouth, or rectum, this is usually a reflection of sexual abuse. It is important to note that gonorrhea infection can spread to other parts of the body; an instance of this would be an eye infection that results from touching infected genitals and then the eyes. Also, those who have had gonorrhea and been treated are still subject to reinfection at another time if they have sexual contact with someone who has gonorrhea.

Symptoms

Symptoms typically appear about two to 10 days after infection, but there are many times, too, when 30 days pass before symptoms emerge. In rare cases, people may not show symptoms for several months, but whether or not infected individuals are exhibiting signs or symptoms, they can spread the infection to sex partners unless they use condoms.

Most commonly, symptoms are a yellowish white or yellow-green discharge from the vagina or penis and/or painful or difficult urination. Men sometimes have swollen testicles that are painful. Men usually show more symptoms than women. They usually have the hallmark discharge from the penis and a burning sensation when they urinate that is sometimes very severe. Rectal infection results in anal itching, discharge, and painful bowel movements.

For women, the primary site of infection is the endocervix, with secondary infection of the rectum or urethra. Early symptoms of gonorrhea can be mild, and many infected women have none whatsoever. Sometimes, a woman's early symptoms of gonorrhea are mistaken for a bladder or vaginal infection. Initial symptoms in women are a painful or burning sensation during urination and vaginal discharge that is yellow or bloody. More advanced symptoms are abdominal pain, bleeding between menstrual periods, vomiting, and fever—symptomatic of pelvic inflammatory disease.

Testing

Several laboratory tests are used to diagnose gonorrhea. This disease is diagnosed by Gram stain, culture, or detection of bacterial genes or deoxyribonucleic acid (DNA), and many doctors use more than one test to obtain an accurate diagnosis. A small specimen of fluid from the infected mucus membrane—rectum, throat, urethra, cervix—can be obtained and sent in for lab analysis.

For men, the Gram stain is accurate, but it is not for women. Only half of women with gonorrhea have positive Gram stain results. This test calls for placing a smear of discharge from the penis or the cervix on a slide and staining the smear with a dye. A lab technician studies the slide under a microscope to find the bacteria. Sometimes a doctor can give test results to the patient during an office visit.

For a culture, a sample of discharge is placed on a culture plate and incubated for up to two days to allow the bacteria to multiply, but the test's sensitivity depends on the site where it was harvested. About 90 percent of the time, cervical samples detect infection if one exists.

A throat culture can be used to determine whether a patient has pharyngeal gonorrhea. If gonorrhea is present in the male or female genital tract, its presence can also be diagnosed with a urine specimen. Urine or cervical swabs are used for a new test that detects genes of the bacteria. These are as accurate as culture.

Complications

Although the cervix is usually the site of infection, the disease can spread and infect the uterus (womb) and fallopian tubes. Women suffer the most serious complications; these can include ectopic pregnancy, infertility, and pelvic inflammatory disease. The latter—a serious infection of the female reproductive organs that affects about 1 million American women every year—is the most serious consequence. Gonococcal pelvic inflammatory disease (PID) usually appears immediately after the menstrual period, and symptoms of PID can be very severe, including abdominal pain and fever. PID can lead to internal abscesses and long-lasting pelvic pain, and it can scar or damage cells lining the fallopian tubes, resulting in infertility in about 10 percent of women affected.

A woman who has gonorrhea can give the infection to her baby during its passage through the birth canal at the time of delivery. This can result in joint infection, blindness, or a serious blood infection in the infant. It is thus extremely important for a woman who is pregnant and has gonorrhea to be treated as soon as possible to stave off these complications. Immediately after a baby is born to a mother who has gonorrhea, the doctor can prevent eye infection (ophthalmia neonatorum) by putting silver nitrate or another medication into the baby's eyes.

In men, a complication of gonorrhea is the painful condition of the testicles called epididymitis. Untreated, this can lead to infertility. Gonorrhea can also affect the prostate and cause urethral scarring that makes urination difficult. In rare cases, gonorrhea spreads to the blood or the joints.

One alarming fact is that having gonorrhea gives an individual a heightened risk—as much as two to five times—of contracting HIV. Furthermore, an individual who has HIV and gonorrhea is more likely to transmit HIV to another person than is an individual who has only HIV.

Treatment

Although penicillin had been the treatment for gonorrhea, since the early 1990s doctors have seen four types of antibiotic resistance emerge. That means that new antibiotics and drug combinations must be used to treat resistant strains.

In fact, it is now common for doctors to encounter gonorrhea strains that are resistant to penicillin, so this common antibiotic is no longer used for gonorrhea treatment. Thus, doctors prescribe other antibiotics, one of the most effective of which is ceftriaxone, injectable by the doctor in one dose. Because it is common for patients to be infected with chlamydia in addition to gonorrhea, doctors usually prescribe a combination—ceftriaxone and doxycycline or azithromycin—in order to treat both infections.

Other effective antibiotics that can be taken orally as a single dose are cefixime, ciprofloxacin, and ofloxacin. One caveat, however: patients 18 or younger and pregnant women cannot take ciprofloxacin or ofloxacin.

In treating gonorrhea, doctors should avoid prescribing fluoroquinolones such as ciprofloxacin if the sexually transmitted disease contact occurred in Asia or the Pacific region, including Hawaii, because of cipro-resistant gonorrhea. Increased levels of fluoroquinolone-resistant gonorrhea were being reported in Hawaii as of 2001, so the CDC now recommends that doctors ask patients infected with gonorrhea whether they or their sexual partners could have acquired the disease in Hawaii, other Pacific islands, or Asia, where this same resistance is common. That would point to treatment for these patients with other drugs—cefixime or ceftriaxone. Also, gonorrhea is beginning to show resistance to azithromycin. All sexual partners should be tested and treated if infected, even if no symptoms occur, and these individuals should be screened for other sexually transmitted diseases as well.

Prevention

At risk is any sexually active person, but sexually active individuals can reduce their risk of contracting gonorrhea by consistent and careful use of male condoms during all sexual activity. It is important to remember that condoms do not convey complete protection because bodily fluids or secretions can flow outside the area the condom covers, thus transmitting infection.

Other ways to reduce likelihood of contracting gonorrhea are: limiting the number of sex partners, not alternating partners, and practicing abstinence. When the possibility of infection occurs, see a doctor and avoid sexual contact until you have been treated and have responded to treatment. Be aware that gonorrhea can even occur in the throat as a result of oral sex. A person who experiences burning during urination or has a discharge or unusual rash or sore should see a health care provider and discontinue all sexual activity for the time being.

When an individual learns he or she has a sexually transmitted disease, it is important to notify all recent sex partners so that they can go in for testing and treatment, if necessary. The sexually active person who is reluctant to inform partners that he or she has gonorrhea should remember that this disease has very serious complications when it is untreated.

Research

Scientists supported by the National Institute of Allergy and Infectious Diseases (NIAID) are working to improve methods for prevention, diagnosis, and treatment. In view of the dramatic rise in antibiotic-resistant strains, there is a need to find a way of preventing gonorrhea. A main priority of researchers is development of a vaccine for gonorrhea.

granuloma inguinale   See DONOVANOSIS.

gum disease   Gingivitis is a condition in which the gums are inflamed. People who have HIV infection often experience problems with gingivitis.

HAART See HIGHLY ACTIVE ANTIRETROVIRAL THERAPY.

Haemophilus ducreyi The cause of chancroid, an ulcerative lesion.
   See also CHANCROID.

health care proxy The authority or power to act for another, or the legal document allowing a person to make medical decisions for someone else when that individual can no longer act in his or her own behalf. The form authorizes access to medical records. In ordinary circumstances, a family member of the patient acts as health care proxy/advocate automatically. Generally, this form is needed in cases in which the sick person wants someone other than a family member to exercise the responsibilities inherent in this role.

health care workers and HIV transmission There is a perceived increased risk to working in health care, insofar as there is greater likelihood of exposure to blood, vomit, and body fluids of an HIV-infected patient. Universal precautions are exercised routinely, however, and even in cases of needlesticks, the probability of contracting HIV from working in a hospital or health care facility is very small.

health maintenance organization A health maintenance organization (HMO) is a group that provides medical services to a set of members for a set fee as well as an annual charge. The HMO, as it is commonly known, is a component of managed care, which differs from the traditional fee-for-service when doctors in private practice were the rule rather than the exception. One downside to

the consumer of an HMO is that there is a list of physicians and hospitals that are covered, and the member cannot diverge from that without shouldering all the burden of the fees. Also, many physicians dislike the fact that HMOs try to keep costs lower by regulating services, hospital admissions, and medications, as well as requiring preauthorization of certain tests and procedures.

Health Plan Employer Data and Information Set (HEDIS) The Health Plan Employer Data and Information Set (HEDIS), developed by the National Committee for Quality Assurance, is a set of measures that are used to evaluate the quality of managed care plans. As of 2003, more than 90 percent of managed care organizations use HEDIS to measure performance. Measures specify how health care plans collect, audit, and report. Then, purchasers use this data for comparison purposes. Chlamydia, the most common bacterial sexually transmitted disease in the United States, comes into play in relation to HEDIS because of the prevalence and high cost of treating chlamydia. The Health Plan Employer Data and Information Set includes screening for *Chlamydia trachomatis* for women 25 and under. As a HEDIS 2000 measure, the group looked at the percentage of sexually active females 15 to 25 who have chlamydia testing each year and emphasized that when this disease is untreated, in about 40 percent of women who have it pelvic inflammatory disease will develop, at a cost of at least $1,167 per patient. Screening in women 21 to 26 increased from 15 percent in 1999 to 19 percent in 2000. Each year, the United States spends about $1.7 billion in direct and indirect costs of chlamydia. Most pelvic inflammatory disease costs could be prevented; in a trial of screening and treatment in an HMO, a 56 percent reduction was seen in the incidence of pelvic inflammatory disease in the year after intervention.

health resources for HIV/AIDS patients Health resources for those with HIV and AIDS vary from place to place, depending on where an individual lives. Basically, though, a person with HIV or AIDS has several choices: treatment by a private doctor, at a clinic, at a public health facility, or in an AIDS clinic. In many cases, those with HIV/AIDS opt to work with a specialist on treating HIV/AIDS in that the treatment plan and regimen for this disease are usually multifaceted and long-term. Also, one's choice of health resources often depends on ability to pay and on the patient's use of public charity facilities or others that are covered by her or his individual health insurance, Medicare, or Medicaid.

Healthy People 2010 The Healthy People 2010 program addresses significant health threats to Americans. Goals that the U.S. Department of Health and Human Services has targeted include those areas that have been deemed in need of improvement: physical activity, obesity, cigarette smoking, substance abuse, responsible sexual behavior, mental health, injury and violence, environmental quality, immunizations, and access to health care.

The specific goal in respect to sexual behavior is to increase the number of adolescents who abstain from sexual intercourse or use condoms if they are sexually active. Among sexually active unmarried adults, the goal is to increase the use of condoms from 23 percent to 50 percent.

Besides these aims, Healthy People 2010 has 28 total focus areas with numerous objectives. The agenda can be viewed on the Web: http://www. Health.gov/healthypeople. For a printed copy of the agenda, call (800) 367-4275.

Helms Amendment Enacted in 1987, this law sought to prohibit people from entering the United States if they were HIV-infected. Immigrants had to be tested for HIV, and a positive result meant they were denied entry. Not surprisingly, civil rights groups were soon up in arms about this. Both human rights and public health authorities were adamant that this policy was extremely unfair, especially because casual contact with travelers with HIV did not pose a health threat. As many people had predicted, Congress repealed the Helms Amendment in 1990. Congress then directed Health and Human Services to produce a new list of diseases that would require exclusion of aliens who had them. Congress asked that the diseases listed be communicable diseases that were of public health significance.

hemophilia A hereditary blood defect (in males) that slows the clotting of blood and sometimes makes stopping bleeding very difficult. The hemophiliac lacks a protein necessary for blood clotting; for this reason, the individual bleeds easily.

In respect to sexually transmitted diseases, hemophiliacs once figured into many discussions of AIDS because they had a high rate of contracting HIV in the years before blood banks began screening for this disease. A high percentage of men with hemophilia A and hemophilia B contracted HIV infection from commercial clotting factors. Since 1985, however, the risk of exposure to HIV in this manner has been reduced practically to zero. Besides the fact that blood is screened routinely for HIV, clotting factors are also heated and purified to kill HIV.

hepatitis A Hepatitis A is a virus that is infectious and contagious and produces inflammation of the liver. Hepatitis A, B, and C can cause acute infections, but B and C can become chronic.

Cause

Typically, hepatitis A infection is person-to-person and fecal-oral, so it is usually spread via contaminated food and water or by oral-anal sex. The latter is seen less often than is transmission via contaminated food and water.

One gets hepatitis A by ingestion of infected fecal matter. A person is most likely to transmit the infection via stool about two weeks before showing symptoms, if there are any, so the individual is unaware of being infected, while being potentially infectious to other people. Many people get hepatitis A by eating food that was prepared by someone who did not wash his or her hands thoroughly after a bowel movement and thus had feces remaining on the skin. This virus is easily transmitted via food contaminated during preparation. Another means of transmission occurs in day care facilities, where children sometimes spread the infection to other children and adults.

Sexual practices that can result in transmission of this virus are oral-anal contact, called rimming or analingus, whereby one partner stimulates the other's anus with the tongue or mouth, and digital-anal contact, whereby one partner stimulates the other's anus with the fingers and then fails to wash them properly. The virus gets into the mouth or on food during preparation. Sometimes there have been outbreaks of hepatitis A among gay men that some believe may have been caused by this kind of transmission.

Health professionals believe that the higher the number of sexual partners a man has, the more likely he is to contract hepatitis A. Also, a woman who engages in the sexual practices of oral–anal or digital–anal contact is at increased risk of contracting hepatitis A. Blood transfusion transmission is very rare because blood banks screen for hepatitis.

Symptoms

Some people have hepatitis A without exhibiting symptoms; most, however, have one or more of the following: fever, loss of appetite, nausea, vomiting, yellowing of the skin and eyes, dark urine, abdominal pain. Young children rarely have symptoms, but adults usually do. Although hepatitis A (usually food-associated) can make someone very sick, infection is temporary and usually resolves within several weeks.

Testing

Testing for hepatitis A is a simple blood test. If someone does have antibodies, these confer protection against getting the infection again. A person who has a negative result on a blood test but has good reason to suspect infection should repeat the test a few weeks later.

Prevention

Doctors often encourage their patients to take advantage of the immunization for hepatitis A, especially for international travel. Many health experts believe that children who live in high-disease-incidence areas should be immunized, along with others at risk.

Whereas formerly the CDC's Advisory Committee on Immunization Practices (ACIP) recommended vaccinating injection drug users and homosexual men, the thrust has changed, and new guidelines from ACIP are based on the findings that most cases in the United States result from person-to-person transmission during community outbreaks, and the most common source of infection is household or sexual contact with an infected person, which accounts for 12 to 26 percent of cases. Other associations are 11 to 16 percent in day care centers; 4 to 6 percent in international travel; 2 to 3 percent via food or waterborne disease; and 50 percent through unknown sources of infection. Native American reservations and Alaskan Native villages have a high rate of hepatitis A: about 30 to 40 percent of the children are infected by age five, and almost all in the community are infected by the time they reach adulthood.

Today the CDC recommends hepatitis A vaccine for the following people: children who live where the rates of hepatitis A are at least twice the national average, travelers to developing countries, homosexual men, illegal drug users, people with chronic liver disease, persons with clotting-factor disorders, and those who have occupational risk factors. Estimates suggest that providing hepatitis A vaccinations for homosexual men at age 20 would save society $10.72 in lifetime economic costs for every $1 spent, according to *Family Practice News* (March 2000). It is believed that savings in treatment costs alone would offset 54 percent of the vaccination costs in five years and 98 percent in 10 years.

Treatment

If someone does contract hepatitis A, a physician usually recommends rest, fluids, and medication to counter nausea. To prevent liver stress, the individual is asked to avoid drinking all alcoholic beverages. In people with liver problems, hepatitis A can be very serious. In some cases, a person with hepatitis A does not recover strength completely for several months.

hepatitis B Sometimes causing infections that last a lifetime, hepatitis B and C are common and often affect those with HIV, because HIV, hepatitis B, and hepatitis C all share the same mode of transmission—blood and sex.

Cause

One way that hepatitis B is contracted is via sexual intercourse, especially anal. Hepatitis B is also transmitted by drug addicts' sharing of needles, by vertical transmission (mother to child), and in health care environments. The more sex partners a person has, the more likely she or he is to get hepatitis B. Also at higher risk are those who have a sexually transmitted disease. This virus is not spread easily and cannot be contracted by sharing of bathroom facilities or casual contact.

Symptoms

Hepatitis B varies greatly, appearing in both mild and severe forms, as well as acute and chronic. Although it is usually symptom-free, hepatitis B can also make the infected person experience any one or a combination of a variety of symptoms: tiredness, anorexia, nausea, vomiting, headache, fever, jaundice, dark urine, and liver tenderness and swelling. A person with hepatitis B may have yellow eyes and skin and brown urine, and symptoms may be similar to those of very severe flu.

Usually if someone does have symptoms, these appear about two to three months after contracting the infection. Symptoms that do occur are often severe and last about six weeks.

Sometimes people who have hepatitis B feel sick off and on for a long time, but most sufferers recover from the infection and cannot be reinfected. However, a small percentage remain chronic carriers of hepatitis B. These are people whose immune systems were not strong enough to rid them of the infection entirely. People with HIV are very likely to become carriers if they get hepatitis B. A child who is infected with hepatitis B will probably become a carrier of the disease. Of special interest is the fact that some individuals whose blood shows evidence of having had this disease in the past were never aware that they contracted or experienced hepatitis B.

Testing

People can have a blood test that is specifically for hepatitis B, but, in fact, most who have acute hepatitis B do not have a positive test finding for the virus when they first visit a health care provider. The blood test result can turn up negative if the individual has recently been infected. A liver biopsy may be necessary to determine stage of infection. A test that measures liver function cannot be used to rule out hepatitis infection. If a person proves to be a hepatitis B carrier, a blood test for hepatitis D (delta hepatitis) should be done, because this can only occur in someone who has hepatitis B—and, together, the two can create a serious health situation.

Complications

Hepatitis B can cause liver inflammation and damage. A small percentage of sufferers have extensive liver damage that eventually results in death.

Treatment

Once a person has hepatitis B, no form of treatment can eradicate it. Fortunately, though, sometimes the body of a hepatitis B carrier eventually manages to clear the infection spontaneously.

As far as treatment goes, people with chronic hepatitis B infection sometimes benefit from alpha-interferon alone or a combination of IV steroids and alpha-interferon. Sometimes, oral medications such as lamivudine or adefovir are used. As a general rule, those who have hepatitis B cannot drink alcohol for about a year after recovery.

In some people who turn out to be carriers, chronic active hepatitis, whereby the virus gradually destroys the liver, leading to cirrhosis, or scarring, of the liver, develops. Liver cancer, which is seen much more often in those who have had hepatitis B than in the general population, can also develop, but most carriers have chronic persistent hepatitis with less debilitating symptoms and livers that are only mildly inflamed. These people are less infectious than carriers of the chronic active variety, and their disease is much less likely to proceed to cancer or cirrhosis.

Prevention

Hepatitis B is transmitted more easily than HIV. The means of transmission of hepatitis B include sexual contact and blood-to-blood contact. Saliva is a means of exposure, too, as is vertical transmission. In respect to blood exposure, a person is at risk of getting hepatitis B through sharing of IV drug equipment or tattooing or body piercing. A needlestick injury and a transfusion with infected blood or blood products are two other possibilities.

If someone knows that his or her sexual partner has hepatitis B, it is imperative to be immunized. Others for whom immunization is advisable are men who have sex with men, men and women recently diagnosed with STDs, people with several sex partners, infants born in the United States or any child 11 to 12 who has not had the series of three shots, those who share a house with a person with chronic hepatitis B, injection drug users, health care workers who are sometimes exposed to body fluids that may be contaminated, dialysis patients and people who receive blood products, people who travel to countries with a high level of hepatitis B, prostitutes, and prisoners. Condoms and barriers such as dental dams can help prevent transmission.

hepatitis C   Formerly known as non-A, non-B hepatitis, hepatitis C is a major health concern worldwide because it is a common cause of chronic liver disease.

Cause

The most common ways this disease is spread are IV drug abuse and transfusions with contaminated blood. It was not until 1992 that screeners began checking the blood supplies for hepatitis C.

According to *Hospital Practice* (January 15, 2000), known risk factors for hepatitis C are a nonautologous blood transfusion before 1992, nonautologous clotting-factor transfusion before 1987, intravenous drug use, organ transplantation before 1992, percutaneous exposure (in a health care worker), long-term hemodialysis, birth to an infected mother, multiple sex partners or history of sexually transmitted diseases, and a long-term infected sexual partner.

Some causes that are suspected but not proved are body piercing and tattooing, shared razors, and intranasal drug use. Further, it is unlikely that casual contact or household exposure that is nonsexual is a risk factor.

Sexual transmission of hepatitis C does occur, but the prevalence of hepatitis C infection in those who have long-term sexual partners is very low. In a long-term monogamous relationship, the risk of transmitting this disease is considered less than 5 percent.

Risk factors are men's having sex with men, presence of other sexually transmitted diseases, needlestick injury, failure to use condoms, needle sharing during drug use, straw sharing in snorting of cocaine, vertical transmission (mother to child), and close contact of mother and child when the mother has hepatitis C. Heterosexuals and IV drug users have hepatitis C more commonly than they have hepatitis B.

Unless saliva has blood in it, it is not a means of transfer of hepatitis C. Risk for transmission grows with duration of exposure to an infected sex partner. Vertical transmission is rare, and breast-feeding has not been shown to transmit the virus to the infant.

Symptoms

The incubation period is 15 to 160 days but averages six to seven weeks. The usual symptoms are fatigue, jaundice (yellowing of skin), diarrhea, and nausea. Early signs during acute infection are malaise, anorexia, and jaundice; typically, these are not diagnosed as signs of hepatitis C. Most cases become chronic, and some progress to cirrhosis or other complications. The symptoms of this illness are often mild, and even more commonly, people with hepatitis C are asymptomatic. Most people with hepatitis C infection do not know they have it because symptoms do not develop.

When donating blood or having liver function tests (blood tests), a person may discover that he or she has hepatitis C. For some, this comes as a shock because their high-risk behavior occurred in the distant past.

Testing

Two licensed diagnostic tests for hepatitis C are ELISA and recombinant immunoblot assay (RIBA). The ELISA test is the initial test done, and it detects antibodies to hepatitis C. Since this test can result in false-positive results, if the ELISA test result is positive, then a confirmatory test is done—usually the RIBA.

The evaluation may include a liver biopsy. Usually, a blood test will yield a positive finding of hepatitis C about six weeks after infection, but it can take months longer than that.

An over-the-counter option approved by the FDA is a telemedicine kit called the Home Access Hepatitis C Check Test Service. The individual testing himself or herself uses a safety lancet to take a blood sample, places it on collection paper, and mails it in an envelope to a laboratory. Ten business days later, the person can learn the results by phone. The client registers an individual ID number by calling a toll-free number before producing the blood sample. Information is available by calling 1-888-888-HEPC.

Guidelines from the American College of Obstetricians and Gynecologists recommend that women who see their doctor for their annual Pap smear be tested for hepatitis C, sexually transmitted diseases, and diabetes. Because about 4 million Americans have hepatitis C, which can be transmitted vertically, it is important to screen women who have high risk for this disease. Some pediatricians believe that children exposed to hepatitis C should be monitored for about 18 months.

Treatment

Recommended treatment for hepatitis C is 48 weeks of combination therapy with the antiviral agents alpha interferon and ribavarin. A patient should be immunized against hepatitis A and B, refrain from consuming any alcohol, and avoid taking any liver-damaging medications. In HIV patients, management of hepatitis C should include screening for hepatitis A and B and immunization against A and B if not immune, and monitoring of liver function test results after HAART. Some doctors believe women 40 and older should be treated for hepatitis C routinely because the disease can stay hidden for up to 30 years.

Prevention

Hepatitis C is infectious, so those who have it should not donate blood or organs. There should be no sharing of toothbrushes or razors. No change in sexual practices is required, although there is a low risk of transmission from a long-term infected sexual partner.

hepatitis D   Also termed delta hepatitis, hepatitis D occurs only in those who have hepatitis B infection. Although hepatitis D can be sexually transmitted, a person is more likely to contract this disease through blood exposure. One can become simultaneously infected with hepatitis D and B or superinfected with D while carrying B.

hepatitis G   Previously seen as an innocuous virus first discovered in 1995, hepatitis G has also been cited as a slower of progression of HIV that serves to prolong the lives of people who are HIV-positive. The findings were reported in two studies in the *New England Journal of Medicine* (September 2001), and the information confirmed earlier studies that suggested patients with HIV and hepatitis G lived longer than HIV patients who did not have hepatitis G. This virus differs from other hepatitis viruses in that it does not cause any disease, including hepatitis. Researchers hope to identify the path that hepatitis G takes to slow HIV.

hepatotoxicity   Destructive to the liver. Sexually transmitted diseases are an important cause of abnormal liver chemical findings, and hepatotoxicity (liver toxicity) is a risk of use of oral therapy (fluconazole) to treat recurrent candidal vulvovaginitis.

herpes   The herpesvirus family includes herpes simplex type 1 (HSV-1) and type 2 (HSV-2). These are different viruses, but they cause similar symptoms. HSV-1 usually causes cold sores around the mouth; HSV-2 typically causes problems in the genital and anal areas. At the same time, infections with both viruses can occur any place on the body (most vulnerable are broken skin and mucosal surfaces). The herpesvirus family also includes vari-cella zoster virus (the cause of chickenpox and shingles), Epstein-Barr virus (the cause of mononucleosis), and cytomegalovirus.

A little-known fact is that a high percentage—perhaps as many as 75 percent—of adults have oral herpes by the time they are in their 40s. HSV-1 usually underlies oral herpes infection; this most often is acquired through nonsexual means when the individual is a young child and is kissed by an adult or child who has oral HSV-1. Although it is less common for HSV-2 infections to occur around the mouth, it does happen. People usually get HSV-2 (oral) as a result of performing oral sex on a person who has genital HSV-2 infection.

Genital herpes is almost always sexually transmitted and is very common in the United States. Of genital herpes cases in the United States, about 70 percent of infections result from HSV-2, and the rest from HSV-1. What many people do not understand is that genital herpes can be caused by either type 1 or 2.

See also GENITAL HERPES.

herpes encephalitis A rare result of oral herpes infections, herpes encephalitis is inflammation of the tissues of the brain caused by herpes simplex virus—almost always HSV type 1. Some of the possible symptoms are headache, fever, vomiting, and irritability, progressing to confusion, seizures, and neurological impairment.

herpes gladiatorum Herpes gladiatorum is a herpes simplex type 1 virus that studies suggest is spread by direct contact, not fomites, according to investigators. Wrestlers investigated in one study had lesions on the head and neck, the most vulnerable parts of the body for wrestling abrasions. The investigation began when there were four confirmed outbreaks of herpes simplex virus type 1 infections in wrestlers in a five-county region in Washington state. That there were three different strains suggests that wrestlers apparently have an increased risk of herpes gladiatorum, although little is known about the spread or proper treatment of this infection. Among the 700,000 wrestlers in

the United States in the year 2001, it was common practice to bench those with suspicious lesions and to sterilize mats. Unfortunately, though, there is little information on the relationship of asymptomatic shedding to the spread of herpesvirus in wrestling.

herpes keratitis An eye infection that is caused by herpes simplex virus. It can be a serious complication because it sometimes leads to blindness.

herpes zoster Also known as shingles, herpes zoster manifests itself in pain along the distribution of a nerve that may be on the face, abdomen, or torso, followed by the development of grouped vesicles on a red base in the same distribution localized to one side of the body. The disease generally lasts a few weeks, after which pain may persist for months in the area of the nerve. The virus that causes herpes zoster also causes chickenpox in children.

herpetic whitlow A disorder characterized by painful, grouped small blisters on a finger that are produced by herpes simplex virus.

heterosexual intercourse Sexual activity between a male and a female in which the penis penetrates the vagina or the anus.

HHV-8 Human herpesvirus 8, also called KS herpesvirus, is reportedly linked to Kaposi's sarcoma (KS).

high-risk behavior Any behavior that increases risk of being exposed to a sexually transmitted disease, including contraction of the human immunodeficiency virus. This includes contact with bodily fluids of an infected person, IV drug use in which needles or paraphernalia are shared, sexual activity without protection, and sexual activity with an IV drug user.

Factors influencing early initiation of high-risk activity are early onset of puberty, sexual abuse, absence of a nurturing parent, low academic achievement, poverty, mental illness, and participation in other high-risk behavior. Behavioral factors leading to an increased risk of STDs are as follows:

- Fear of diagnosis is a deterrent to seeking medical care.
- It is easier to have sex than to talk about it.
- People with sexually transmitted diseases sometimes demonstrate a marked lack of compliance with their treatment regimens and have a high risk of reinfection.
- Partner notification is problematic.
- Substance use tends to impair judgment and to increase the risk of multiple partners.

The following are biological factors that lead to increased risk (to oneself or one's partners): the lack of symptoms of 50 to 80 percent of infections; long lag time between initial infection and complications; the vaginal ecosystem can be altered by vaginal douching; use of IUDs, which increases risk of complications; cervical squamocolumnar junction susceptibility to STDs; and high prevalence of human papillomavirus (HPV), which can be the cause of neoplastic transformation (HGSIL 0.5 percent, cancer, 0.1 percent).

High-risk groups can be extrapolated by considering the following information from the *2001 Update on Sexually Transmitted Diseases:* average age of first intercourse for Americans is currently 15 to 17 years old; 37 percent of high school freshmen have had intercourse; 65 percent of seniors in high school are sexually active; 20 percent of seniors have had four or more partners; and oral sex is increasingly common among teens and viewed by many participants as "not real sex."

It is abundantly clear that the lack of knowledge about sexually transmitted diseases in very young people is a large contributor to the high rate of STDs. According to a 1999 survey of American teens, only 20 percent recognize that there is a risk of contracting an STD with one sexual encounter. Furthermore, about 45 percent think the risk of sexually transmitted diseases is not significant until they have had about seven or more partners. About 25 percent think risk is not significant until a person has had 20 or more partners. Another

belief in this group is that a series of monogamous relationships exposes a person to less risk for sexually transmitted diseases.

high-risk sex   Several aspects of an individual's behavior that increase his or her risk of contracting a sexually transmitted disease. These include numerous sex partners, unprotected sex, and other forms of sex that cause contact with bodily fluids of a partner who may be infected with an STD.

Hispanics and HIV   The number of U.S. Hispanics reported to the CDC as having AIDS as of December 2000 was 141,694. In 2001, according to the Centers for Disease Control and Prevention, 14 percent of the U.S. population (including those who live in Puerto Rico) were Hispanic; Hispanics had 19 percent of the total number of new HIV cases in the United States reported that year. It is also notable that AIDS incidence per 100,000 population among male Hispanics in 2001 was 42.8, a figure that is more than three times the rate for white men (13.8) but lower than the rate for African-American men (106.7). In women, AIDS cases per 100,000 in 2001 were 11.2 in Hispanics compared to 2.2, white; and 46.1, African American. Of the Hispanics reported with AIDS in 1999, 57 percent were U.S.-born and 43 percent Puerto Rican–born.

From the outset of the AIDS epidemic through December 1999, of Hispanic men reported with AIDS in the United States, 43 percent were men who have sex with men; 36 percent, injection drug users; and 6 percent, men who had heterosexual contact. About 7 percent of these were Hispanic men who had two risky behavior factors: sex with men and drug injections. For Hispanic women, 47 percent of cumulative AIDS cases were attributed to heterosexual contact, and most of these were associated with sex with a person who was an injection drug user. Among U.S. Hispanic women, injection drug use accounts for an additional 40 percent of AIDS cases.

Health care experts believe that prevention messages need to be tailored to fit affected communities, because it appears that risk for infection among Hispanics may be heightened by higher poverty rates, greater likelihood of substance abuse, limited access to or use of health care services, and language or cultural factors. The idea is advanced that the most effective prevention programs must feature activities that will help build skills that enhance changes in sexual behavior. Cultural aspects must also be taken into consideration. For example, in Hispanics born in Puerto Rico, high-risk behavior associated with drug abuse such as participation in "shooting galleries" is more prevalent; thus, in these cases, the use of shooting galleries must be discouraged, as must the sharing of needles.

For Hispanics who were born in Mexico, Cuba, and Central and South America, CDC data show that male–male sex is the number one mode of HIV transmission. This means prevention messages that target these populations must be shaped with a view to their attitudes toward homosexuality and bisexuality.

In some parts of the United States, groups are forming to try to affect the trend of Hispanics contracting HIV at a rapid rate. Union Positiva, founded in South Florida to help Spanish speakers prevent and treat AIDS, is one such group. Originally the goal was to disseminate AIDS prevention information to Latin America, but in recent years, the nonprofit has changed its primary focus to homeland problems, offering anonymous testing and counseling, prevention efforts, street outreach, treatment education, and referrals.

The group's representative, Dr. Eddie Sollie, indicates that Hispanics lagged behind African Americans and gays in demanding to be heard by the U.S. government. Dr. Sollie attributes this to cultural taboos among Hispanics concerning discussions of sex and emphasizes that the taboo must be broken because the "AIDS virus doesn't make any exceptions." Since joining Union Positiva as political adviser, the activist Luis Penelas, Jr., the brother of the Miami-Dade mayor, Alex Penelas, has spoken on radio shows and received an excellent response to his efforts.

HIV (human immunodeficiency virus) First reported in the United States in 1981, AIDS is caused by the human immunodeficiency virus (HIV), which destroys the body's ability to fight off infection. Thus, those who have AIDS are very susceptible to some forms of cancer and to life-threatening diseases, called OIs—opportunistic infections.

The most common modes of transmission are sexual activity and sharing of needles used to inject IV drugs, when a syringe is contaminated with small quantities of blood from an HIV-infected person. During sexual activity, the virus enters the body via the lining of the vagina, vulva, penis, rectum, or mouth. Contact with infected blood also spreads HIV. Before blood was screened for evidence of HIV infection and before heat-treating techniques began to be used to destroy HIV in blood products, HIV was transmitted more frequently by means of transfusions with contaminated blood or blood components. Now, when a person gets a transfusion, the probability of acquiring HIV in that manner is extremely small.

Soon after being infected with HIV, a person has a 50 percent chance of development of flulike symptoms. During this time, in the plasma, there are high levels of replicating virus—until the immune response kicks in, and the high levels of infectious plasma viremia disappear and then, for several years, stay at a very low detectable state. More than half of those infected do not have symptoms during the latency period. When years pass and there is a reemergence of high levels of replicating virus in the plasma, 50 percent of those with HIV will experience clinical symptoms. Researchers now know that even during the period that the HIV-infected person has no symptoms, the virus is still replicating at very high levels. Better tests to examine viral ribonucleic acid (RNA) revealed that the replication at that time was occurring primarily in lymphatic tissue. A hallmark of HIV is its ability to replicate well in parts of the body where immune activation occurs—such as lymph nodes. The upshot of these findings is that researchers now understand that HIV follows a highly dynamic road, with extremely high-level viral replication and potentially high-level cellular turnover.

The antiretrovirals have had great success, which led some to predict that a person with HIV could be treated for three years with HAART and eradicate all virus, but it became clear that long-lived memory CD4 T cells harbor the virus in its latent state and spring back to restart the infection when HAART is stopped. Researchers are now trying to activate the latent virus form in order to make it susceptible to treatment with chemokines and cytokines.

As for the future of HIV in the United States, some researchers think it is clear that the virus is going to mutate and become resistant to the treatment drugs now being used. The virus's error-oriented reverse transcriptase continues to complicate the effort to develop therapies as well as a vaccine. Researchers seek to develop many drugs to battle HIV so that these can be used in powerful combinations with the potential to stomp out the virus before it manages to mutate or replicate.

Acute Retroviral Syndrome

According to estimates, at least 50 percent and up to 90 percent of patients newly infected with HIV will experience at least some symptoms of the acute retroviral syndrome and are thus candidates for early therapy. Symptoms of acute retroviral syndrome are fever; lymphadenopathy; pharyngitis; rash on the face, trunk, and extremities and/or ulceration involving the mouth, esophagus, or genitals; diarrhea; headache; nausea and vomiting; weight loss; thrush; and neurologic symptoms, including: facial palsy, Guillain-Barré syndrome, brachial neuritis, cognitive impairment or psychosis, peripheral neuropathy or radiculopathy, meningoencephalitis, or aseptic meningitis. Also, acute primary infection can occur without any symptoms. Unfortunately, the similarity of these symptoms to those of the flu sometimes makes it easy for doctors to miss the diagnosis of HIV initially.

Most health care professionals endorse the course of treating acute HIV infection, but this course is based primarily on a theoretical rationale, experience of HIV clinicians, and limited but supportive clinical trial data. Early intervention in cases of acute retroviral syndrome seems prudent for several reasons: to suppress early viral replication and decrease the virus dissemination throughout the body; to decrease disease severity; to alter the viral setpoint, which may tend to affect rate of progression; to reduce, perhaps, risk of transmission of the virus; and to preserve immune function insofar as possible. Risks, on the other hand, include the adverse effects of drug therapy, resulting from toxicities and dosing constraints.

Persons at Risk

Those at risk for contracting HIV are people who have sexual contact with HIV-infected partners, those who have blood or bodily fluid contact with a person who has HIV, anyone who shares needles or drug paraphernalia that is being reused without being sterilized, an infant who is born to a mother with HIV or who is breast-fed by her, and, very rarely, those who receive transfusions of blood or blood products.

Early Symptoms

Early symptoms of HIV infection can include fever, night sweats, weight loss, anorexia, eye floaters, thrush, problems with teeth, difficulty or pain with swallowing, shortness of breath, oral thrush, pneumonia, abdominal symptoms, genital or perirectal ulcers, vaginitis, cough, and weakness. Skin signs of primary HIV are hair loss, mucocutaneous ulcers, skin peeling, hives, and most commonly, a roseola-type rash on the chest.

Primary HIV infection syndrome produces symptoms in up to 90 percent of those infected, and these occur about six to eight weeks after exposure. This is a mononucleosislike illness—pharyngitis, rash, hepatitis, aseptic meningitis.

One of the most difficult aspects of knowing whether one has contracted HIV is that in some people, infection with HIV has no early symptoms, whereas in others a flulike illness that may cause fever, headache, malaise, enlarged lymph nodes in the neck and groin, all of which disappear in about a week, occurs. At this time, though, the HIV infected individual is extremely infectious because large quantities of HIV are in genital secretions.

Not surprisingly, physicians may easily miss clues to a diagnosis of HIV infection or AIDS because primary acute retroviral syndrome has the symptoms of common viral infections: fever, pharyngitis, generalized lymphadenopathy, arthralgia, myalgia, lethargy, malaise, anorexia, weight loss, headache, and retroorbital pain.

Other conditions that should raise a physician's suspicion of HIV are meningoencephalitis, brachial neuropathy, radiculopathy, brachial neuropathy, and Guillain-Barré syndrome. At the same time, in some people who are infected with HIV, the only signs of infection are depression and irritability.

In intermediate HIV disease and AIDS, the patient can be asymptomatic a great deal of the time, and this period can last more than 20 years. Even so, it is most important to arrive at a diagnosis as early as possible in order to start drug therapy and prevent transmission of the infection to other people.

Frequently a person has candidiasis (thrush) and oral hairy leukoplakia—white plaques in the mouth. Though it is also seen in people without HIV disease, oral hairy leukoplakia is an almost sure sign of HIV infection. Positioning of oral hairy leukoplakia is usually on the lateral borders of the tongue, but it can occur anywhere in the mouth. Severe gingivitis and dryness of the mouth are not unusual. Other manifestations are the following:

Gastrointestinal: acalculus cholecystitis, *Candida* species esophagitis, heartburn, hemorrhoids
Neurologic: neuropathies, meningoencephalitis, dementia
Dermatologic: eosinophilic pustular dermatitis, Kaposi's sarcoma, psoriasis
Pulmonary: *Pneumocystis carinii* pneumonia, other lung infections
Endocrine: hypogonadism, adrenal insufficiency, hypertriglyceridemia

Later Symptoms

The severe symptoms and those that persist often do not appear for a decade or more after an adult first contracts HIV. In children, the period is about two years after they are born with HIV. On the other hand, some people begin to experience symptoms a few months after they are infected with HIV.

Even during the period in which no symptoms are evident, the disease is continuing to multiply, and it is infecting and destroying immune-system cells. The most obvious change is a decline in blood levels of CD4+ T cells, which are also referred to as T4 cells. These are critical infection fighters, so as these are disabled or killed, the body is rendered less capable of warding off other collateral diseases. Along with the breakdown of the immune system, the patient sees one of the first symptoms experienced—"swollen glands." These lymph nodes can remain enlarged for three months or more.

Other symptoms that HIV-infected individuals experience before actual onset of AIDS are reduced energy, weight loss, sweats and fever, yeast infections (oral or vaginal), skin rashes and/or flaky skin, pelvic inflammatory disease that does not respond to treatment, and memory loss (short-term). Shingles and severe herpes outbreaks resulting in sores in the mouth, genital area, or anus are other possible results of HIV. In HIV-infected children, health experts see slow development and a failure to thrive.

The specific immunologic profile that is typical of AIDS is a progressive reduction of CD4+ T cells resulting in persistent CD4+ T lymphocytopenia and profound deficits in cellular immunity, and this is very rare in the absence of HIV or other factors that cause immunosuppression.

Testing

HIV can be detected early by a blood test that ascertains the presence of antibodies to HIV. HIV antibodies usually do not reach levels that make them detectable for one to three months after infection. In some people, it takes six months for large enough quantities to allow standard blood tests to produce an accurate result to appear. It is important to note that saliva and urine samples can also be used for HIV testing.

If a person suspects that he or she has contracted HIV, testing is encouraged as soon as there may be antibodies to the virus. This allows initiation of early treatment. It is also important to determine whether HIV infection exists before continuing high-risk behavior that could spread HIV further.

Doctors' offices and health clinics offer HIV testing and counseling. Some sites offer anonymous testing, which should be sought if a person has concerns about confidentiality. People can also get test kits through pharmacies and phone order and use these at home.

The antibody tests ELISA and Western blot are used to diagnose HIV infection. The ELISA test is used first, and if it produces a positive result, then the Western blot test is done for confirmation. If someone thinks she or he is infected yet both test results prove negative, the doctor may test for the presence of HIV itself in the blood. Then that individual is told to repeat the antibody testing at a later date when antibodies have had time to develop.

In the case of vertical transmission, a baby may or may not be HIV-infected, but he or she will carry the mother's antibodies to HIV for several months. In symptom-free infants, a definitive diagnosis cannot be made until the child is at least 15 months old. At that point, the child's immune system will have produced antibodies if indeed the child is HIV-infected, but it is unlikely that the baby would still have the mother's antibodies.

New HIV detection technologies enable doctors to determine more accurately HIV infection in babies from the time they are three months old to age 15 months. Researchers are working on blood tests that can detect HIV infection even earlier in infants.

Complications

Complications usually take the form of opportunistic infections. *Update in Sexually Transmitted Diseases 2001* alludes to current issues related to opportunistic infections in the highly active antiretroviral therapy (HAART) era: the changing epidemiologic characteristics of opportunistic infections, identification of risk factors for development of opportunistic infections during HAART, new clinical presentations ("immunorestoration syndromes"), and determination of whether to continue primary or secondary prophylaxis for specific opportunistic infections (some findings suggest secondary prophylaxis or OI suppression should be discontinued after recovery of CD4 cells).

The U.S. Public Health Service and the Infectious Disease Society of America offer revised guidelines for preventing opportunistic infections

in HIV patients, with the following major changes and additions:

- Discontinuation of prophylaxis against specific opportunistic infections when the CD4+ T lymphocyte count increases in response to HAART
- Recommendations for short-course chemoprophylaxis against TB in HIV-infected individuals with positive tuberculin skin test results
- Changes in secondary prophylaxis (chronic maintenance therapy) recommended to prevent the recurrence of *Mycobacterium avium* complex and cytomegalovirus disease
- Caution against using fluconazole during pregnancy

Elaborating on these recommendations published in *Hospital Medicine* (October 1999), *Consultant* (November 1999) looks at various aspects of lifestyle that can be monitored to limit exposure to opportunistic infections for HIV-infected patients:

- Safe-sex emphasis is on the use of a latex condom during every act of sexual intercourse to reduce risk of exposure to cytomegalovirus (CMV), herpes simplex virus, genital warts, and other STDs. It is believed that condom use can reduce the risk of human herpesvirus 8 infection as well as superinfection with an HIV strain that does not respond well to HAART drugs. It is also recommended to avoid sexual practices that may result in oral–fecal exposure, which can lead to intestinal infections.
- Injection drug use was once again on the list of taboos, and health experts emphasized that it exposes users to hepatitis C virus, drug-resistant strains of HIV, and other pathogens.

Set Point

An important discovery is that the viral set point of an individual, the balance between the effectiveness of the immune system against HIV and the vigor with which the virus is replicating, is critical. It is the set point that indicates the clinical course that person's disease will take years down the road when the virus "reactivates." It has been seen that individuals who have a low viral set point progress to a clinical disease state much more slowly than persons with HIV who have a higher viral set point.

Seroprevalence

Seroprevalence is an indicator of how far-ranging a disease is at a given time. In respect to HIV, seroprevalence points to the incidence of infection in a certain population. The CDC assembles this information.

HIV/AIDS facts

Activist Groups

Activist groups such as amfAR are known for their work to ensure that all rights of being an American are guaranteed for those with HIV/AIDS, as well as resources and opportunities. The group ACT UP (AIDS Coalition to Unleash Power) has promoted the idea that HIV/AIDS patients should take proactive roles in their health care. ACT UP is best known, though, for pressuring the FDA to approve drugs in much less than the usual period required. Initially, many Americans viewed ACT UP as a radical group because of its advocacy of condom distribution and needle exchange programs. In recent years, new chapters have been formed with the thrusts of reemphasizing safe sex and lobbying Washington, D.C., for sufficient budgetary expenditures for HIV/AIDS services.

Adolescents and HIV

Two prongs of the adolescents–HIV connection are prevention and education. With sexually transmitted diseases looming large as an overwhelming scourge of society, the need persists for parents to communicate with their adolescents about sexuality. Two barriers to communication, according to parents surveyed in a study done in Iowa, are that parents do not feel they have adequate information and that they feel uncomfortable talking to their children about sex. Findings from the study documented in the publication *Adolescence* suggest that parents and young people turn to the media as a source of information on sexuality and use articles as a launching pad for productive discussions. According to the National Campaign to Prevent

Teen Pregnancy, programs that focus on sex and some that do not address sex have shown some positive effects: delaying onset of sexual activity, increasing the use of contraception, and preventing pregnancy among adolescents. One intensive three-year program, which included sex education, health care, and activities, was reported to have affected the behavior (sexual and contraceptive), pregnancy rate, and birth rate of the young women who participated in it. Abstinence-only programs often show inconclusive evidence, although the results do not look very promising. In some cases, the evaluation techniques appear to be questionable. Better results were found in federally funded evaluation of abstinence-only programs. Released May 30, 2001, the report showed good news for those communities that were seeking to reduce the rate of teen pregnancy. Activities sponsored by communities appear to go a long way toward convincing teens that pregnancy and parenthood are not good choices for teens.

Findings from the report "Emerging Answers" included the following:

- Eight programs posted strong successes.

- Evidence shows that sex education that discusses contraception does not make teens begin having sex sooner, increase their frequency of sexual activity, or cause than to sample a greater number of partners.

- Family planning clinics that provide high-quality educational materials, discuss sexual and contraceptive behavior, and offer clear messages are reportedly responsible for increasing the rate of use of contraceptives.

- The act of making condoms or other contraceptives available to adolescents does not increase the rate of sexual activity or hasten its onset.

CDC surveillance data from 25 states with integrated HIV/AIDS reporting systems for January 1996 to June 1999 showed that young people (ages 13 to 24) accounted for a much larger percentage of HIV (13 percent) than of AIDS cases (3 percent). This shows an important trend: even though AIDS incidence is declining, there has not been a comparable decline in the number of newly diagnosed HIV cases among young people. Because this age group has more recently started high-risk behavior, scientists think that cases of infection in this age group reflect overall trends in HIV incidence. Females accounted for almost half (49 percent) of HIV cases in this age group, reported for 32 places with confidential HIV reporting in 1999. In teens 13 to 19, a much greater proportion of HIV infections was seen in females (64 percent) than in males (36 percent).

Overall, it is also important to note that young African Americans are most at risk: 56 percent of all HIV cases were reported in this age group in the 32 areas.

In 1999, there were 1,813 teens aged 13 to 24 reported with AIDS, making the total AIDS cases in this age group 29,629. Among young men 13 to 24, half of all AIDS cases reported in 1999 were among men who have sex with men; 8 percent, injection drug users; and 8 percent, young men infected heterosexually. That same year, among women in the same age group, 47 percent of all reported AIDS cases were acquired through heterosexual activity, and 11 percent through injection drug use.

According to the Centers for Disease Control, data suggest that many adolescents who indulge in oral sex do not consider it sexual intercourse. They believe they can remain abstinent by not having anal or vaginal sex and seem unaware that STDs, including HIV, can be transmitted via oral sex.

Of the total number of AIDS cases reported to the CDC through December 2000, patients' ages at time of diagnosis were as follows: below age five, 6,872; five to 12, 2,036; 13 to 19, 4,061; 20 to 24, 27,232; 25 to 29, 101,494; 30 to 34, 172,310; 35 to 39, 173,512; 40 to 44, 128,177; 45 to 49, 74,724; 50 to 54, 39,625; 55 to 59, 21,685; 60 to 64, 12,023; 65 and older, 10,711.

Confidentiality Issue

A patient's right to confidential medical records is an issue that encompasses disclosure of information about that individual's medical problems, including sexually transmitted disease, from HIV to genital herpes. An American has the right to prohibit the release of his or her records and any information regarding medical history. At the same time, with the proliferation of HIV, this became a hotly debated matter in that state constitutions do not always expressly specify this right to privacy of one's medical records. Typically, there are provisions requiring disclosure of information to health departments, to the subjects of the tests, and to the doctors involved in ordering the tests. Some states also have mandatory testing and disclosure rules.

Counseling

The work of a counselor or therapist in providing guidance is generally viewed as a much-needed part of the treatment program for a person with a sexually transmitted disease.

Decline in Deaths

Decline in deaths is a term used in epidemiologic studies to refer to the decreasing number of deaths attributed to a particular disease. An example in the framework of sexually transmitted diseases is HIV/AIDS, which has seen a decline in death rates that is usually attributed to HAART.

Epidemiology

Greatly increased life expectancy in people with HIV is the most remarkable aspect of the changing disease management in the new millennium. From 1996 to 1997, the age-adjusted mortality rate of HIV infection in the United States declined by 47 percent, as reported in *Patient Care* (October 1999). The number of deaths in people with AIDS continued to decline each year through 2001.

In the past, patients with AIDS who had advanced disease with opportunistic infections, very low CD4+ lymphocyte counts, or both, would live two to three years. New medications, however, now enable these individuals to live for many years.

At the end of 2002, there were 42 million people worldwide estimated to be living with HIV/AIDS; 38.6 million were adults. Twelve million young people (ages 15 to 24) were living with HIV/AIDS worldwide at the end of 2001. About 3.2 million children younger than 15 years were living with HIV/AIDS. As of 2002, an estimated 28 million people had died from AIDS since the epidemic began. During 2001, AIDS caused the deaths of an estimated 3.1 million people. Women were increasingly affected by HIV: worldwide, about 50 percent were women at the end of 2002. Most people with HIV/AIDS (about 95 percent of the global total) were living in countries in the developing world.

During 2002, of about 14,000 new infections that were occurring daily, 95 percent were in the developing world. In 2002, 6,000 new infections were in young adults ages 15 to 25 worldwide. About 2,000 children were also infected daily in 2002. Total U.S. spending on HIV/AIDS for fiscal year 2002 was $14.7 billion; U.S. spending on HIV/AIDS in low- and middle-income countries for 2002 was $1 billion.

What has increased the longevity of those with HIV/AIDS is HAART, highly active antiretroviral therapy; researchers, however, continue to search for even better medications that are less toxic with long-term use. With the use of protease inhibitors (PIs), the frequency of major opportunistic infections fell by about 80 percent over five years.

An ironic twist to the changing HIV picture is the possibility of reduced vigilance about preventing transmission. If therapies result in undetectable viral loads, an individual may consider it safe not to use condoms. However, it is important to note that the risk of transmission still exists, and having another sexually transmissible disease can make HIV progress more rapidly.

A CDC study in 2000 revealed a trend toward relaxed sexual practices among young gay men in San Francisco. Women with HIV in another study reported risky behavior, but a survey of 7,000 New York City sexually active gay and bisexual men in 1998 revealed several promising trends: rates of HIV infection were relatively low; sexual practices were relatively safe; and frequent HIV testing occurred. Of those surveyed, 73 percent said they were HIV-negative, and half of them either used condoms or refrained from anal sex.

AIDS prevalence has increased steadily over time. By the end of 2001, about 362,827 people in the United States were living with AIDS. The CDC also estimates that about 200,000 to 250,000 Americans have HIV but do not know it. This underscores the belief of experts that prevention strategies must target the goal of making sure that more people learn early that they are HIV-positive,

because that is the time when there is greatest potential for transmitting the disease to others—and that is also the time when the need for treatment is critical. Infected people also must learn to practice safe behavior and undergo comprehensive care that will make them more likely not to transmit the disease to sex partners and will help infected individuals avert progression to AIDS.

Preventing new HIV infections has proved difficult because of the growing complacency inspired by HAART treatment. Some communities have reported increasingly lax attitudes toward sexual behavior, which are based on the view that AIDS is now more of a chronic illness than a death sentence. This makes people forget that the longer survival rates of those who are HIV-infected also imply an ever-larger population of people who are living with HIV and AIDS. At the same time, those at risk for HIV have become a diverse group.

An estimated 900,000 people in the United States are infected with HIV. Minority populations have experienced the largest growth of this epidemic, which is the leading killer of African-American men. The CDC reports that AIDS is six times more prevalent among African Americans and three times higher among Hispanics than among whites.

Most affected by the AIDS epidemic are the following populations:

- African Americans: in this population, the rate of AIDS deaths and AIDS incidence is 10 times higher than among whites. According to the CDC, overall half of all HIV infections, AIDS cases, and AIDS deaths occur in those who are African American. Of all women with AIDS, almost two-thirds are African American. Of reported pediatric AIDS cases, about two-thirds are among African Americans.

- Latinos: about 20 percent of new HIV infections and AIDS cases occur in Latinos. In Chicago, for example, Latinos of Puerto Rican ancestry have the highest cumulative AIDS case rate of any racial or ethnic group: 511 cases per 100,000. The rate for whites is 349 per 100,000; African Americans post 423 per 100,000.

- Gay men: gay men remain at high risk of HIV infection and make up 60 percent of all HIV infections among men in the United States. Rates of infection are highest in gays who are Latino and African American. Although some communities have made tremendous strides in reducing high-risk behavior, a recent trend in some areas is resumption of risky behavior, based on people's belief that HIV is "less serious" simply because it is now more treatable. The bottom line is that all people who are sexually active should still remember the indisputable fact: AIDS is a terminal disease. That has not changed.

• Injection drug users: about 36 percent of all AIDS cases ever reported in the United States have been among injection drug users, their partners, and their children, according to the Centers for Disease Control. The one promising note on this front is that prevention efforts seem to be resulting in a slowing of HIV infection rates in this population.

• Young people: one of the most jarring statistics is discovered in reviewing this population. At least half of new HIV infections occur in those who are 25 or younger. Most of these are young gay men who are infected homosexually and young women who are infected heterosexually. While the country sees the overall number of new AIDS diagnoses declining, thanks to HAART, no comparable decline in newly diagnosed HIV infections is being seen in youth, according to CDC studies.

• Children: the number of reports of new pediatric HIV (not AIDS) cases increased sharply from 224 children younger than 13 in 2000 to 543 in 2001. The cumulative total almost doubled, from 2,134 to 3,923.

Geographic Areas of Affinity

According to information from the CDC, the 10 leading states or territories reporting the highest number of cumulative AIDS cases among residents as of December 2001 were as follows: New York, 149,341; California, 123,819; Florida, 85,324; Texas, 56,730; New Jersey, 43,824; Pennsylvania, 26,369; Illinois, 26,319; Puerto Rico, 26,119; Georgia, 24,559; Maryland, 23,537. The

10 leading metropolitan statistical areas reporting the most cumulative AIDS cases (as of December 2001) were New York City, 126,237; Los Angeles, 43,488; San Francisco, 28,438; Miami, 25,357; Washington, D.C., 24,844; Chicago, 22,703; Philadelphia, 20,369; Houston, 19,898; Newark, 17,796; Atlanta, 17,157.

Interventions for High-Risk World Populations

According to the Joint United Nations Programme on HIV/AIDS, the trends worldwide, as of December 2002, were that 42 million were estimated to be living with HIV/AIDS, and the majority of those with HIV—about 95 percent of the global total—lived in countries in the developing world. People newly infected with HIV in 2002 totaled 5 million. AIDS deaths in 2002 were 3.1 million.

The Centers for Disease Control and Prevention's programs work to promote the prevention of the spread of HIV/AIDS worldwide. Research, technical assistance, and training are devoted to gaining a greater understanding of the dynamics of HIV transmission and to improving prevention technologies and plans to control the spread of sexually transmitted diseases for high-risk world populations, as well as in the United States. For many of the world's high-risk populations, CDC researchers have collaborated with host countries to improve or begin HIV prevention interventions among injection drug users, female sex workers, and other populations at risk. Many interventions have had good results, particularly those designed to increase condom use and treat STDs of female sex workers.

HIV/AIDS Research

The *Journal of the American Medical Association* Women's Health Sexually Transmitted Disease Information Center reports that there are a few people—fewer than 50—who have been infected with HIV for 10 or more years yet have not seen the disease progress to the point that they have shown symptoms. This has been an area of extreme interest to scientists, who want to determine whether it can be attributed to specific traits of these people's immune systems, to infections by a less aggressive strain, or to whether their genetic material is protective. This lack of progression to

AIDS is an anomaly that, with extreme study, may spawn ideas for HIV vaccines.

Investigators are doing a huge volume of research on HIV infection, which encompasses work on developing vaccines and creating new therapies for HIV and related conditions. More than a dozen HIV vaccines are being tested in people. Also, there are numerous drugs for HIV- and AIDS-associated opportunistic infections that are being developed, as well as others undergoing testing.

Significant breakthroughs in uncovering the biological characteristics of HIV are pointing researchers toward new therapies. One of these trail-blazing discoveries is the way in which HIV enters the CD4 cell. The chemokine receptor is the principal receptor for HIV, and all transmission seems to be mediated through CCR5, so researchers are studying the potential of the first chemokine receptor CCR5 and envelope interactions with it. Those people who do not express CCR5 are believed to be completely resistant to HIV; that finding has spawned the creation of companies that offer CCR5 genotyping. (Many people want to be genotyped for CCR5.) It is thought that drugs against CCR5—drugs that would essentially block HIV interaction with CCR5—would block infection and that inhibiting the CCR5 function would not be detrimental to health, because the five people in the world known to have this mutation are alive. Today, pharmaceutical companies are trying to develop a chemokine receptor antagonist to block HIV entry.

Researchers want to unravel the 15 proteins and ribonucleic acid (RNA) that make up HIV. Fathoming the interfaces of those proteins with cellular components may put researchers in a good position to interfere with the virus and block replication. Three regulatory proteins of the 15 are tat, rev, and nef.

What makes vaccine development difficult is that the virus can be transmitted from cell to cell in the human body and targets exactly those cells in the immune system appointed to eliminate the virus. HIV also can establish latent infections in T cells and macrophages and can infect parts of the body that are immunologically privileged (the central nervous system). Of chief importance, researchers know that the virus can replicate as a swarm of numerous antigenic variants. Some researchers think that the most promising approach to a vaccine is the live attenuated vaccine, which can protect against HIV or simian immunodeficiency virus (SIV) infection in a way that no other vaccine can—but has the downside of being unsafe. These nef-deleted viruses are weakened but can still cause disease. There is a great deal of research on using interferon and interleukin-2, which are both natural substances that enhance the body's ability to fight viruses. Information on studies on new HIV therapies is available from AIDS Clinical Trials Information Service, (800) TRIALS-A, or (800) 243-7012 (TDD/Deaf Access).

See also NONPROGRESSORS.

HIV-associated dementia A problem associated with late-stage HIV infection, dementia is the condition in which a person's intellectual abilities have deteriorated. Thus, the individual loses some memory and ability to focus. Symptoms of HIV-associated dementia are slow thought processing, unfocused motor movement, lethargy, and difficulty in concentrating and remembering.

HIV explosion in Russia A tidal wave of HIV hit Russia in 2000–01. Officially, Russia reported the diagnosis of 129,261 new cases of HIV over a period of a year and a half, which ratcheted up its infection rate to the highest in Europe. However, many experts predict that the real number could be as much as 10 times greater. Dr. Alex Gromyko, HIV adviser to the World Health Organization, calls the development a major catastrophe, citing the fact that Russia went from the bottom of the list to number one in only two years. More than 63,000 new cases were documented during the first five months of 2001: three times the rate two years before and double the total for the years 1987 to 1999. Reasons cited as contributing to the soaring rate of transmission are that Russians do not routinely use protection against STDs, rampant needle sharing occurs among drug users, and a staple of birth control is abortion, which makes the use of condoms less likely.

However, despite the dismal health situation for the sexually active in Russia, the Health Ministry of Russia chose to reject an offer of a $150 million World Bank loan to treat TB and AIDS because the powers that be viewed the money as a pittance. Unfortunately, the sad state of affairs means that only a handful of people in Russia are receiving adequate drug therapy.

HIV patients' risks Having HIV puts people at risk for developing other health problems. Thus, it is wise for the HIV-infected person to take special precautions in regard to travel, hobbies, environment, pets, and food and water.

Travel Precautions

An HIV-infected person should be highly aware of the dangers inherent in traveling to developing countries, where the risk of exposure to opportunistic infections may be greater. Before traveling, an HIV-positive individual should check into the risks that prevail in the country and take appropriate proactive measures. As a general rule, skin contact with soil and sand can be prevented by shoes and clothing and using towels on beaches.

Patients are advised to consult their doctors about the advisability of vaccinations. In general, an HIV-positive person must avoid all live virus vaccines; however, nonimmune persons who are not severely immunosuppressed can have measles vaccination, and nonimmunosuppressed children with asymptomatic HIV can have varicella vaccination. Cholera vaccine is not recommended, but the yellow fever vaccine can be offered to asymptomatic patients who must travel to places where they could be exposed to this disease.

When traveling, it is important to keep in mind that the risk of infections carried in water and food is substantially increased. To steer clear of contaminated options, one can opt for foods that are steaming hot; fruits that the person peels before eating; bottled carbonated beverages, beer, wine, hot coffee, or tea; and water that has been boiled for one minute. It is important to avoid swimming in contaminated water and swallowing any water when swimming.

To ward off traveler's diarrhea, HIV patients should take along an antimicrobial agent for use if diarrhea develops. One should go to a physician in the country where traveling if one or more of the following occurs; diarrhea that is so severe that an antibiotic does not help, bloody stools, fever and shaking chills, or dehydration. If there is high fever or blood in the stool, an HIV patient should not take antiperistaltic agents—diphenoxylate (Lomotil) and loperamide (Imodium). It is also important to note that antimicrobial prophylaxis for traveler's diarrhea is not routinely advised for HIV-infected persons who plan to travel to developing countries because of the risk of adverse effects, but when the risk is high and the travel period is short, it may be required.

Workplace/Environmental Risks

- On the subject of workplace and environmental risks, those who work in health care environments, homeless shelters, and correctional institutions are often at greater risk for TB exposure. Extent of exposure depends on type of duties, which should be the determinant of whether an HIV-positive person should continue working in such an environment.

- A worker in a child-care setting can do thorough hand washings to prevent infections borne by saliva, urine, and feces, for there are risks inherent in such environments: CMV infection, cryptosporidiosis, hepatitis A, and giardiasis.

- Working with animals is not considered risky enough to justify making it off limits for those with HIV, but vets and farmworkers do run risks of several types of infection: cryptosporidiosis, toxoplasmosis, salmonellosis, and others.

Garden Risks

- Gardeners should also practice frequent hand washing to lessen the likelihood of cryptosporidiosis and toxoplasmosis infection.

- If someone is living in a place where histoplasmosis is endemic, that person should avoid cleaning chicken coops, disturbing soil under bird roosts, and exploring caves. He or she should also avoid extensive exposure to disturbed soil in excavation sites in spots where coccidioidomycosis is endemic.

Pet Precautions

For a person with HIV, the pros and cons of cat ownership should be weighed carefully because cats are potential sources of toxoplasmosis, bartonellosis, and enteric infections. If a person with HIV has a pet that has diarrhea, contact should be avoided until the problem is resolved. By the same token, it is wise to avoid contact with stray animals and cats younger than a year old. Overall, a general pattern of hand washing should be observed when an HIV-infected person lives with pets. Caregivers for children with HIV should be advised to make sure children wash their hands before eating. As a rule, an HIV-infected patient should avoid exotic pets and reptiles and use gloves when cleaning aquariums.

Food and Water Cautions

Those with HIV would do well to avoid raw eggs and raw-egg preparations such as some hollandaise sauces; raw or insufficiently cooked meat, poultry, and seafood; and dairy products that are not pasteurized. Produce should be washed thoroughly before eating. All individuals with HIV (and without) should be sure to cook meat and poultry until no pink is visible in the middle.

It is important to reheat food until it steams to reduce the risk of the disease listeriosis, which soft cheeses and ready-to-eat foods (hot dogs, cold cuts) can sometimes cause. One should be wary of cross-contamination of foods via hands, cutting boards, kitchen countertops, and cooking utensils and knives.

An HIV-positive individual should not drink water from lakes or rivers or inadvertently ingest it during swimming. During outbreaks of cryptosporidiosis, water should be boiled for at least one minute, or bottled water should be used.

HIV Postexposure Prophylaxis Registry A key surveillance program to collect safety information on using antiretroviral drugs in non-HIV-infected health care workers who receive postexposure prophylaxis (PEP) for occupational HIV exposure is important because much remains to be learned about the management of exposure to HIV. Little information is available on use and toxicity of anti-retroviral drugs (other than zidovudine) by persons who do not have HIV. When a health care provider does prescribe HIV postexposure prophylaxis to a health care worker for occupational exposure to HIV, he or she should contact the registry, which will want information at the onset of treatment, after completion, and six months after the exposure. The health care workers who participate are volunteers whose names are kept confidential. For information on the HIV PEP Registry Protocol, see the Centers for Disease Control and Prevention website: http://www.ama-assn.org/special/hiv/preventn/pepflybw.htm, or call (888) PEP-4HIV.

HIV prevention Three goals of HIV prevention from the Centers for Disease Control and Prevention are as follows:

1. Increase the number of HIV-infected people who know their serostatus.
2. Ensure that the additional people identified each year have access to prevention services and are linked to appropriate care and treatment.
3. Reduce the cumulative number of new HIV infections through support of science-based prevention interventions.

So far in the history of HIV/AIDS, prevention efforts in the United States have been very effective, greatly reducing the incidence of HIV infection. The CDC points to the fact that prevention initiatives were factors in slowing the rate of new HIV infections in the United States from more than 150,000 in the late 1980s to about 40,000 per year in 2001–2002. It appears clear that these efforts contributed to

- A decline by 50 percent in HIV prevalence among white gay men (1988–93)
- A 73 percent drop in vertical transmission of AIDS (1992–98)
- A drop in HIV prevalence in the New York City injection-drug-user population: 34 percent in 1990 to slightly more than 4 percent in 1998
- Five states were funded in 2002 to conduct pilot studies of Serologic Testing Algorithm for Recent HIV Seroconversion (STARHS) of serologic specimens from new HIV diagnoses. This is because

close monitoring of HIV incidence is key to evaluating progress on the CDC's goal of reducing new infections in the United States from 40,000 to 20,000 by 2005.

As for the future of prevention, CDC goals are achievable with adequate resources, such as partnerships of local, state, and community groups. The idea advanced is that the U.S. epidemic can be stopped by effective prevention programs and a significant increase in outreach efforts for the HIV-infected who have not become aware of their disease status. Researchers actually contend that U.S. infections could be nearly eliminated in four years with sustained preventive efforts aimed at at-risk populations and much-increased efforts to reach (with testing and prevention services) those who are unaware of their infection. Once that goal is reached, the nation will be responding only to outbreaks rather than to ongoing, sustained transmission. The CDC emphasizes that a substantial investment would be necessary to attain that goal, but it is also true that significant reductions in HIV infection can be achieved.

The downside of the picture that the CDC presents is that a state of level funding will probably not produce a stable HIV U.S. epidemic. A growing population of people living longer with HIV has more opportunity to infect others, and that could eventually lead to an increase in HIV infections and AIDS. Health experts worry that if current complacency continues, the upshot could very well be the first upswing in HIV infection rates in many years. Many health care experts have expressed concerns about the degree of complacency that seemed to be in evidence at the dawn of the new millennium—a result of the many success stories of HIV treatment with antiretroviral drug therapies. The Centers for Disease Control and Prevention reports that even though the annual rate of HIV infections has been relatively stable since the mid-1990s, there is still reason for concern considering late 1990s era outbreaks of gonorrhea and other sexually transmitted diseases, which could be indicative of potential future increases in HIV.

A December 1999 CDC update looks at HIV prevention programs that have proved effective, reviews the state of the epidemic in the United States, and outlines the goals, steps, and investment that will be required to reduce the annual U.S. rate of HIV infections. Fortunately, intervention programs have had successful outcomes. The Centers for Disease Control and Prevention research programs in communities across the country have met their goals of reducing high-risk sexual behavior and drug use among those at great risk.

The Compendium of HIV Prevention Interventions with Evidence of Effectiveness reviewed 24 scientifically evaluated HIV prevention programs that target specific groups: men who have sex with men, heterosexual adults, young people, and drug users. This report underscores a great deal of scientific evidence on the HIV intervention measures that proved effective in all four populations.

The compendium highlights the following efforts:

- Heterosexual adults: a clinic in Los Angeles, California, sponsored group sessions led by a health educator. These lasted 30 minutes and were made available to heterosexuals who were waiting for clinic appointments. The aim was to make those participants more likely to use condoms by giving them knowledge about and skills for proper use. The findings gave reason for optimism about this form of intervention: at one-year follow-up, the adults who took part in the half-hour session were much less likely to return to the clinic in the year that followed with a new sexually transmitted disease than were those in the comparison group. The difference was 20 percent versus 11 percent.

- Men who have sex with men: Popular Opinion Leader was a three-city project in which gay-club bartenders singled out peer leaders, who were trained to promote reductions in risky behavior in those communities. The leaders also discussed HIV risk reduction when they were in gay bars with their peers. The results were staggering. The men in the intervention communities were 34 percent less likely to have unprotected sex compared to men in the control communities. In these cities, nearly 1,300 gay men were surveyed. Pinpointing the intervention factor as the single factor that accounted for this one-third reduction is, perhaps, a bit simplistic, but even so, it points up reason for optimism. Implementing opinion leader programs would clearly be a way to reduce the likelihood of gay men having unprotected sex.

- Young people: considerable strides in improved self-care behavior were seen as a result of an inner-city program that targeted African Americans aged 14 to 18. For two months, program directors spaced weekly sessions of one to two hours that sought to help these young people gain a better understanding of HIV-related behavioral issues. To make it seem relevant, the teachers used video games and rap music for information delivery. At the outset, the youngsters received basic education on AIDS, then the curriculum progressed to discussions and skill building. The teens learned how to use condoms properly if they were already sexually active, and if they were not having sex yet, they were briefed on ways to resist pressure to have sex. The program also tried to help these young people form supportive social networks, whereby they could share information and boost the idea of risk reduction. The program netted very positive results. Participants reported much higher rates of condom use during intercourse than did peers who did not participate in the program, 82.9 percent versus 62.1 percent, after two months. Those who were abstinent reported a greater delay in becoming sexually active than did youth who had been abstinent but were not participants (a year later, 11.5 versus 31.1 percent initiated sexual activity).

- Drug users: group sessions focusing on reducing the incidence of drug use and high-risk behavior, were conducted. Participants were 567 adults who had been drug users; the setting was an inpatient drug detoxification and rehabilitation center. Two approaches were sampled for effectiveness. One format was a basic education session that used lectures to disseminate information on HIV prevention. The other participants received training via an "enhanced intervention" program that focused on individual susceptibility, situation analysis, and skills-building practice. Those who participated in the second form of education—the enhanced intervention—showed much greater benefits. Obviously reacting more favorably and openly to the practical "real-life" scenarios encountered in training situations, they showed gains, reporting significantly lower rates of cocaine use (33 percent versus 47 percent) and a 59 percent reduction in drug-injection frequency 10 to 18 weeks after the intervention. Those who were "lectured" were less moved to change their lifestyles by the information they received in the all-too-traditional mode.

Other programs are detailed in the CDC compendium, which includes information on how to access CDC materials and expertise in order to conduct any of these programs. Elements are outlined to enable others who want to do their own programs to modify them according to their preferences. The CDC's HIV/AIDS prevention activities are vital parts of the prevention strategies, which include monitoring the spread of the disease in order to target activities of care and prevention, researching effectiveness of the methods and programs that are used, funding local programs aimed at prevention in high-risk areas, and fostering cooperation between care and treatment programs.

The CDC collaborates with governmental and nongovernmental partners in casting a wide net of informational strategies, all of which go a long way toward preventing infection and helping those already infected. In this respect, the CDC provides HIV antibody counseling, testing, and referral services; financial and technical support for disease surveillance; outreach programs; risk-reduction counseling; case management; prevention/treatment of other STDs that heighten the risk of HIV transmission; public information and education; school-based education on AIDS; international research studies; technology transfer systems; and program-relevant epidemiologic, sociobehavioral, and evaluation research.

As far as distribution of CDC funds, nearly 80 percent of fiscal year 1998's funds were dispersed via cooperative agreements, grants, and contracts, most of which went to state and local agencies. The largest portions of HIV prevention resources go to state, local, and territorial health departments. Most of these funds support about 200 local and regional groups that do HIV prevention planning for communities.

The CDC's internal organization for prevention efforts has two divisions in the National Center for HIV, STD, and TB Prevention—the Division of HIV/AIDS Prevention–Intervention Research and Support (DHAP-IRS) and the Division of HIV/AIDS Prevention–Surveillance and Epidemiology (DHAP-SE).

DHAP-IRS is in charge of conducting behavioral intervention and operations research. It evaluates these programs and provides financial and technical assistance for HIV programs that are run by health departments (state, local, territorial); national minority groups; community-based organizations; business, labor, and religious groups; and training agencies. DHAP-IRS has five branches:

- The Behavioral Intervention Research Branch uses theory, practice, and empirical findings to plan and carry out research on state-of-the-art interventions that are aimed at HIV-infection prevention. Researchers look at determinants of risk behavior and collect and analyze data.

- The Community Assistance, Planning, and National Partnerships Branch is in charge of providing technical assistance, policy guidance, and human resources to 65 health departments (state and selected locals); 22 national and regional minority organizations; 10 national business, labor, and faith partnerships; and 94 community-based groups to conduct HIV prevention services among high-risk populations.

- The Program Evaluation Research Branch does studies to check the effectiveness of prevention strategies and programs. This branch also conducts economic evaluations of HIV prevention, including assessments of alternative prevention strategies to encourage best use of resources and develops outcome measures.

- The Technical Information and Communications Branch disseminates information on HIV/AIDS via electronic media and printed materials.

- The Training and Technical Support Systems Branch supports those who provide HIV/AIDS prevention services with ongoing upgrades in technical support, program development, and training.

DHAP-SE is responsible for surveillance and epidemiologic and behavioral research in evaluating trends and risk behavior (HIV/AIDS-related). The data gleaned help to evaluate programs and target prevention resources. DHAP-SE also helps developing countries with HIV/AIDS activities: surveillance, research, prevention, evaluation, and technology transfer. The division has five branches:

- The Epidemiology Branch designs and conducts studies (epidemiologic and behavioral) in the United States to determine risk factors, cofactors, and modes of HIV transmission.

- The International Activities Branch plans and implements epidemiologic and intervention studies of HIV infection and associated illnesses in other countries in collaboration with host nations, the United Nations AIDS Program, the U.S. Agency for International Development, and numerous nongovernmental organizations. They conduct studies of risk factors for AIDS and HIV transmission, studies of HIV genotypic variants, seroprevalence studies, and surveys and evaluations of AIDS prevention and control activities. Two research field sites are in Bangkok, Thailand, and Abidjan, Côte d'Ivoire.

- The Prevention Services Research Branch works on research designed to help improve HIV prevention strategies; studies identify and evaluate specific at-risk populations, determine risk for HIV infection in specific populations, review HIV counseling and testing, and investigate HIV genotypic variations and antiretroviral drug resistance. This branch also collects data on HIV prevalence and incidence in the United States and is in charge of assisting other centers within the CDC in evaluating new HIV-related tests and maintaining a repository of stored sera and cells for studies of HIV infection.

- The Statistics and Data Management Branch provides data management and statistical support for HIV/AIDS surveillance, HIV serosurveys, epidemiologic studies, and other studies conducted within the two divisions; creates mathematical models to project the incidence of AIDS and HIV infection; and develops and rates projects to construct mathematical models of the spread of AIDS and HIV infection and other HIV and AIDS studies.

- The Surveillance Branch coordinates with state and local health departments in surveillance of HIV/AIDS. This provides population-based data for research, evaluation, and prevention. This branch also maintains the national confidential registry of HIV/AIDS cases, monitors HIV-related mortality and morbidity rates, and conducts (population-based) surveillance of risk behavior.

Other offices of the CDC also conduct certain prevention activities:

- The National Center for Infectious Diseases (NCID) provides laboratory research on HIV and lab support for the surveillance, epidemiologic, and clinical activities of NCHSTP. It also conducts studies of HIV-infected and uninfected people who have hemophilia and assists in programs for them and their families. The Hospital Infections Program, also located in NCID, helps the U.S. Public Health Service and other organizations worldwide with the prevention and control of nosocomially acquired HIV infection.

- The National Center for Chronic Disease Prevention and Health Promotion (NCCDPHP) includes the Division of Adolescent and School Health. NCCDPHP provides support to agencies and groups that address adolescent health. NCCDPHP's Division of Reproductive Health conducts research on prevention of HIV in women at risk for both HIV and unintended pregnancy.

- The National Center for Environmental Health's Clinical Biochemistry Branch runs a quality assurance program for labs testing dried blood spots for HIV antibodies and offers consulting services for emerging concerns in lab quality assurance.

- The National Center for Health Statistics collects HIV- and AIDS-related data, including HIV-related deaths, from the National Vital Statistics System; use of health services from the National Health Care Surveys; and data on HIV-related knowledge and HIV testing behavior from the National Health Interview Survey and the periodic National Survey of Family Growth.

- The National Institute for Occupational Safety and Health's HIV Activity develops, implements, and evaluates strategies for the prevention of occupational transmission of HIV. The emphasis is on protective equipment, engineering controls, and evaluation of factors that influence prevention strategies.

- The Public Health Practice Program Office contributes to prevention of HIV/AIDS in communities by training, improving quality of lab testing, developing computing and telecommunications tools, and doing research into effective public health practice.

To receive the CDC HIV/STD/TB Prevention News Update by e-mail each day, one can subscribe to the PreventioNews Mailing List. This features news updates, conference announcements, funding opportunities, articles, and other announcements. A person can be added to the list by sending a blank message to the address preventionews-subscribe@cdcpin.org. For more information on CDC programs and studies, call the CDC National AIDS Hotline: (800) 342-AIDS; Spanish: (800) 344-SIDA; deaf: (800) 243-7889.

Partner Protection

A sexual partner who has frequent HIV tests and has not engaged in risky behavior would still be wise to use protection. The CDC recommends abstinence or protection with male latex condoms during sexual activity whether oral, anal, or vaginal. It is important to use male condoms made of latex, and those who are sexually active should use water-based lubricants with these latex condoms.

In certain clinical trials, there has been evidence that spermicides killed HIV organisms, but these products should not be considered preventive or protective. Their ability to prevent HIV has not been shown.

In one study presented at the 12th World AIDS Conference, one factor associated with increased risk was use of amyl nitrate (poppers). Sexual activity with many partners, unprotected receptive anal sex with an HIV-infected man or partners of unknown HIV serostatus, drug use, oral sex to ejaculation with an HIV-positive partner, and being uncircumcised were also associated with a greater risk of infection.

A widely disseminated myth is that oral sex is safe sex, lacking the risks of anal and vaginal sex. The truth is, oral sex does have an element of risk when one partner is infected with HIV, when one partner's HIV status is unknown, when a partner injects drugs, or when one partner is not monogamous. The Centers for Disease Control attests that many studies indicate that oral sex can result in the transmission of HIV and other STDs. The only ways that a person can be completely protected from HIV is to abstain from oral, anal, and vaginal sex or have sex exclusively with an uninfected partner who the first partner can be absolutely 100 percent sure is monogamous.

At the same time, the risk of contracting HIV from an infected partner by having oral sex is much smaller than the risk posed by anal or vaginal sex. But remember, too, that it is hard to assess the exact risk since most people who are sexually active tend to indulge in oral sex as well as vaginal and/or anal sex. So, which form of sexual activity is responsible when HIV is transmitted?

Factors that make oral sex with an HIV-infected partner very risky behavior are oral ulcers, bleeding gums, and genital sores. Furthermore, the presence of another sexually transmitted disease increases the likelihood of transmission of HIV from an infected partner.

In describing this kind of risk, the term *theoretical risk* is used by scientists, who mean, in essence, that the possibility exists that the infection could be passed from one person to another via this kind of behavior. This does not mean that infection is likely; it translates as "possible." This is in contrast to *documented risk,* which is applied to transmission that has occurred, been investigated, and documented in the scientific literature.

Unfortunately, many people do not believe that they can get HIV if they refrain from anal and vaginal sex and have only oral sex. In a national survey of teens that was done for the Kaiser Family Foundation, 26 percent of sexually active young people aged 15 to 17 believed that a person "cannot become infected with HIV by having unprotected oral sex." An additional 15 percent admitted they did not know whether infection is possible in that way.

Oral sex is giving or receiving oral stimulation—sucking or licking—to the penis, vagina, and/or anus. The technical term for oral contact with the penis is *fellatio.* Oral–vaginal sex is termed *cunnilingus.* Oral–anal contact, sometimes called "rimming," is *analingus.*

The Centers for Disease Control reports the following comparisons of risk in various types of sexual contact:

- Documented: HIV has been transmitted to receptive partners during the act of fellatio, even in cases in which insertive partners did not ejaculate. The risk is much smaller in fellatio than it is in anal or vaginal sex. Theoretical: The receptive partner—the one doing the sucking—can theoretically be infected with HIV because the HIV-infected preejaculate fluid or semen can enter that person's mouth. The insertive partner—the one being sucked—has a theoretical risk of infection from infected blood transferred from the partner's bleeding gums or open sore, which could enter the skin by means of a penis sore, cut, or scratch.

- Documented: HIV transmission during cunnilingus is unusual, but there have been a few cases in which oral–vaginal sex was the mode of transmission. The risk is quite low compared to that of vaginal and anal sex. Theoretical: There is transmission risk for a person licking or sucking a woman's vagina because blood and fluids infected with HIV can enter the mouth. There is even a risk for the person who is being licked or sucked because the individual performing cunnilingus may have oral sores or bleeding gums, and the infected blood can come in contact with a vaginal or vulvar cut or sore.

- Documented: One case of HIV transmission associated with oral–anal sexual contact has been published. Theoretical: The person licking or sucking the anus is at risk if he or she is exposed to infected blood (bloody fecal matter) or anal cuts or sores. The person whose anus is being licked or sucked is at risk if infected blood in saliva comes in contact with anal or rectal lining.

Oral sex has also been a factor in the transmission of other STDs: herpes, syphilis, genital warts, gonorrhea, intestinal parasites (amebiasis), and hepatitis A. To decrease the chances of contracting HIV or another STD during acts of oral sex, sex partners should use latex condoms every time. In performing cunnilingus or analingus, one can use plastic food wrap, a cut-open condom, or a dental dam. The bottom line is this: no one should view oral sex as safe sex, because it is not.

HIV testing   The consensus among doctors who care for those with HIV and AIDS is that all doctors should investigate the possibility of HIV/AIDS more frequently, especially when one considers that the symptoms of acute retroviral syndrome mimic those of other common viral diseases. A physician's clues as to whether a patient merits further evaluation are often based on risk behavior and a complete physical examination and medical history.

Often the first signs of acute primary infection are neurologic (headache or meningoencephalitis) or dermatologic, and these signal that HIV testing should be initiated. Markers of intermediate HIV disease and AIDS that are often missed by doctors are oral hairy leukoplakia, oral candidiasis, neuropathies, hypogonadism, and eosinophilic pustular dermatitis.

Doctors who primarily care for HIV/AIDS patients are always concerned when they observe that certain markers of HIV disease were overlooked in early diagnostic opportunities. Unfortunately, the patients in such cases have probably been less than forthcoming about their medical history and their risk factors, and they may even be unwilling to reveal what they suspect—that they are HIV-infected. This puts the onus on physicians to find clues, because the course of HIV can be greatly improved, in most cases, by instituting early drug therapy.

Diagnostic Testing for HIV-1 and HIV-2

The standard screening test to detect the presence of antibodies to HIV is the enzyme immunoassay (EIA) or enzyme-linked immunosorbent assay (ELISA), which should be accompanied by another test for confirmatory purposes. The Western blot is often the choice.

Other tests available include the following:

- Radioimmunoprecipitation assay (RIPA): this blood test is used to confirm the diagnosis when antibody levels are very low or hard to detect or when the results of Western blot are not definitive. The RIPA is expensive, is time-consuming, and requires expertise.

- Rapid latex agglutination assay: this simple, cheap blood test is a useful option for areas that are medically disadvantaged and have high HIV prevalence.

- Dot-blot immunobinding assay: this cost-effective rapid-screening blood test may eventually supersede EIA and Western blot.

- HIV-1 (or p24) antigen capture assay: the Food and Drug Administration added this blood test as an interim measure to HIV antibody testing in 1996 to protect the blood supply further until other tests were available to detect early HIV infection before antibodies are fully developed. This is not useful for determining whether someone has HIV because p24 antigen activity is very unpredictable.

- Polymerase chain reaction (PCR): this expensive and labor-intensive blood test looks for HIV genetic information but has the great advantage of being able to detect the virus in a person who has only recently been infected. The FDA wants more tests for HIV genetic material developed.

Rapid HIV tests produce results in five to 30 minutes, whereas results from the EIA take one to two weeks. The FDA has licensed a rapid HIV test for use in the United States, and it is rated as reliable as is the EIA. Both the rapid test and the EIA detect the presence of antibodies to HIV in an individual's blood, but every screening test needs a confirmation by a second test in order for the diagnosis of HIV infection to be official.

One of the most difficult aspects of HIV testing is that these tests look for antibodies that the body produces to fight HIV—but the antibodies can develop in varying lengths of time. The average, according to the CDC, is 25 days, but development can occasionally take six months. Most people have detectable antibodies three months after infection or earlier.

The CDC recommends that an individual who has been exposed to HIV undergo testing six months after last exposure, whether that exposure was needle sharing or oral, vaginal, or anal sex. However, during the six-month period from exposure to testing, this individual absolutely must protect herself or himself against other exposure to HIV and protect others as well.

A person cannot tell whether he or she has been infected with HIV without an HIV blood test. This can be done at an AIDS testing facility, doctor's office, or clinic. The possibility of having anonymous testing should be considered. This means the individual has an identification number and is the only recipient of test results.

Home test kits are available. To find a testing site in your area, call the CDC National AIDS Hotline, (800)342-AIDS.

Mandatory Testing in Pregnant Women

An issue hotly argued is whether women should be required to have HIV testing when they are pregnant. In view of the fact that vertical transmission of HIV has been reduced by nearly 70 percent through the administration of zidovudine to HIV-infected pregnant women, the numbers of advocates for such testing are growing steadily. The Institute of Medicine takes the stand that this testing should be a routine part of prenatal care, and both the American Academy of Pediatrics and the American College of Obstetricians and Gynecologists have come out in favor of testing for pregnant women.

In October 1998, the Institute of Medicine of the National Academy of Sciences reported to Congress that they were recommending routine testing of all pregnant women in order to reduce vertical transmission. Under this recommenda-

tion, the mother would be told that the test was going to be done and would be informed that she could opt not to take it. This recommendation was adopted by the American Academy of Pediatrics and the American College of Obstetricians and Gynecologists in July 1999. The two organizations asserted that pretest HIV counseling could be provided but that lacks thereof should not be a barrier to HIV testing.

Universal HIV counseling and voluntary HIV testing are now the standard of care for all pregnant women, according to the Health Care Financing Administration. A woman who has already been tested for HIV nevertheless needs to have an HIV test on confirmation that she is pregnant.

People are also cautioned that up to six months from time of infection may pass before a test can detect HIV. So if a woman does not test HIV-positive when she is newly pregnant, she should be careful to avoid unprotected sex, sex with multiple partners, and sharing of drug needles. If she has had or continues to have unprotected sex or shares drug needles during pregnancy, it is very important that she have an HIV test during the last three months of her pregnancy.

A mother-to-be should seek to be in prime health in order to be ready to take care of her baby. A woman who discovers that she does have HIV can find out what kind of medications she will need by consulting her doctor on this matter. Also, the knowledge that she is HIV-positive enables a mother to enlist her doctor's help in reducing the risk imposed on the infant. Certain drugs can greatly reduce the chance of an HIV-positive mother giving her baby HIV infection.

A woman who is HIV-infected can reduce the probability of infecting her baby with HIV when her doctor performs a cesarean delivery, according to some studies. However, a cesarean section is not routinely recommended for HIV-positive women unless medically necessary.

Even those who doubt that they are HIV-positive may not be aware of the real risk for infection. Transmission via male–female sexual activity was the most rapidly increasing group of new HIV infections as of 2003, but many people remain unaware of their susceptibility and thus do not take proper precautions.

Home Testing

Those at risk for HIV appear to be taking advantage of home testing kits. In the first year these were on the market (1996–97), most of those who used them were people who had not been tested. Most were white men between the ages of 25 and 34. One home HIV test—the Home Access—is approved by the Food and Drug Administration and sold at many drugstores. (Other home tests have not been verified as accurate.)

Proper Timing for First Testing

Because HIV tests look for antibodies produced by the body to fight HIV, it is key for an individual who suspects infection to be tested—and then retested. Most people have antibodies that are detectable within three months of initial infection; the average period is about 25 days. However, there have been documented cases in which about six months elapsed before antibodies appeared. Thus, the CDC recommends testing six months after the last possible exposure to unprotected sex (vaginal, anal, or oral) or sharing of needles (in drug users). During the six months between exposure and the test, a person who suspects HIV should protect himself or herself and others from possible exposure to HIV.

Anyone seeking an HIV test can go to any one of the many facilities that provide HIV testing: private physicians' offices, clinics, local health departments and agencies, and sites designated for HIV testing. HIV/AIDS counseling is another vital element, so it is important to find a testing facility that has AIDS counselors who can answer questions and provide guidelines. They can also steer an infected individual toward appropriate local resources. For questions about testing, anyone in the United States can call the CDC National AIDS Hotline; (800)342-2437 (English). (800)344-7432 (Spanish); and (800)243-7889 (TTY).

HIV transmission According to the Centers for Disease Control and Prevention, HIV is transmitted by sexual intercourse with an HIV-infected person. Intercourse can be anal, vaginal, or oral. Other common means of transmission are sharing of needles or injection materials with an injection drug user who is HIV-infected and passing of infection to babies before or during birth or through subsequent breast-feeding by HIV-infected mothers. HIV enters the body through a vein, as in injection drug use; through the anus or rectum, vagina, penis, mouth, or mucous membranes (eyes or inside of nose); or through cuts and sores.

Transfusions of infected blood or blood clotting factors can also transmit HIV, and needlesticks have infected some health care workers through HIV-infected blood. Rumors of environmental transmission are untrue, and this appears to be an unlikely eventuality in that HIV does not survive well in the environment.

The Internet has spread frightening rumors, such as those alleging that people have been stuck by needles discarded by HIV-infected drug users who left them in theater seats, phone booth coin returns, gas-pump handles, and other miscellaneous spots. The CDC's response to inquiries on these rumors is that it is false that the CDC confirmed the presence of HIV in the needles. In fact, most of the reports have no foundation in fact. The CDC was told of a needlestick from what was believed to be an insulin needle, which occurred when it was left in a pay phone coin return. HIV, however, was not contracted.

What is fact is that needlestick injuries can transfer blood and blood-borne pathogens, such as hepatitis B, hepatitis C, and HIV. A person's risk of contracting one of these diseases from a discarded needle is low. A person who does receive a needlestick should go to an emergency room or call a physician. Other than in a health care setting, however, the CDC has no documented cases of HIV transmission by needlestick.

Biting

Although biting rarely transmits HIV, the CDC notes that reports in the medical literature suggest that HIV appeared to have been bite-transmitted, and there has been a state health department investigation of a blood-to-blood transmission of HIV by a human bite. In each of these cases, the biting involved tissue damage and blood. Also, for many bites that have been reported one partner had HIV but the infection was not spread.

Breast-feeding

A baby born to an HIV-infected mother can contract the disease before birth, during birth, and through breast-feeding subsequent to delivery.

Casual Contact

It is generally agreed among experts that HIV is not transmitted via casual contact: shaking hands, hugging, using a toilet, sharing a glass, sneezing, or coughing. A person cannot get HIV from a toilet seat, drinking fountain, doorknob, drinking glasses, food, pets, or dishes.

However, in a few cases, people have reported transmission as a result of casual household contact with the blood or body secretions of an HIV-infected household member. This type of transmission is very rare. Studies of families with HIV-infected members show that casual contact—sharing food utensils, towels, bedding, swimming pools, toilet seats—does not spread HIV.

Infected individuals have had HIV detected in their saliva, but there is no proof that a person can contract HIV via saliva contact. According to lab studies, saliva's natural compounds serve to curb the infectiousness of HIV. Scientists have also not illustrated spread of HIV through sweat, tears, urine, or feces.

What can increase the likelihood of acquiring HIV is the existence of another STD in an individual, which weakens the immune system and makes it less resistant to transmission during sex with an infected partner. Having unprotected sex (sexual activity without the use of male condoms) and sharing needles are two ways to spread HIV infection.

Contaminated Blood

HIV can be transmitted through transfusions of infected blood or blood clotting factors, but such transmission is very rare now that all blood in the United States is tested for HIV. The U.S. blood supply is rated among the world's safest.

Contaminated Needles

Some health care workers have become infected with HIV by needlesticks when these exposed them to HIV-infected blood. An HIV-infected health care worker has infected patients in one instance only—a dentist with HIV transmitted it to six patients.

Also, sharing syringes and other drug paraphernalia is a well-known means of HIV transmission, but people are less likely to know the startling fact that far beyond the circle of injectors themselves, the epidemic is spread because these people transmit HIV to partners who do not inject drugs. The sexual transmission of HIV is a risk for those who have sex with injection drug users. The children of mothers who contracted HIV through needle sharing or having sex with an injection drug user are also at risk of infection.

From the outset of the AIDS epidemic, more than a third of AIDS cases in the United States have been attributed to injection drug use. In 2001, AIDS cases attributed to injecting-drug-use transmission were a total of 201,326. Men who have sex with men and inject drugs totaled 51,293 AIDS cases. It is a trend that continues. Consider the fact that of new HIV infections reported in 2001, 25 percent were injection-drug-user-associated. In 1999, racial minorities were the groups most affected. Injection drug users were 33 percent of all AIDS cases among African Americans and 35 percent among Hispanics. This is contrasted with the figure for whites, which was 23 percent.

Also, since the outset of the epidemic, 58 percent of all AIDS cases in females have resulted from injection drug use or from sex with partners who inject drugs. In men, the figure is 31 percent of cases.

In many cases, health experts have seen that effective substance abuse treatment not only helps the injection drug user stop drug use but often eliminates the risk of HIV transmission from needle sharing and from behavior that spreads STDs. In the case of injection drug users who continue their habit, the emphasis must be on persuading them to use sterile needles and syringes only one time: the only way to limit HIV transmission. Users need advice on using sterile paraphernalia; never reusing needles, syringes, and other equipment; and never using syringes cleaned with bleach or other disinfectants.

To disseminate information and help prevent HIV, the CDC recommends several strategies: preventing initiation of drug injection, using community outreach programs to reach street drug users, improving access to substance abuse treatment programs, instituting HIV prevention programs in correctional facilities, providing health care for injection drug users who have HIV, and making HIV risk-reduction counseling and testing widely available for injection drug users and their sex partners.

Man to Man

From 1996 to 2001, AIDS incidence in men who have sex with men declined sharply and then leveled. Of 282,250 adult and adolescent men with AIDS in 2001, 57 percent were men who have sex with men and eight percent were MSM and injection drug users. Men who have sex with men still constitute the largest group reported with AIDS each year.

It is clear that major emphasis on prevention efforts for each generation of young gay and bisexual men is necessary, according to the CDC. Recent data on risk behavior and HIV prevalence underscore experts' beliefs that these men are still at high risk for HIV and other sexually transmitted diseases.

The CDC reports that in the 32 states with confidential HIV reporting, large numbers of men who have sex with men continue to be infected. In 1999, male-to-male sexual contact was believed to be the cause of 46 percent of reported HIV diagnoses in men aged 13 to 19 and 51 percent of cases in men 20 to 24.

Research is indicating that a more cavalier attitude concerning sexual activity has developed in recent years, thanks to better medications that have allowed individuals with HIV/AIDS to live longer. Some, gay and bisexual men admit that they are more inclined to take risks because they are less worried than they once were. This fact is supported by the increases in incidence of gonorrhea in gay men in several large U.S. cities in the period between 1993 and 1996.

The information that must be disseminated is that HIV infection remains a serious, usually fatal disease, as well as one that requires expensive and complex treatment. Plus, the new drug therapies are not effective for all who have HIV. Better prevention programs for African-American and Hispanic gay and bisexual men are definitely needed, because denial prevails at times in their cultures because of homophobia. For many of these men, there is still a huge stigma attached to gay sexual activity.

One type of gay sexual activity—oral sex—has been studied to determine the likelihood of transmission by this route. A study that is a component of an HIV infection study called the Options Project is funded by the Centers for Disease Control and Prevention at the University of California, San Francisco. The study was conducted to determine the extent of HIV transmitted by oral sex among homosexual men who were identified with HIV infection within 12 months of becoming infected. To date, this is the most definitive study. Findings showed that the probability of transmission from an infected person to an uninfected person depends on the type of exposure or contact; as a result, the probability varies. A person has a lesser risk of contracting HIV through unprotected oral sex than through unprotected anal or vaginal sex, but it is important to note that even a lower-risk activity, if done frequently, becomes a significant mode of infection.

Those researchers handling the Options Project reported that eight of 102 (7.8 percent) of recently infected men who have sex with men in San Francisco were probably infected via oral sex acts. Most of those who contracted HIV through oral sex reported that they had believed the risk of HIV transmission by this route was minimal or nonexistent.

This raises the obvious question: how did they get HIV? In half these cases of transmission, the one who transmitted HIV reported the presence of bleeding gums. Almost all (seven of eight) had oral contact with presemen or semen.

Admittedly, researchers know that it is hard to authenticate oral transmission of HIV as the single cause of transmission because it is unusual for sexually active people to indulge in oral sex exclusively. A trained evaluator posed the study questions, and all participants' risk behavior was assessed. Of the eight cases, four had had protected anal intercourse with people who did not know whether they had HIV or who were HIV-infected. (The condoms used had not broken.)

Researchers found a risk of transmission via oral sex that was higher than they expected to find and higher than that seen in other studies. It is believed that more men are opting to have oral sex, supposedly with lower risk, over anal sex.

The upshot of the study findings is that anytime someone has sexual contact with a person who has HIV, this is not going to be a risk-free activity. Protection requires that individuals who do want to engage in sexual activity take precautions: limit sexual activity to sex with only one uninfected partner, use a condom in every instance of sexual intercourse and oral sex, and consider mutual masturbation as a lower-risk option.

Occupational

Among health care workers, the likelihood of acquiring HIV from an inadvertent needlestick is very small, yet many health care workers continue to worry about their susceptibility to HIV transmission. In fact, their risk of on-the-job transmission is extremely low, according to the CDC, if they follow universal precautions. Everyday contact with an HIV-infected person does not expose health care workers to HIV. The main risk for this profession is an accidental needlestick or skin puncture by some other instrument contaminated with HIV. Researchers believe that even then, the risk of infection from a needle jab is less than 1 percent; this figure is based on studies of health care workers who have been punctured by HIV-contaminated needles or otherwise exposed to blood with HIV.

In studies of 22,000 patients of 63 health care providers who had HIV, researchers saw no evidence of provider-to-patient transmission in the health care setting except in one well-documented case. In 1999, the CDC reported on a Florida dentist whose HIV infection was transmitted to six patients during dental work on them. The means by which the disease was passed to the patients has never been established.

No known risk of transmitting HIV exists in restaurants; however, food-service workers (with or without HIV) should not work if they have infections or illnesses such as diarrhea or hepatitis A, according to CDC recommendations. Otherwise, they need not be restricted from work. Precautions from the CDC issued in 1985 advocate that per-sonal-service workers (hairdressers, barbers, massage therapists, cosmetologists) take routine precautions despite the lack of evidence of HIV transmission in these professions. Careful handling and sterilization of instruments are important.

Open-Mouth Kissing

Studies have yielded no evidence that people have given others HIV by kissing, but the risk from French, or "deep," kissing, in which large amounts of saliva are exchanged, is unknown. The CDC reports that open-mouth kissing is a very unlikely mode of transferring HIV infection. At the same time, it is important to note that prolonged kissing of this nature could allow HIV to pass from one partner to another in the event that lips become damaged and vulnerable because of cuts or sores. *Morbidity and Mortality Weekly Report (MMWR)* (July 17, 1997) documents a case in which a woman who contracted HIV from a sex partner was exposed to contaminated blood via open-mouth kissing. After informed consent from both partners, in 1992 these individuals were participants in a study involving couples with one HIV-infected partner and one noninfected. Study participants were counseled and tested periodically for HIV. While blood drawn from the woman cited on July 19, 1994, was HIV-negative, later serum specimens from her (taken on July 24, 1995, and September 11, 1995) produced positive results on both enzyme immunoassay and polymerase chain reaction tests. According to the article in *MMWR*, the woman denied any HIV risk exposures during the interval since her previous "uninfected" test result, including other sex partners, drug use, STDs, blood transfusion, artificial insemination, occupational exposure to HIV, acupuncture, tattoos, body piercing, or other injections. Furthermore, the couple used condoms for sex and did not have anal sex. The man reported mouth sores and gum disease. Researchers concluded that blood in the man's saliva infected mucus membranes in the woman's mouth. He admitted that his gums bled often after he brushed his teeth, and subsequently the couple engaged in deep open-mouth kissing. She also had used his razor and toothbrush, neither of which had visible blood. Also, the female partner had dental records that noted "poor condition of gums." When she began to show symptoms of infection that suggested onset of acute retroviral syndrome, the couple's lab results were compared, and these underscored a "high degree of relatedness" between the viruses infecting the man and the woman, supporting the conclusion that HIV was transmitted from the HIV-infected man to the uninfected female partner.

In an editorial note to this article, researchers stated that exposure to saliva uncontaminated with blood is a rare transmission mode for several reasons: saliva inhibits HIV-1 infectivity; HIV is rarely isolated from saliva; none of the 500,000 cases of AIDS reported to the CDC have been attributed to saliva exposure; levels of HIV are low in the saliva of HIV-infected persons; transmission via children has not been documented in studies of nonsexual household contacts of HIV-infected people; and bite-related cases of HIV transmission from saliva exposure (when saliva contained HIV-infected blood) have rarely been reported. Further, the summary points out that they could not rule out the possibility that the woman was exposed to the man's blood or semen, particularly during oral sex.

One important finding of this case was the recognition of the many routes of possible exposure to HIV that are inherent in being sexually intimate. A person who is embarking on an intimate relationship with a partner who has HIV should be aware of the possibility of infection through mucous membrane exposure, should use condoms correctly and consistently, and should prevent exposure to all body fluids.

Truths and Rumors (Sports, Sanitary Pads, Insects, and Other Means of Transmission)

Dispelling rumors is one of many tasks of health care workers who deal with HIV on a regular basis. Basically, there are no documented or reported cases of an individual contracting HIV from exposure to a soiled feminine pad containing the blood of an HIV-positive woman. At the same time, good sense would suggest that one should avoid touching these; simply wrap and dispose of them so that the blood is not a risk factor to anyone's health.

Sports transmission of HIV has not been documented. The only risk of transmission during participation in sports activities appears to be body contact involving bleeding, and thus exposure to contaminated blood.

Contrary to rumors, HIV is not airborne or foodborne. Outside the body, the virus does not live very long.

Tattoos and body piercing do present a risk of HIV transmission in that instruments may be contaminated by blood or may not be disinfected or sterilized after use from one client to the next. The CDC recommendation is that those who work in these businesses use disposable instruments or clean and sterilize equipment. Before getting a tattoo or piercing, it is wise to inquire about staff procedures concerning instruments used and ask what is done to prevent transmission of HIV, hepatitis B, and other disorders. Some health departments can also offer information on various local businesses that do tattoos and body piercing and the sterilization procedures that they follow.

Mosquito infection is often a concern, but not one that is founded on reality. In truth, no insect could transmit HIV via HIV-infected blood on its mouth because HIV-positive people do not have consistently high levels of HIV in the bloodstream, insects have minute amounts of blood on their mouths, and biting insects fly to a resting place to digest the blood they have imbibed—not to another person for another meal. Plus, HIV lives for a very short time inside an insect, and HIV does not reproduce in insects.

Saliva, Tears, Sweat

Thus far, contact with the saliva, tears, or sweat of an HIV-infected person has not spread the disease to anyone. The rumor that this is a means of transmission probably stems from the fact that HIV has been noted in saliva and tears in very small amounts. However, finding HIV in a body fluid does not automatically mean that the body fluid will transmit HIV. Sweat of HIV-infected individuals has not shown HIV.

Superinfection and Reinfection

The HIV organism has been shown to be too diverse to be viewed as a single entity. The issues of reinfection or superinfection are unresolved. *Reinfection* is defined as new infection after viral load is reduced; *superinfection* is defined as infection of an individual by a resistant strain.

Transplantation-Associated Transmission

One case has been documented of a person contracting HIV through organ transplantation. Although the blood of the deceased was, of course, negative for HIV, researchers believe that the problem stemmed from the fact that the person who died had been infected recently and had not yet reached the point of having enough HIV antibodies to yield a positive result.

Vertical Transmission

HIV can be vertically transmitted to infants during pregnancy or birth. About one-quarter of untreated pregnant women with HIV pass the infection to their babies. The breast milk of mothers who have HIV can also spread HIV to babies.

Mothers who take AZT during pregnancy can greatly reduce the probability of giving their babies HIV. When the doctor performs a cesarean section on the mother with HIV who has also been treated with AZT, the infection rate is reduced to 1 percent.

Women are a fast-growing HIV-infected population. The estimate is that about 110,000 to 155,000 women are living with HIV today, and in the United States alone, about 15,000 children now have HIV. This is one of the top 10 causes of death in children of ages one to four. Most of these children are infected by vertical transmission, from mother to child.

A mother can transmit HIV to her child in any one of three periods: intrauterine period, intrapartum period, and postnatal period. Positive HIV culture findings are seen in aborted and miscarried fetuses after only 12 weeks of gestation. Most, though—about 75 percent of infections—occur during the intrapartum period, according to the AIDS Clinical Trials Group classification of intrauterine transmission: a positive viral culture result within 48 hours of childbirth. The definition of intrapartum transmission is a negative or positive culture result in week one of the infant's life, followed by a positive finding within the next three months. Postnatal HIV transmission is accomplished when a mother breast-feeds her infant, but the percentage of transmissions occurring in this manner remains unknown.

Vertical transmission rates (30 to 40 percent) are highest in Africa—a statistic widely attributed to long-term breast-feeding. Lowest rates of vertical transmission are seen in Western Europe, where the figure is 15 to 20 percent.

How HIV is transmitted via the intrauterine route is not known, but it appears that it may involve the exposure of the infant's thin skin and mucosal surfaces to the mother's blood and secretions.

A 1994 study conducted by the Pediatric AIDS Clinical Trial Group showed that a three-part regimen of zidovudine given during pregnancy, during labor, and postpartum could reduce vertical transmission from 25.5 percent to 8.3 percent.

The HIV-infected mother and her fetus must be monitored carefully. The newborn should have a baseline blood cell count and differential before zidovudine use, and repeated hemoglobin measurements should be obtained after the six-week regimen and at 12 weeks. Six weeks after birth, these infants should receive *Pneumocystis carinii* prophylaxis.

Woman-to-Woman

Cases of female-to-female transmission of HIV appear to be quite rare. But they occur, as does female-to-male transmission. Clearly, vaginal secretions and menstrual blood are potentially infectious. Through December 1998, 109,311 women were reported to have AIDS. Of these, 2,220 had sex with women, but also had other risk factors: sex with high-risk men, receipt of blood or blood products, and injection drug use. Of the 2,220, 347 said they had sex with women exclusively, but 98 percent of them had another risk factor (usually IV drug use). In follow-up, women with AIDS whose only reported risk is sex with women have been carefully investigated; as of December 1998, there were no confirmed cases of female-to-female HIV transmission. Women refused interviews or had other risks that complicated pinpointing their mode of transmission.

Patient Care (October 1999) described a trailblazing research study that is looking at several aspects of lesbian sexuality: the causes of transmission of HIV between female sex partners, sexual behavior between women, and lesbians' adherence to safe-sex guidelines. At any rate, women who have sex with women are advised to follow certain precautions to reduce the likelihood of contracting HIV: preventing exposure of the mouth to vaginal secretions and menstrual blood; using condoms for all sexual encounters with men or use of sex toys; avoiding sharing of sex toys; avoiding contact with body fluids during oral sex; knowing each sex partner's HIV status.

Changes in U.S. population trends of new cases of HIV infection indicate that the rate is increasing in women, in people of racial and ethnic minorities, and in adolescents and older people. At the same time, newly diagnosed AIDS cases are increasingly attributed to heterosexual transmission and injectable drug use. Cases among homosexual men are declining in number. As of 1999, at least 20 percent of people living with HIV disease were 50 or older. Perinatal transmission is also on the decline. It is believed that the reason for this decline is prenatal administration of antiretroviral agents.

Heterosexual Transmission

As of September 2000, it was believed that heterosexual contact presents the greatest risk of contracting HIV, and sex with drug users plays a large role in this process. Unfortunately, HIV infection among U.S. women has increased greatly over the last decade. The CDC estimate is that the United States has 120,000 to 160,000 adult and adolescent women living with HIV or AIDS. It is significant that in 1992, women were 14 percent of adults/adolescents with AIDS, but by 1998, that had exploded to 20 percent. In a little more than one decade, the percentage of all AIDS cases reported among women more than tripled; it was 7 percent in 1985 and 23 percent in 1999. In 2002, about half of adults living with HIV/AIDS worldwide were women. Three-fourths of AIDS cases reported to date in the United States are in women who are African American and Hispanic. For women in the United States who fall in the age group 25 to 44, HIV/AIDS is one of the leading causes of death.

In 1999, heterosexual exposure to HIV explained how most women (40 percent) contracted AIDS, whereas 27 percent of cases were attributable to injection drug use. In 2001, new infections in women in the United States were through heterosexual sex (75 percent) and injection drug use (25 percent).

To improve these statistics, prevention efforts are focusing on developing and making widely available effective prevention methods that can be initiated by females. These need to be provided for women whose partners refuse to use condoms. The CDC is studying the prevention effectiveness of the female condom, as well as working on topical microbicides that can kill HIV and the pathogens that cause STDs.

Around the world each day, more than 6,500 new cases of HIV infection in women are diagnosed, and this figure does not even take into account vertical transmission. Oddly, though, these women have trouble accessing medical care.

Unbelievably, in Africa, more than 50 percent of women in the age group 15 to 25 are HIV-positive. These women in particular are often ostracized and face a life of poverty and little hope of drug therapy for the disease. In Africa, huge social taboos, which stand in the way of curbing the epidemic, remain.

Furthermore, in the United States, of newly reported cases, 40 percent are women. The CDC reports that most of these are in the South, followed by the northeastern states. In 2001, of newly HIV-infected women, about 64 percent were black, 18 percent were white, 18 percent were Hispanic, and a small percentage come from other racial/ethnic groups.

HIV treatment For a long time, it has been the general belief that the individual who tests positive for HIV should immediately begin a program that will protect his or her health. It is generally believed that early intervention can delay the onset of full-blown AIDS and help to ward off opportunistic infections. As soon as possible, it is critical to see a doctor—if possible, one with plenty of experience in treating HIV. The CDC also recommends that the person who has just learned of HIV-positive status have a TB test and try to eliminate habits that will serve to weaken the immune system: smoking cigarettes, drinking a great deal of alcohol, and using illegal drugs. For an HIV-infected person who has an addiction, this is a good time to look for a program to help with cessation of the habit.

Interestingly, the year 2002 ushered in a different idea about the rush to treatment for those recently diagnosed with HIV. Two new studies in *JAMA* underscored the new belief that people with symptom-free HIV can hold off starting drug regimens without causing themselves extra problems. Whereas the 2002 revised guidelines suggested that drugs could still work well if they were begun when CD4 levels dipped to 350 cells per cubic millimeter (versus the previous figure of 500), new theories based on latest–greatest studies indicated that the drugs will work even when a patient's CD4 is as low as 200, and even with high virus levels in the blood. Delaying treatment did not appear to hurt a number of patients who were observed.

It is important to entrust treatment to a health care provider who has treated a large patient base of HIV-infected individuals or a physician who works in consultation with an AIDS specialist. The treatment modalities are a rapidly changing area, and the patient's long-term outcome depends greatly on the right choice of therapies. Also, if a physician prescribes the wrong choice in early treatment, that mistake sometimes may preclude some future therapies because of problems with viral resistance.

Planning for Care

It is best to find a doctor who specializes in HIV to set up a treatment plan as soon as possible. For an HIV specialist, check with a local HIV/AIDS group that can make recommendations. Other tips for the person who has just received an HIV-positive test result are the following:

- Seek psychological counseling. Most people need a great deal of support in dealing with this diagnosis, especially at the outset.

- Try to develop a matter-of-fact attitude; ask yourself what you can do, and work to stop beating yourself up about the past. Think positive thoughts such as "Yesterday is history; tomorrow is a mystery; today is a blessing."

- Promise yourself that you will take a proactive approach. Become well informed about HIV and AIDS, and choose from the options that health care specialists recommend to you. The more you know, the better off you are. Armed with knowledge, you will feel more in control of your destiny.

- Do not be afraid to speak your mind. If a treatment strategy does not appeal to you, say so. You are not compelled to follow every aspect of a plan that your doctor proposes. Try to set yourself up as a partner in the treatment process. You need to be in sync with your doctor in order to maintain the level of compliance that will enhance your day-to-day health.

- Think assertive, and think positive.

- Be a smart consumer in sorting through the vast array of information that is available on HIV and AIDS: rumors, the Internet, magazines, newspapers, and books. Also, be wary of groups that advocate "living with the disease," promoting the idea that the AIDS epidemic is a figment of the health care establishment's imagination. By taking a no-treatment vow, you are taking the enormous risk of letting the disease run rampant in your body, unscathed by moderating medications. Remember that many major advances are being made in treating HIV, and staying as healthy as possible will make you more likely to benefit from new drugs that appear on the market.

- Set yourself up for success. HIV can cause serious regression in your progress if you do not take medications as prescribed. In some cases, the virus has time to mutate so that the drugs will no longer be effective in stemming its movement. Timing of taking medications is important; never missing a pill is important, too. Do not attempt improvisations on the plan you have devised with your doctor. If you start taking medications and are tempted to eliminate one that has nasty side effects, check with your doctor first. He or she may be able to replace it with something you can tolerate better.

- Find out what you need to know about your prescriptions. You need to know which ones have to be taken with food, which one requires the elimination of grapefruit juice from beverage consumption, and which side effects are normal. Do whatever it takes to remind yourself to take each pill. Think of it as mounting a defense in your body, which will require a high level of all the fighters. Take your drug therapy seriously.

As of 2002, the recommendation for treating asymptomatic HIV in adults was as follows:

- Treatment is begun when the CD4 count falls below 350 cells/mm^3 or viral load exceeds 30,000.
- An individual with HIV usually takes a combination of at least three anti-HIV drugs in highly active antiretroviral therapy (HAART).

Rationale for treatment should be based on preservation of CD4 counts, preservation of CTL response, and prevention of opportunistic infections and death. In primary HIV infection, the clinical course is loss of CD4 count over several weeks; increase in CD8 count; decreased viral load to set point; normalization of CD4 and CD8 counts; loss of CTL response over six months.

An understanding of what occurs in HIV is key. The human immunodeficiency virus gets inside T cells, which are part of the immune system. For self-monitoring, one needs information on T cell count (or CD4 count), which indicates number of T cells, whereas viral load points to the amount of existing virus within a person's body. The best-case scenario is a high T cell count with a low viral load. The way that antiviral treatment helps is by keeping virus out of healthy T cells and preventing an infected T cell from releasing new virus cells. Treatments also serve to boost the immune system, making it more stalwart in fighting the disease.

At the outset of the disease, the HIV-positive person's immune system fights so well that symptoms (apart from those of the initial acute retroviral syndrome) typically do not appear for years. Usually, antiviral drugs provide a way to attack the virus in those individuals whose immune system is virus-ridden. Opportunistic infections come into play when the T cell count drops too low, because the immune system is, in short, no longer able to fight off these diseases. So, the name "opportunistic infections" makes sense in that the infections basically "seize" the window of opportunity. This is why a death from AIDS is actually a death resulting from an opportunistic infection, because HIV has weakened the immune system to the point that the disease can wreak havoc.

Alternative Therapies

Of growing interest to some HIV-infected patients are the options in alternative remedies and herbal supplements. Many use these in addition to traditional drug regimens. About 30 to 50 percent use alternative therapies. Herbal preparations include cat's claw, echinacea, ginseng, and aloe vera. Other options are vitamins and special foods thought to be helpful, shark cartilage, acupuncture, and ozone. The HIV-infected person who does choose to use supplements should consult his or her physician on the use of alternative therapies because there is always the possibility that mainstream therapies may not interact well with some herbal treatments.

Although it is unconscionable that people would prey on those who are HIV-positive, it does, of course, happen. Scams are not unusual, nor are snake-oil sellers. However, most physicians do not discourage a patient from using a therapy or herbal supplement that does no harm.

One of the most recent upgrades in information on supplements is the discovery by researchers that garlic supplements can impede HIV medication. There is a potentially harmful interaction when garlic supplements are combined with a type of medication used to treat HIV/AIDS. Investigators from the National Institutes of Health reported that garlic supplements sharply reduce blood levels of saquinavir, an anti-HIV drug. The study's senior coauthor, Judith Falloon, M.D., an AIDS clinical researcher at the National Institute of Allergy and Infectious Diseases, reported that blood concentrations of saquinavir, in the presence of garlic supplements, were decreased by about 50 percent among study participants. Researchers saw a definite and prolonged interaction, which indicates that doctors and patients should use garlic supplements with caution during HIV therapy. Also of interest was that even after a 10-day "wash-out" period (no garlic supplements), the volunteers' blood levels of saquinavir still averaged about 35 percent lower than the expected baseline amount, when the volunteers were again using only the protease inhibitor for three days. Researchers concluded that it is clear that anyone who is using saquinavir as the sole protease inhibitor should not use garlic supplements. Also, in this team's first study, they uncovered a potentially dangerous interaction between Saint John's wort and the protease inhibitor indinavir.

Early Therapy

In the early days of AIDS, patients had no drug options to address immune deficiency. Furthermore, they could turn to few treatments for the opportunistic diseases that afflicted them, but years of dealing with this disease generated a great deal of research that developed medications that fight HIV infection, associated infections, and cancers. This is a huge step forward for those who have HIV infection.

A study of patients with a one-year or shorter history of HIV infection found evidence that early treatment may lead to the fastest recovery of the naïve cell repertoire and may also limit establishment and expansion of latent HIV reservoirs. According to a report on the medical literature published in *Hospital Physician* (January 2000), 10 patients were put on a drug regimen of hydroxyurea, didanosine, and indinavir, before complete Western blot seroconversion. Complete Western blot seroconversion eventually occurred in most, but progression was very slow.

HAART (Highly Active Antiretroviral Therapy)

The literature inevitably lags behind what is late and great in the fast-changing HAART area. Basically, the gold standard is a combination therapy that usually calls for three medications from at least two drug families. The following classes of antiretroviral drugs are now at the forefront:

- PIs: indinavir, nelfinavir, ritonavir, saquinavir, and amprenavir. These protease inhibitors interrupt virus replication at a later step in the life cycle. The fact that HIV can become resistant to

each class of drugs makes combination therapy necessary to achieve virus suppression.

- Nucleoside analog reverse transcriptase inhibitors (NRTIs): zidovudine (AZT), didanosine, zalcitabine, stavudine, lamivudine, and abacavir. These interrupt an early stage of virus replication and may slow the spread of HIV in the body.

- Nonnucleoside reverse transcriptase inhibitors (NNRTIs): delavirdine, efavirenz, and nevirapine. They inhibit synthesis of viral DNA by binding to reverse transcriptase.

- The newest class, the nucleotide reverse transcriptase inhibitors, of which tenofovir is the first available. As do nucleoside agents, the nucleotides compete with normal DNA precursors. None of these classes of medications prevents transmission of the disease.

For physicians, timing the initiation of drug therapy is extremely important in that the wrong timing has an effect on the later course of treatment. Equipped with the broadest base of knowledge, HIV specialists are best informed for making specific drug determinations. The rule of thumb is that symptomatic patients receive drug therapy, as well as asymptomatic patients with a CD4+ cell count less than 350 cells/mm3 or a plasma viral titer of HIV RNA exceeding 30,000 copies/mL indicated by bDNA (branched DNA) testing or 55,000 copies/mL by reverse transcriptase–polymerase chain reaction testing.

The hard reality of how difficult these drugs are for patients to tolerate has changed the aggressiveness and haste with which physicians have initiated therapy. The thinking is now that because the side effects of the drugs may become less well tolerated as time passes, the timing of the initiation of drug therapy is crucial.

Patients who are on drug therapy must be attuned to their own bodies and act as participants in their treatment regimens. A patient who has a preference for one of two drug regimens that are equivalent should express that preference. Certainly, most people are more likely to be compliant in taking 30 pills per day if they have a voice in the decision. A patient should let the health care professional know her or his desires: does he or she want medication designed to extend life or medications that will make him or her comfortable?

Also affecting the individual are other health problems, lifestyle, and medication toxicity and side effects. Patients must be careful to inform their doctors about any complementary therapies, such as herbal supplements, they are taking.

It is important to emphasize that these drugs do not constitute a cure for HIV or AIDS. Also, patients may encounter side effects that often prove severe, such as AZT's possible depletion of red or white blood cells, and dideoxyinosine's (ddI's) possible inflammation of the pancreas and painful nerve damage.

In many patients, protease inhibitors cause bouts of nausea, diarrhea, and other gastrointestinal symptoms. They also have to be monitored carefully because there is a possibility of serious side effects of interactions with other drugs. Another recent discovery is abnormal body-fat distribution in some people who take protease inhibitors.

Besides receiving antiretroviral therapy, those adults whose T cell count is below 200 cells/mm3 are usually treated for prevention of PCP, a common and deadly opportunistic infection that affects HIV-infected individuals. In children, PCP therapy is administered when the T cell count drops below a level that is the norm for their age group. Regardless of T cell count, HIV-infected children and adults who have survived a bout with PCP will be given medication lifelong to prevent recurrence of the pneumonia. In those with HIV infection, Kaposi's sarcoma and other cancers are usually treated with radiation, chemotherapy, or alpha-interferon injections.

A high percentage of antiretroviral drug–naïve patients experience maximal viral load suppression about six to 12 months after start of therapy; it has also been observed that only about half of patients in a city clinic setting achieved similar results. The predictors of success are low baseline viremia and high baseline CD4+ T cell count, rapid decline of viremia, decline of viremia to below 50 HIV RNA copies/mL, adequate serum levels of antiretroviral drugs, and adherence to the drug regimen.

Other ways to heighten HAART benefits are smart sequencing of drugs and preservation of future treatment options. Current thinking in 2003 is that a class-sparing regimen will preserve or retain one or more classes of drugs for future use. This way, the overall effectiveness of HAART ideally will extend over a longer period. The effectiveness of PI-containing HAART regimens has been shown to include durable viral load suppression, partial immunologic restoration, and decreased incidence of AIDS and death.

Early results of drug therapy in women with HIV seemed to indicate that women were not responding as well as men, but now it is clear that women have the same rate of disease progression when they are submitted to the same drug regimens. One difference documented in studies is that women have lower median viral load than do men with similar CD4 counts—and half the viral load of men with similar rates of disease progression.

Reactions to HAART differ in men and women. Whereas men experience more diarrhea, increased levels of triglycerides and cholesterol, and increased abdominal fat and loss of peripheral fat, women are more likely to experience vomiting, stomach pain, itching, rashes, and nausea. Also more common in women than in men (yet still rare) is lactic acidosis, which can lead to organ damage and death.

Structured Intermittent Therapy

The seven-day-on, seven-day-off regimen—new in the treatment of HIV as of December 2001—had notable results in a pilot study at the National Institute of Allergy and Infectious Diseases (NIAID) that suggested that some people with HIV may benefit from a seven-day-on, seven-day-off regimen of anti-HIV therapy. This cyclic approach differs from the usual method, which depends on continuous administration of HAART drugs.

In the NIAID study of structured intermittent therapy, 10 patients had repeated on–off cycles of therapy, including seven days of treatment with potent combinations of HIV medications, followed by seven days off these drugs. When these people were enrolled in the program, they were being treated with continuous HAART and experiencing success with the therapy. However, switching to the intermittent HAART regimen showed no adverse effects on the course of the disease—plus, there was a significant reduction in some of the side effects of HAART treatment.

Researchers believe that structured intermittent therapy has many advantages: it halves the total time that patients receive HAART and thus reduces costs and side effects of these drugs. Cost is a very important issue in third world countries. At the same time, researchers emphasize that patients should not self-medicate in a structured intermittent fashion. The results of randomized and controlled clinical trials that are now under way must verify the benefits of this experimental approach before it will be recommended to patients outside the clinical trial setting.

The NIAID researchers also assert that HAART has benefited many HIV-infected people greatly in that this therapy has substantially reduced HIV-related morbidity and mortality rates. The downsides, though, are that HAART's usefulness is limited by significant toxicities (short- and long-term); dosage regimens that are complex, producing adherence difficulties; development of drug resistance; and high costs that make it nonviable for widespread use in resource-limited countries.

The NIAID director, Anthony S. Fauci, M.D., has contended that structured intermittent therapy may well be adapted for use in developing nations, where more than 95 percent of the world's HIV-infected live. Currently, few of these people have access to HAART because these medications are expensive.

The *Journal of the American Medical Association* looked at all English-language articles published from January 1999 to August 2001 regarding those who had been treated with HAART for whom treatment interruption was studied. They found that structured treatment interruption (STI) may offer more benefit during acute infection when a patient's immune system is still nearly intact. The jury is still out as to whether STI works in long-term management by decreasing the problem of the toxicity of the drugs and improving the individual's life without ruining treatment effectiveness. The authors suggest that what is needed is a safer approach; therapeutic immunization or vaccination would be preferable for spurring vigorous T cell–mediated immune responses and control of HIV during treatment interruption.

Experimental Therapy

Experimental therapy is a form of treatment regimen in which participants are informed that the therapy being used is "experimental," and thus its benefits and risks are largely unknown, and the subjects agree to be exposed to a particular drug therapy in order for researchers to weigh the effect on a dependent variable. Doctors sometimes try experimental therapies in treating diseases (such as cancers and AIDS) for which no known cures exist.

Pain Management

The term *pain management* is pertinent to the study of sexually transmitted diseases in that the end stage of AIDS can be very painful, and medications are often administered to make the patient comfortable and ease pain. Physicians, in handling the pain-management aspect of AIDS, must take into consideration several aspects of the picture: maintaining quality of life, allowing basic functioning of the individual, and keeping side effects of the drugs to a minimum. Early in the treatment of a person with HIV, a doctor usually prescribes acetaminophen or ibuprofen for pain relief; if and when pain escalates, management may employ codeine or morphine or another opiate. In administering pain medication, the doctor who is treating a person with HIV or AIDS must also carefully monitor the route of administration, because some patients are hampered by vomiting, dehydration, and difficulty in swallowing.

Periodic Testings

Patient Care (October 1999) suggests that physicians recommend that patients with HIV have periodic tests to monitor their health status. This is because their immunosuppression makes them more vulnerable to infections. Testing for the following is recommended:

- Cytomegalovirus antibodies
- Hepatitis B and C serologies
- Pap smear for women one to two times a year
- Purified protein derivative test for tuberculosis once a year
- *Toxoplasma gondii* serology
- Test for syphilis (annually for patients who are sexually active)

Prolonged Hospitalization

Some treatment programs for HIV address the psychosocial factors associated with prolonged hospitalization of a population with advanced HIV. One study reported in May 2001 looked at a group of HIV patients at risk for adverse psychosocial outcomes and in need of more targeted hospital resources. *Prolonged hospitalization* was defined as length of stay that exceeds 90 days in a 33-month period. Reasons included mania, psychosis, and anxiety; HIV dementia; housing issues; and need for social work interventions.

Prophylaxis for Opportunistic Infections

Using prophylaxis means planning ahead and taking a medication before a disease develops. In the case of HIV, doctors prescribe primary prophylaxis to prevent infection. Secondary prophylaxis, then, is meant to prevent recurrence of an infection the patient has already had. The latter is often used for long-term suppressive treatment of incurable infections (toxoplasmosis).

For the HIV patient, it is important to emphasize the importance of using a latex condom during every act of sexual intercourse to reduce that person's risk of exposure to cytomegalovirus (CMV), herpes simplex virus, human papillomavirus, and other sexually transmitted pathogens. It is believed that condom use can decrease one's risk of superinfection with an HIV strain that is resistant to the drugs used to treat HIV. People with HIV should also avoid oral–anal contact, which gives them a heightened risk of development of intestinal infections: hepatitis A and B, shigellosis, cryptosporidiosis, campylobacteriosis, amebiasis, and giardiasis.

Those with HIV should also be highly aware of work-related and environmental risks. For example, the HIV-infected person who works or volunteers in a health care facility, homeless shelter, or jail is at extra risk of contracting TB.

In child care settings, there should be an awareness of the risk of being infected with CMV infection, cryptosporidiosis, hepatitis A, and giardiasis. Thorough handwashing should be a frequent practice. That rule also applies to those who work with animals, because there is risk of contracting cryptosporidiosis, toxoplasmosis, salmonellosis, campylobacteriosis, and bartonellosis.

Good handwashing after any exposure to soil is also important to prevent contracting toxoplasmosis or cryptosporidiosis. An HIV patient who lives where histoplasmosis is endemic should stay away from chicken coops, caves, and sites where birds roost. Pets, food, and water also bear risks, so regular vigilant handwashing and avoidance of any contaminated fluids are extremely important for someone who is HIV-infected.

Injection drug users have extra risk of exposure to hepatitis C, drug-resistant strains of HIV, and other pathogens that are borne by blood. Strategies that HIV-infected drug users should employ include avoiding reusing or sharing syringes, needles, water, and drug-preparation equipment (which should be carefully cleaned with bleach and water); using only sterile syringes from a pharmacy or syringe-exchange program; using sterile water to prepare drugs (or fresh tap water if sterile water is not available); preparing drugs with a new or disinfected "cooker" and a new filter; swabbing the site before injection with a new alcohol swab; and disposing of a syringe safely after using it once.

Psychosocial Issues

When a person is informed that he or she has HIV, this information is always interpreted as a death sentence. Anyone who has received this diagnosis needs to understand that it is certainly normal to feel sad and dejected for a few days. On the other hand, it is important to emerge from the reaction to become proactive in fighting the disease.

Those who counsel individuals newly diagnosed with HIV are quick to inform them that, thanks to advances in drug therapy, many people with this disease live decades past initial diagnosis. Furthermore, a diagnosis of HIV does not have to mean the end of intimate relationships forever, endurance of shunning by others, or being immersed in depression. Counselors inform a person with HIV that this disease—like any other—is what the afflicted individual decides it will be. Being well informed can help an HIV-positive person cope more effectively.

Counselors also urge those who are ill not to focus on the fact that HIV leads to death. Rather, they should be comforted by knowing that every person dies—and each day is a gift, just as it is for someone who is disease-free.

The decision about sharing the information on one's HIV status is personal. Some people do inform, and others keep it to themselves. Most people do better psychologically when they share their grief and are reassured to find that friends and family are supportive. (As is true of other sexually transmitted diseases, there are many people walking around with the same disease you have, but they keep this information to themselves.)

The enormous emotional stressors inherent in HIV should be dealt with because they make life difficult and can impair medical treatment. The depression, anxiety, stress, and substance abuse associated with HIV disease require treatment. Important aspects of HIV care are support groups and counseling, which can be fashioned to fit the needs of patients.

Resistance to HAART

In the early days of treating HIV, it was soon found that single-drug therapy did not work well, because the virus can quickly develop resistance to antiviral agents. Mutating, the virus changes genetic code to produce enzymes unaffected by drugs. It may take a number of these mutations to allow the virus to produce high-level resistance to a certain drug, but consider the fact that the body daily produces tens of millions of viruses. Hence, it does not take long for a drug-resistant version of HIV to develop.

For the patient, it is important to understand that the resistance persists even after the particular drug is no longer being used; adding insult to injury, the virus adds a layer of cross-resistance to drugs that are similar. The upshot is that the viral load must be suppressed in order to prevent resistance. Experts tell us, however, that even at viral loads of 500 copies/mL, there is enough viral reproduction to allow development of resistance.

When someone takes HAART drugs inconsistently, HIV is allowed to regain a foothold and begin multiplying again. As more resistance is developed, the antiretroviral drugs are rendered impotent against the multiplying virus.

Roger Spitzer, M.D. ("Living with HIV," April 1, 2001), contends

- That multiple drug therapy should be used to suppress viral load to undetectable levels
- That adding drugs one at a time sequentially and using single-drug therapy are less effective than the multidrug approach
- That if the viral load continues to increase, despite the drug regimen, one's health care provider should change at least two drugs at a time, replacing these with drugs with little cross-resistance
- That the patient must take all HAART medications all the time exactly as prescribed
- That those who have been thoroughly treated with HAART drugs and have not had complete viral suppression may have the unfortunate circumstance of development of so much resistance that no regimen that employs the drugs available will be effective in knocking down the viral load to undetectable levels

To find therapy regimens that have minimal probability of drug resistance emerging, researchers must uncover more detailed information on the evolutionary dynamics that lead to the emergence of drug-resistant strains of HIV. It is believed that either drug-resistant strains evolve during therapy or drug-resistant strains exist in the virus population before therapy is even begun. Some researchers think that the dosage of treatment should be increased in order to minimize the residual replication of the sensitive virus during treatment—if, indeed, these drug-resistant strains do develop during therapy. But if the resistant strains are preexisting entities, the drug's effect on the wild-type virus is basically irrelevant because a potent drug will make resistant mutants escalate quickly and wild-type virus decline quickly, whereas the opposite—a weak drug—will do the reverse. In the case of preexisting strains that are able to resist one or more drugs, researchers suggest that the strategy could be to combine more drugs with different resistance profiles, in hopes of diminishing the likelihood that any virus strain could have resistance to all drugs.

According to a report from the American Foundation for AIDS Research, a December 2001 symposium sponsored by the National Cancer Institute underscored a dire situation related to frequent emergence of drug-resistant HIV strains. An observational cohort study by Douglas Richman, Sam Bozzette, and colleagues from the University of California, San Diego (UCSD) and the RAND Corporation (RAND) saw a widespread prevalence of treatment failure and drug resistance, as researchers looked at blood samples taken in 1999 from a cohort established by Bozzette in 1996. The group was representative of Americans receiving any sort of HIV medical care at that time. It was the same year that highly active antiretroviral therapy (HAART) became the gold standard for treating HIV. Of a quarter of a million Americans receiving HIV-related care, researchers initially interviewed 2,864 patients. They took blood samples in 1999 from 1,906 of these patients (only two-thirds were still alive and could be found). Of the follow-up group, only 37 percent had viral load below 500 copies/mL. As for drug resistance in the HIV in those with viral load above 500 copies/mL, they found that 79 percent had HIV that resisted at least one of the medications.

A separate study by Richman cited continuing increase in transmission of drug-resistant HIV; from 1999 to 2000, a national survey found that 14 percent of newly acquired HIV was highly drug-resistant (14 percent to at least one HIV drug and 5.5 percent to two or more). So, in the United States, some people who are acquiring HIV for the first time receive a strain that is drug-resistant, meaning that these people start out with a built-in history of past drug exposure and failure.

At the same time, researchers point out that this UCSD–RAND cohort experience may not be completely representative when one considers that people now starting HAART for the first time may do better as a result of the improved medical management available. Note that 60 percent of those in the treated cohort already had AIDS; therefore, they were already at the point where their response to drug therapy was reduced. Also, 79 percent had previously used anti-HIV drugs that were almost entirely single- or dual-nucleoside analogs. The serial addition of new drugs to regimens that were failing may have put the UCSD-RAND group at a disadvantage when encountering HAART. Also confusing matters were the partici-

pants' "drug holidays." These people reported going on and off drug therapy, a practice that has been shown to lead to drug mutations.

Unfortunately, the number of new AIDS cases rose slightly in the year 2000, and in early January the CDC's preliminary figures for 2001 showed a further 8 percent increase in the number of AIDS cases in the United States. In New York City alone, the rate of AIDS was up 47 percent. Sadly, these increases are on the heels of the 1990s' sharp decline, which almost halved the AIDS incidence as a result of HAART therapy.

Subsequent Treatment

Therapy that is begun when an individual has advanced HIV disease is approached differently than is HAART begun early after initial infection. Health care professionals typically urge all who have advanced HIV disease, including patients with symptomatic HIV infection (thrush and unexplained fever) without AIDS, to be treated with antiretroviral agents. Extra factors to be taken into consideration in the treatment regimen are the patient's acute illness with an opportunistic infection or another complication of HIV, drug toxicity, ability to adhere to a regimen, drug interactions, and lab abnormalities insofar as determining timing of starting HAART.

After the doctor begins the patient's therapy, a maximally suppressive regimen should be used. Also, advanced-stage patients who are on an antiretroviral regimen should not discontinue therapy during an acute opportunistic infection or malignancy, unless their doctor has drug concerns (toxicity, intolerance, interactions).

Complicated drug combinations are often used when the patient's disease has progressed to AIDS. Factors that complicate the treatment of advanced disease are wasting and anorexia, because certain protease inhibitors require that the patient be following certain dietary requirements for effective absorption. Further, ZDT-associated bone marrow suppression and the neuropathic effects of dideoxycytidine (ddC), starudine (d4T), and ddI—combined with the direct effects of HIV—may render drug therapy intolerable to the patient.

Some recovery in immune function can be achieved by potent drug therapy even in advanced

HIV. At the same time, the patient with advanced HIV and an opportunistic infection may have new symptoms in response to a new immunologic response to the pathogen. It is important not to presume, then, that this means the antiretroviral therapy has failed, and new opportunistic infections should be treated appropriately. The patient's viral load measurement at this point can shed light on the entire situation.

Treatment of Syphilis in HIV Patients

When doctors treat syphilis in HIV patients, there may be inadequate or no response to treatment. *Cortlandt Forum* (November 1999) reported a study of 64 HIV-positive patients that matched them with an equal number of patients who were HIV-negative and found that 56 percent of the HIV-positive patients did not experience the desired fourfold decrease in their syphilis test results, compared with 38 percent of the other patients. This was after six months of standard treatment as recommended by the Centers for Disease Control and Prevention. Coinfection presents unique treatment considerations.

HIV type 2   According to the Centers for Disease Control and Prevention, HIV-2 was the second type of HIV documented when, in 1986, it was found in AIDS patients in West Africa. HIV-1 and HIV-2 are transmitted in the same ways, and both have links with opportunistic infections and AIDS. Those with HIV-2, however, seem to experience a progression of immunodeficiency that is slower and milder. Those with HIV-2 are also less infectious early on. However, with the progression of HIV-2, infectiousness increases (but in a shorter period than for HIV-1).

The United States has few reported cases of HIV-2. Because the possibility of contracting HIV-2 in the United States is remote, the CDC does not recommend routine testing at U.S. HIV counseling and test sites or in settings other than blood centers. On the other hand, when HIV testing is done, tests for antibodies to types 1 and 2 should be done if there is reason to believe that HIV-2 could be present.

Those at risk for HIV-2 are sex partners of a person from a country where HIV-2 is endemic (Cape Verde, Ivory Coast, Gambia, Guinea-Bissau, Mali, Mauritania, Nigeria, Sierra Leone, Benin, Burkina Faso, Ghana, Guinea, Liberia, Niger, São Tomé, Senegal, Togo, Angola, Mozambique), sex partners of a person who is HIV-2-infected, people who have received a blood transfusion or a nonsterile injection in one of the HIV-2-endemic countries, people who have shared needles with someone from an HIV-2-endemic country or with someone who has HIV-2, and children of women with risk factors for HIV-2 or known to have this disease. Others for whom HIV-2 testing is advisable are people with an illness that suggests HIV infection but who are posting a negative HIV-1 test result and people with an indeterminate test-band pattern in the HIV-1 Western blot finding.

Also of note is that all U.S. blood donations since 1992 have been tested for both HIV-1 and HIV-2. Of course, a donation detected with either is excluded from clinical use, and the donor cannot donate again.

The best approach to treating those with HIV-2 is unknown. Some of the drugs used to treat HIV-1 are not as effective in dealing with HIV-2. Also, researchers cannot tell whether HAART treatment slows progression in view of the fact that HIV-2 shows a slower development of immunodeficiency anyway.

Another factor is that monitoring treatment of those with HIV-2 is more difficult, and there is no FDA-licensed HIV-2 viral load assay available. The tests for HIV-1 are not reliable for monitoring HIV-2.

Fortunately, HIV-2 infection is rarely seen in children, and it seems to be less transmissible from mother to infant. But there have been documented cases of transmission from infected mother to fetus or newborn when the women had primary HIV-2 infection during pregnancy.

To make sure HIV-2 does not spread in the United States, the CDC recommends continued surveillance and programs especially aimed at those most at risk: injection drug users and those who have multiple sex partners.

home care for the AIDS patient   Gone are the days when a person with AIDS routinely was hospitalized. Today most of those who have AIDS can live at home and enjoy the freedoms and comforts of a setting that is familiar and convenient. According to the Centers for Disease Control and Prevention, people who have AIDS-related illnesses often improve more quickly when friends and family care for them in a home setting. Complaints of discomfort are also fewer. For the caregiver, it is important to remember that AIDS has unique repercussions for each individual, so he or she must seek frequent updates on treatment and care information from the person's doctor. Many times, those who assist AIDS patients at home provide helpful services such as bill paying, housekeeping, and grocery shopping.

See Appendix III.

homosexual intercourse Acts of sex that take place between two people of the same sex.

hospice care The delivery of health care that is primarily supportive in nature and targets the terminally ill patient. The patient is kept comfortable and the family is provided support. Covered by Medicare, Medicaid, and some health insurance plans, hospice care is provided in a facility, in the patient's home, or in both. The team of health care professionals may include a social worker, a nurse, a physician, and a spiritual adviser. Many people who have been through the experience of caring for a relative who had a terminal illness view hospice care as the most humane way to handle the final months of life of a person with AIDS or cancer because the individual can be at home, surrounded by loved ones, yet still receive proper care.

hospital An institution where the ill and injured receive medical care.

host factors The factors in a patient's body that affect the rate at which a disease progresses. In the case of HIV, host factors influence the rate of virus replication and affect the rate at which full-blown AIDS will develop. Factors include a person's immune response and genetics. Host factors combine with viral factors to make up the events that

eventually wreak havoc with the HIV-infected individual's immune system and lead to death.

housing Because of the stigma that lingers, families with a person who has HIV/AIDS sometimes face ostracism when seeking housing. An example of new thinking in this respect is provided by a Los Angeles, California, townhouse community that was developed for homeless and low-income families affected by HIV/AIDS. Having opened its doors in 2001, this facility is Salvation Army–sponsored and is one of the first and largest nationwide.

Focus on security and comfort for the families was central to the program, according to its executive director, Douglas Loisel, who was concerned that many of the families had been ostracized by other family members and by the larger community, leaving the HIV-positive person no place to go. The townhouse project gives people a place to live where there is no stigma attached to an HIV diagnosis. There are 16 units of one- and two-bedroom transitional housing, which residents can use for up to two years. The community also has permanent housing: 28 two- and three-bedroom townhouses.

Rounding out the convenience of the neighborhood is a licensed 60-space day care center that serves residents and families in the surrounding community. Services for those who live in transitional housing are medical support, treatment for substance abuse, vocational services, meals, and medications. This housing development stemmed from strategies spawned at Bethesda House, a Salvation Army–run facility in downtown Los Angeles that was also established to meet the needs of low-income people with AIDS.

HPV See HUMAN PAPILLOMAVIRUS.

HSV-1 (herpes simplex virus 1) See GENITAL HERPES.

HSV-2 (herpes simplex virus 2) See GENITAL HERPES.

human immunodeficiency virus See HIV.

human papillomavirus   See GENITAL WARTS.

hypnosis   A state of heightened awareness that can be used to manipulate perceptions. A technique used by many medical professionals to help patients deal with pain, anxiety, or phobias; explore various aspects of repressed thoughts; and handle their feelings about various issues, from cancer to smoking cessation to weight loss. In respect to fighting a serious disease such as HIV/AIDS, the individual may consider the option of hypnosis in hopes of improving the ability to cope with the disease. Some cancer and AIDS patients listen to audiotapes that further underscore the messages received during hypnosis, so that they are able to imagine themselves as proactive participants in fighting the deadly diseases that are ravaging their bodies.

idiopathic thrombocytopenic purpura An autoimmune disorder characterized by a low platelet number that results in bruising and spontaneous bleeding. The term idiopathic means that the exact cause is unknown. Doctors suspect idiopathic thrombocytopenic purpura (ITP) when they have excluded other causes of low platelet count, such as drugs that are known to cause thrombocytopenia. In the autoimmune disorder ITP, a person may appear to be healthy except for having a low platelet count that may cause him or her to bruise or bleed easily. The person's body forms antibodies that bind to platelets. High-dose steroid therapy is usually the initial treatment, but many adults with ITP eventually need to have the spleen surgically removed.

immune system The complex system that enables the body to fight off disease.

immunity The result of the immune system's prevention or limiting of infection by microorganisms (viruses, bacteria, fungi, parasites). Antibodies serve to neutralize toxins and microorganisms. Cell-mediated immunity fights bacteria, fungi, and parasites and is involved in killing of virus-infected cells and tumor cells. Immunity is induced when an individual is given a vaccine (immunization) or has exposure to the antigenic marker on an organism that invades the body.

A baby is born with certain innate immunities; acquired immunity results from development of active or passive immunity. In active immunity, there is production of antibodies (either after vaccination or after exposure to the disease) that fight infectious agents. Passive immunity occurs when a mother passes her fetus immunities through the placenta or through breast-milk. Cell-mediated immunity results from activation of sensitized T lymphocytes.

immunocompromised An immune system that is not functioning properly, with the result that an individual is more susceptible to disease.

immunodeficiency disorders In immunosuppression, the immune response either has been reduced or is entirely deficient. In a healthy individual, the immune system capably protects the body from toxins, cancer cells, microorganisms, and other elements. T and B lymphocytes are types of white blood cells. B lymphocytes are responsible for production of antibodies. T lymphocytes are responsible for cell-mediated immunity.

Immune system disorders are the result of failure of the immune system, which shuts down or semi–shuts down and becomes ineffective as a defense against invasion of harmful organisms or tumors. The person can be plagued with recurring infections, faulty response to treatment, opportunistic infections, and increased incidence of cancers such as non-Hodgkin's lymphoma and Kaposi's sarcoma. HIV patients, for example, can fall prey to opportunistic infections—the term for ordinarily controllable infections that can turn severe in those with a compromised immune system. To prevent immunodeficiency, a person can make a point of following a good nutrition regimen and using safe sex practices to prevent HIV transmission.

A person who does have an immunodeficiency disorder should avoid contact with people who have contagious diseases and avoid those who have had recent immunizations. If a disease is contracted, it must be treated aggressively. Preventive treatments may be necessary. In some cases, bone marrow transplantation is the best option for treating immunodeficiency disorders.

immunosuppression   The state in which the body's immune system is "downsized" in its ability to fight infection or disease. It is clear that individuals whose immune system is not functioning normally are at greater risk for development of disease.

The term *immunosuppressed* can apply to people who have immunodeficiency as a result of medications; this condition is desired when someone is being treated for disorders such as autoimmune disorders. Immunosuppression also results from chemotherapy, cancers, aging, and malnutrition. For example, a person may have a temporarily low white blood cell count after chemotherapy.

impotence   The inability of a male to have sexual intercourse; this may be caused by inability to have or sustain a hard erection for sexual intercourse, or it may be an ejaculatory dysfunction—in other words, the penis is erect and hard, and penetration does occur, but the man does not ejaculate semen. Impotence can be caused by a problem that is physical or psychological. There are a number of treatment options, and a man who frequently experiences impotence may want to seek medical evaluation so that he can look into the possibility of being treated.

impotent   A term sometimes used to describe the sexual function of a man who has problems with impotence. A man who is unable to get or keep an erection or unable to ejaculate semen over a period of time may be termed impotent. Often, however, impotence is simply a temporary problem that is related to illness or stress. Sometimes, though, it can be a long-term condition.

incontinence   A state in which an individual cannot control the bodily functions of defecation and/or urination (more often, the term is used to refer to the latter). In the context of sexually transmitted diseases, incontinence may be a problem for someone who is experiencing dementia related to AIDS. The human immunodeficiency virus can affect the brain in a way that diminishes the sensation of needing to void one's bladder. This can result in bedwetting, and eventually, loss of control of the bowel and bladder. Bedpans and adult diapers may prove necessary for people with advanced AIDS who do experience incontinence.

incubation period   The time span between when a person becomes infected and the first symptom of disease appears. This varies in sexually transmitted diseases. In herpes, for example, the first symptoms may show up a few days after infection or weeks later—or may not show up at all. In HIV, the first symptoms of an individual's weakened immune system often do not appear for several years. For the usual incubation period of a specific sexually transmitted disease, see the entry in this book on the disease.

infected sex partners   In the context of sexually transmitted diseases, it is important to know that any person who is sexually active may have clear intentions of staying healthy and consistently avoiding sexual contact with STD-infected sex partners. Unfortunately, however, all these good intentions can be futile when one confronts the reality one faces in being sexually active—and that is the silent nature of many diseases. It is clear that in the United States today, there are many people who are already infected with sexually transmitted diseases who have no knowledge of having an STD at all and, thus, have the potential to infect any sex partner with whom they have sexual contact.

A new partner with whom someone wants to be intimate may appear perfectly healthy and safe because he or she is symptom-free and has had no reason to seek medical evaluation. Granted, a new sex partner who says that he or she has always used condoms in every sexual contact is less likely to be infected with a sexually transmitted disease (if that person is telling the truth). Still, though, a sex partner's disease-free status cannot be considered 100 percent certain because most sexually transmitted diseases can sometimes be spread even when a condom is being used.

Thus, an excellent approach to safe sex is for an individual to insist on sexually transmitted disease testing of both partners before having sex or becoming physically intimate in any way. If the tests show that both people have no diseases, it is still wise to be retested in six months—it takes at least three months in most people for antibodies to register after an exposure to HIV. This is especially true in cases in which a partner (or both) can be considered at high risk; in that case a third HIV test should be considered at six to 12 months after a worrisome exposure (see HIGH-RISK). However, even if both parties prove to be free of STDs, each must remain careful and observant and use latex condoms consistently, because it may be impossible to be sure that the other person is not involved with other sex partners.

Also, in the interest of maintaining one's health, it is extremely important to be alert and after noting any rashes, sores, or discharge in a partner, to refrain from sexual contact until the health condition is evaluated by a doctor. Sometimes one partner who is starting an intimate relationship with another person does a visual sizing up of the other person's genitals, and perhaps can spot a problem before the individual himself or herself has noticed it.

If a sexually transmitted disease is diagnosed in a partner, a physician can start treatment and advise both partners as to when it would be safe to resume sexual activity, if that is the goal. In the case of herpes or HIV, both partners need counseling on how they can help prevent transmission of the disease to the uninfected partner. Certainly, it is not unusual at all for couples to deal with chronic sexually transmitted diseases and have normal sex lives apart from taking certain precautions.

Another scenario is the discovery of an infected partner after an individual has already begun a sexual relationship with that person. Either the information is purposely withheld and finally revealed or the disease is transmitted without the uninfected partner's ever knowing she or he was risking exposure. This kind of problem can be a major stumbling block in a relationship (and a major health issue for the newly infected person), and an infected partner with a chronic disease is far

wiser to discuss the matter early rather than after the fact.

infection An instance in which the body is invaded by microorganisms that go on to multiply and produce disease. When the person's immune system is functioning well, an infection is often fought off successfully by the automatic immune responses of a healthy immune system. Otherwise, in cases when the body does not succeed in fighting off infection, disease can thrive and spread. There are many possible symptoms of infection, which vary according to type of infection. Examples of symptoms of infection include fever, chills, sweating, diarrhea, cough, sore throat, and skin lesions.

For specific symptoms of sexually transmitted diseases, see Appendix VI.

infectious A state of an illness in which an infected person can infect another individual. Often, in the case of sexually transmitted diseases, people are infectious at times when they are not yet aware they have a disease. This is one factor that has made the spread of sexually transmitted diseases an enormous public health problem. It is a mistake to think that a person can know whether a sex partner has a disease simply by looking at the person or the genitals; often, sexually transmitted diseases have no obvious symptoms.

See information on each specific sexually transmitted disease in this book.

infectious mononucleosis An acute viral infection that causes fever, sore throat, and swollen lymph glands in the neck. Usually caused by the Epstein-Barr virus (EBV), infectious mononucleosis is typically transmitted by saliva exchange, which is why this disease is often called the "kissing disease." (A mononucleosislike disease also may be caused by the cytomegalovirus.) Commonly referred to as "mono," infectious mononucleosis can be transmitted via blood transfusion, too, but this route is relatively rare.

The age bracket of 10 to 35 years is the population group most often affected by mononucleosis; the majority of cases occur in people younger than 19. In some lower-income population groups, this disease is a common early childhood infection. Incubation period, from time of infection to development of infectious mononucleosis, is about five to seven weeks; children have a shorter incubation period.

When someone has infectious mononucleosis, typically it affects lymph nodes in the armpits, neck, and groin, and the symptoms last for a number of weeks. Most people have fever, sore throat, swollen lymph nodes, fatigue, and headaches, and some have an enlarged spleen. In the majority of those who have infectious mononucleosis, abnormal liver function test results are noted. For physicians, the hallmark trait of mononucleosis is a sore throat that becomes progressively worse, with enlarged tonsils that are covered in whitish yellow exudate. Some people have a pink rash that resembles that of measles.

People with symptoms of mononucleosis should see their health care providers as soon as possible. In particular, however, if someone experiences a sharp, sudden pain in the left upper abdomen, that individual needs to call 911 or ask someone to take him or her immediately to a local emergency room. (A doctor will perform emergency surgery if the problem is a ruptured spleen.)

The classic test for mononucleosis is the demonstration of heterophil antibodies. A rapid slide test (Monospot) uses the latex agglutination technique. The test is not accurate for children four years old or younger because false-negative results often occur. In those younger than age four, serologic testing is used to determine the presence of antibodies to EBV. About 90 percent of adults in the United States have EBV antibody.

While the individual with mononucleosis has an enlarged spleen, she or he should not take part in vigorous workouts or contact sports. Treatment for infectious mononucleosis includes recommendations for reduced activity, bed rest, and avoidance of contact sports and intense exercise for at least one month and until the person has seen the doctor for follow-up to confirm that the spleen is no longer enlarged. A person can take analgesics to relieve pain and fever and gargle with salt water for sore throat. Symptoms of mononucleosis usually subside over time—weeks

to several months. Four to six weeks is the norm. Fever should recede in a week or so, and the spleen and swollen lymph glands usually take about a month to normalize. In many mononucleosis sufferers, a tired feeling lingers for several months. As for measures to prevent contracting mononucleosis, people should avoid kissing or sharing utensils or drinks with those who have this infection because it is contagious and believed to be spread by saliva.

Complications are rare; they may include secondary throat infection, aplastic anemia, hemolytic anemia, rupture of the spleen, cranial nerve palsy, encephalitis, hepatitis with jaundice, Reye's syndrome, myocarditis, transient arrhythmias, upper airway obstruction, Guillain-Barré syndrome, and "Alice in Wonderland" syndrome, which is distortion of the sizes, shapes, and spatial relations of objects. Chronic Epstein-Barr virus infection has an association with several types of malignancy. Mononucleosis can even lead to death in those who are immunocompromised, but rarely in others. Children with X-linked lymphoproliferative syndrome often contract fatal infectious mononucleosis.

infertility   The inability to have children, a health condition that may arise from a physical problem that affects either partner. Most often, *infertility* is a term used to refer to a woman's inability to become pregnant and a man's inability to induce conception in a woman. There are many possible causes of infertility. A woman may be infertile as a result of obstruction of the fallopian tubes, lack of ovulation, or endometriosis. Infertility can result from prior pelvic inflammatory disease. A man may have semen that lacks sufficient motility or numbers of sperm; another possibility is an absence of sperm. Gonorrhea, which is a common cause of pelvic inflammatory disease in women, can also result in fertility problems in men who have had the infection in the past. There are several ways to treat infertility.

One of the potential solutions for infertility—in vitro fertilization—carries the very rare hazard of obtaining sperm from a source that does not screen for HIV properly and thus has the potential for transmission of the disease. This is very unlikely, of course, but anyone who is investigating the in vitro fertilization option should inquire about the particular facility's policies on screening of donor sperm and find out how the screeners make sure that any man who has donated sperm is not in an early stage of HIV (when testing cannot reveal his true HIV status).

inflammation   A condition that is characterized by redness, swelling, pain, and heat in bodily tissue as a result of infection or injury.

information   In the context of STDs, a person who wants to become engaged in sexual activity with a new partner may lack information on sex and may be entirely unaware of the need for a safe-sex discussion. Also, many people (young and old) are not at all sure what they can do with a sex partner that constitutes safe sex.

Many health agencies do disseminate tips and guidelines on preventing transmission of sexually transmitted diseases, but often this is general information that is not specific enough to be helpful. As a result, many people pick up misinformation about sex from magazines, friends, the Internet, and television. Furthermore, when everything related to sex is packaged in "sexy" wrapping, as is often done in our culture, it is easy for people to forget that unsafe sex is anything but sexy when it results in an unwanted pregnancy or a sexually transmitted disease.

Seeking good, reliable information can start with a sex education class at school, a physician, a parent, a church counselor, a teacher, or another person who is in a position to have correct information. The education process needs to start when children are very young (eight or nine), as soon as questions about sex arise and information is sought. Young people should be told about the option of abstinence—not having sex, usually until the individual marries and/or is older. A person who is sexually active, however, needs valid, practical information on protection from transmission or contracting of a sexually transmitted disease and on prevention of unwanted pregnancies.

informed consent   A legal requirement that a patient must give permission for a health care professional to perform a treatment, surgical procedure, or test. Informed consent can be given only after the person has been briefed on all risks and benefits of the procedure, test, or treatment and, typically, has signed documents to that effect.

inguinal   Relating to the groin.

insect bite   A bite on a person's skin that is inflicted by an insect. Lab research has shown that transmission of HIV or any other sexually transmitted disease by means of an insect is extremely unlikely because of the low levels of HIV in blood and the small amounts that can be ingested by insects such as mosquitoes. Experts consider the belief that HIV can be spread by insects "urban legend."

insurance   In respect to sexually transmitted diseases, health insurance is an especially important factor to consider because prolonged treatment is not unusual. Also, some proposed treatments for a disease such as HIV may be experimental and thus less likely to meet insurers' requirements for coverage. In the early days of the AIDS epidemic, many health insurers sought ways to avoid paying for diagnosis and treatment of their insured who had HIV or AIDS because it was clear that these people would require expensive and extensive treatment and health care. This quickly turned into a matter that was resolved in U.S. courtrooms; some patients had to sue to retain coverage when insurance companies sought to drop them after discovering their diagnosis. Ultimately, U.S. government agencies became more involved in regulating the insurance companies' practices, with the goal of ensuring fair treatment to all.

For a person facing a long-term disease such as HIV, the worry and anxiety concerning the expenses involved in years of treatment can be enormous. Expensive medical care is a given, and some experts estimate that medical care for a lifetime of fighting HIV could easily exceed $1 million for an individual.

Unfortunately for those who are fighting a sexually transmitted disease, medical care in the United States has become complex and unwieldy. An individual with HIV may have to finance his or her own care (self-pay), may qualify for a state or federal health program, or may have private health insurance coverage. Private insurance and public programs are all called third-party payers. Private payers are managed care groups and commercial insurance companies. Medicare, Medicaid, and the Veterans Administration are huge public third-party payers. A large number of those people receiving Medicaid are people with HIV or AIDS.

Most Americans who have insurance have a combination of self-pay and third-party insurance. Sometimes a person's insurance pays some of the costs and the individual is required to pay all of the fees that exceed the base that will be paid—or she or he may have to pay all costs for treatment options the insurance plan does not view as "approved." Third-party payers may not fully reimburse costs of some services for those who are suffering from HIV and AIDS. To receive public funds (state and government), a diagnosis of full-blown AIDS may be required.

In the realm of managed care, an individual may have a group plan or an individual plan of a third-party payer. An insurance company offers group plans to companies, which then offer the health insurance coverage to their employees. A person who has an individual plan is working directly with the third party, with no go-between; an example would be a self-employed person who buys his or her own health insurance. Typically, if a person is signing up for a group plan (when beginning a new job, for example), there is no physical examination or health-status inquiry required. A person with HIV who works for a company of that kind would automatically be covered along with everyone else who works for that company, but there may be a rule about any preexisting conditions, and there will usually be a waiting period of a few months before coverage kicks in.

A person may also find that a health insurance policy has limits on coverage. Often this means that the coverage is about 80 percent of hospital expenses and about 60 percent of physician expenses. After the insurer pays, the amount that is left over and not paid by the insurer must be paid by the individual. It is important to note, too, that there are limits to the lifetime coverage of a policy and a limit on the drug coverage, so a person with HIV may use up her or his entire coverage (or "cap") of a lifetime limit of $1 million and be left to foot the bills after that.

In the case of preferred provider organizations (PPOs), certain participating physicians agree to charge lower fees so that the cost is lower for the individual, and the insurance company saves money, too. The benefit of a PPO is that a patient does not need a referral in order to see a specialist.

The downside of HMOs is that they do not allow the patient a wide and liberal selection of physicians or hospitals; they provide a list of doctor and hospital choices. Further, a patient may need to obtain a referral from the primary care practitioner in order to see a specialist.

An individual who quits a job, is fired, or is a victim of company cutbacks can continue with the group plan that has covered him by taking advantage of a continuation-of-benefits federal law called the Consolidated Omnibus Budget Reconciliation Act (COBRA) of 1985, an option that must be offered if a company has more than 20 employees. The former employee pays the insurance premiums and is allowed to continue coverage for a period of up to 18 months, at his or her own expense. (If a person is terminated for "gross misconduct," COBRA may not apply, however.) Often, one's spouse and dependent children are also eligible for COBRA coverage, sometimes for up to three years. It is important to remember, though, that COBRA does not apply to individual plans that a person buys; once that coverage is lost, an extension via COBRA is not allowed.

Eligible for COBRA are employees or former employees (retirees) in private business, those employees' spouses, and their dependent children. The qualifying event for COBRA coverage can be any of the following: you quit your job; you were terminated from your job; or your hours were reduced. In all of these instances, maximum coverage would be for 18 months. Qualifying events for a spouse and dependent children of someone who was granted COBRA are that the employee is entitled to Medicare, that there was a divorce or legal separation, or that the employee died. In all of these instances, the coverage can last for up to 36 months. If a dependent child loses dependent-child status, he or she qualifies for COBRA for up to 36 months. Note: no one has to take advantage of COBRA; also, a spouse or child may enroll in COBRA even if the employee herself or himself decides to forgo coverage by COBRA.

The COBRA eligibility umbrella extends to state and local governmental workers and workers who are classified as "independent contractors." The law exempts, however, the District of Columbia, federal employees, some church groups, and firms that employ fewer than 20. Check on individual state laws that are known as mini-COBRA. COBRA coverage ends when premiums are not paid on a timely basis, the term of maximal coverage ends, the employer stops maintaining a group health plan, the employer goes out of business, a beneficiary is entitled to Medicare, or an individual gets coverage via another employer group health plan that does not contain exclusion or limitation with respect to preexisting conditions of a beneficiary. Being eligible under a spouse's group health plan does not count.

A person who does choose to continue health insurance under COBRA usually finds that the premiums are steep. The employer no longer pays for part of the premiums, and the individual also must pay an administrative fee of up to 2 percent.

To get COBRA instituted, a person must follow the rules. An employer must notify the health plan administrator within 30 days after a death, job termination, reduction in hours, or Medicare eligibility. The family has the responsibility to notify the health plan administrator within 60 days of the event in cases of divorce, legal marital separation, or a child's loss of independent status. Then, after the notification, the plan administrator must alert the employee and family within 14 days about the right to continue coverage via COBRA. This can take place by mail or in person. An administrator who does not do this can be held personally liable for breaching duties, but he or she must have in hand the person's correct mailing address.

An employee, the spouse, and children have 60 days to decide whether they will go the COBRA route. This period begins on the date a person was notified of eligibility or the date health coverage ended. Even a person who waives the right to COBRA can change his or her mind during the election period. Also, a health plan can be extended beyond the specified COBRA period if the insurer wants to offer that option.

If a person relocates out of the COBRA health plan's coverage area, the COBRA benefits are lost, and the employer is not required to offer a plan in the new location. It is important to remember that neither the health plan office staff nor the employer is required to send a notice that the premium is due, so it is important to record due dates on a monthly planner. Those who are eligible for Social Security Disability benefits may receive COBRA coverage for 29 months.

Unrelated to the COBRA issue, if someone decides to apply for an individual health insurance plan that is offered by a third-party payer, he or she can opt for a large deductible ($1,000, for example) to keep the monthly fee lower. Sometimes, these plans deny coverage by deeming applicants uninsurable, meaning that they have medical risks that are unacceptable. These are individuals who have diabetes, HIV/AIDS, cancer, and heart disease. Typically, an applicant is asked to take a medical exam and provide a detailed medical history and is required to report any existing diseases that have been diagnosed, such as HIV/AIDS. Previous medical records are requested, and these records will include HIV status. In some states, an HIV test is required.

Insurers try to pinpoint any preexisting medical conditions, which are those for which a person has received medical advice or treatment from a physician in the last five years. There are preexisting conditions that do not prevent insurers from accepting an applicant. In the case of HIV, a person who tests positive for HIV but is asymptomatic does not, according to insurance definition, have a preexisting condition. However, these people with HIV are still unlikely to be approved for individual policies. Insurers can reject a person completely or offer to cover her or him while excluding the coverage of all treatments and diagnostic measures related to the preexisting condition. For specific information, refer to your policy or contact an insurance representative. Those who are denied health insurance because they are deemed to be in an "unacceptable risk" category can buy insurance at very high prices from a state's high-risk insurance pool, available in some states, or take advantage of insurance companies' "open enrollment" for high premiums.

Note: before you decide not to opt for COBRA or buy any health insurance at all, consider that a gap in insurance coverage of more than 63 days (in the United States) causes a loss of health insurance rights. Under the federal Health Insurance Portability and Accountability Act, it is guaranteed that anyone who has continuous group health coverage without a gap of more than 63 days cannot be denied group health insurance even if that person has a preexisting condition such as HIV-positive status. Another insurance issue that relates to STDs and, in particular, HIV/AIDS, is life insurance. A person who wants to apply for life insurance is administered a health exam, which invariably includes an HIV/AIDS test.

See also MEDICAID; MEDICARE.

intercourse   See SEXUAL INTERCOURSE.

interferon   This antiviral protein that can modulate a person's immune response has come into play in various arenas, from treatment of some cancers, to use in eradicating genital warts, to treatment for Kaposi's sarcoma. Interferons are made by the body when cells are stimulated by a virus and other agents, they can also be genetically engineered. The three main groups are alpha-interferon, beta-interferon, and gamma-interferon. All have been synthesized.

Studies are under way to gauge their effectiveness in treating HIV and AIDS. It is known that interferons have antitumor activity and can stifle nonviral parasites' growth in cells. The FDA has approved a manufactured alpha-interferon for treatment of Kaposi's sarcoma, hepatitis B virus, and hepatitis C virus.

interleukin   Any of several compounds produced by lymphocytes, monocytes, and macrophages that help regulate the immune system. Interleukin-2 (IL-2) is a compound produced by helper T cells that causes proliferation of immune cells. It has been tested in various doses and regimens as a way to boost the immune system of those with HIV. Experience has generally been limited to use in experimental protocols, and as of October 2001, IL-2 had not moved into standard therapies.

Some researchers believe that interleukin-2 may augment the immune response in individuals with HIV. Highly active antiretroviral therapy (HAART) suppresses replication of HIV, but it does not promote rapid restoration of normal immunoreactivity, nor does it eliminate the pool of residual latent proviral DNA. That characteristic has led to a search for ways to accelerate recovery of the immune system, treatments that can purge the latent viral reservoir—or maintain viral latency and thus allow discontinuation of antiviral drugs.

interstitial pneumonia   An acute inflammation that involves the connective tissues of the lung. Of interest in respect to sexually transmitted diseases is the fact that when a child below age 13 is diagnosed with interstitial pneumonia, this diagnosis suggests the presence of the AIDS virus in his or her body.

intervention   An action of someone who seeks to advocate for, help, or advise a person who has an STD or is at risk for one. Health care professionals seek to make their intervention efforts serve as long-term advocacy for reducing high-risk activities with high-risk and/or multiple partners. Forms of intervention include those involving families, one-on-one efforts, and community programs. The goals are to educate the individual(s) in question and promote the idea of changing behavior to reduce the likelihood of contracting diseases. Public health agencies, private health facilities, hospitals, and the media often partner in trying to disseminate messages of health interest to target audiences—the sexually active public.

intrapartum transmission The transmission of a sexually transmitted disease during childbirth or delivery.

intrauterine device (IUD) A device that a doctor inserts into a woman's uterus for contraception; it is not intended to prevent sexually transmitted diseases.

intravenous drug user An individual who injects drugs into the body for a purpose that is not medicinal (probably recreational). When people share their drug paraphernalia such as needles and syringes, they put themselves and perhaps others at risk for contracting viruses such as HIV or hepatitis. Viruses can be transmitted to other people through the contaminated blood that is still in the syringe or the needle. IV drug users continue to have a huge role in spreading HIV.

introitus The entrance to a hollow organ or body cavity, such as the vaginal introitus.

investigation The process of looking at drugs for possible use in treating various diseases.

Investigational New Drug Program A U.S. program that investigates new experimental drugs. Investigational New Drug (IND) is a Food and Drug Administration–approved program that is pivotal in some physicians' treatment regimens because they can procure a drug that they believe will help gravely ill patients and, in exchange, provide feedback data on the drug. The idea is to allow use of promising drugs as early as possible, in order to benefit patients who are in need of the drug therapy. Sometimes after researchers can declare a drug safe and likely to be effective, it is granted IND status before final approval and completion of paperwork, so that doctors can use it. In the era of fast-changing treatments for HIV and AIDS, the Investigational New Drug Program has become extremely important because of the urgency physicians feel in their roles as health care givers who may be able to help HIV-positive patients extend life. Finding new ways to squelch the stealthy invasion of HIV via drug therapy continues to be a much-discussed topic in health care circles and at international conferences on HIV and AIDS.

in vitro fertilization Fertilization of an ovum (an egg) outside the body—in vitro fertilization—in a procedure that is done because a woman has blocked fallopian tubes or there is some other reason that the sperm and ovum cannot be united successfully in the reproductive tract. In the realm of sexually transmitted diseases, it is important for a woman who is receiving donor sperm to make sure that it has been screened and rescreened for HIV.

In the procedure of in vitro fertilization, the woman undergoes hormone therapy so that several ova will mature at the same time. The ova are mixed with sperm from a partner and incubated in a culture medium until the blastocyst is formed. The blastocyst is then implanted in the mother-to-be's uterus, and the pregnancy proceeds normally. The person who donates the sperm may be the woman's husband, a friend, a life partner, or an anonymous donor.

irregular bleeding Bleeding between a woman's menstrual periods and after intercourse can be the result of an inflamed or irritated cervix. This can happen when there is an infection such as mucopurulent cervicitis, herpes, trichomoniasis, gonorrhea, or chlamydia. Vaginal infections and pelvic inflammatory disease can also cause spotting between periods. Other conditions that can result in irregular vaginal bleeding are menopause, pregnancy, fibroids, uterine cancer, bleeding disorders, anovulation, and starting of birth-control pills.

Jarisch–Herxheimer reaction   A worsening of symptoms (visual and neurologic) of patients with syphilis that can occur immediately after the inception of antibiotic therapy. Symptoms are mild fever, malaise, headache, muscle aches, and chills. Some believe that the symptoms result when killed organisms release a fever-producing enzyme. It most commonly occurs in early syphilis but has also been seen in all phases of syphilis and with therapies other than penicillin.

jaundice   A medical condition that manifests itself in yellow skin and eyes, as a result of excess bilirubin in the blood and body tissues. The disorder that results when bile made in the liver does not reach the intestine because of bile-duct obstruction is termed *obstructive jaundice*. Diseased liver cells (as in hepatitis) impair the body's ability to get rid of bilirubin, resulting in excess bilirubin in the blood, and this condition is called hepato-cellular jaundice. Excessive destruction of red cells in the blood leads to hemolytic jaundice. In several sexually transmitted diseases, such as hepatitis, jaundice is a symptom.

Johnson, Magic   In 1991, the basketball great Earvin "Magic" Johnson announced to the world in a televised news conference that he had con-tracted HIV through heterosexual sex. In the years subsequent to his startling announcement, how-ever, he has gone on to live a vital life, complete with TV sports commentary, intense workouts, and the appearance of exuberant health. Clearly, he stands out as a prime example of the benefits of HIV drug therapy. His wife and his son, who was conceived shortly before Johnson's announce-ment, are both HIV-negative.

Kaposi's sarcoma   A rare cancer, Kaposi's sarcoma occurs in the United States almost exclusively in people who have AIDS. It is common in Africa.

Kaposi's sarcoma is a malignant tumor that arises from blood vessels in the skin and is manifested in purple to brown nodules or blotches. The purple blotches proliferate and also can appear on internal organs. Kaposi's sarcoma in the lungs can cause pulmonary fluid buildup and obstruct airways and sometimes can cause bleeding and breathing difficulties. When lymph tissues are involved, the disease can spread quickly to other organs and devastate the person's health.

This is a cancer that evolves slowly and also one that is a hallmark of AIDS. Evidence suggests that Kaposi's sarcoma is virus-caused (herpesvirus 8). The *New England Journal of Medicine* reported that herpesvirus 8, once thought to be transmitted through sexual intercourse, can also be spread by kissing. Early research suggested that oral–anal sexual activity can heighten a man's chance of development of Kaposi's sarcoma. In a test of 39 gay men who did not have Kaposi's sarcoma but did have herpes, researchers found herpesvirus 8 in 30 percent of saliva samples and mouth swabs and only 1 percent of anal and genital samples. Virus levels found were also higher in the saliva than in the semen. Men who reported they had deep-kissed, exchanging saliva, were shown to be at higher risk of contracting the virus. This finding points to the fact that safe sex (condom use) helps prevent other sexually transmitted diseases but perhaps not herpesvirus 8. A high percentage of HIV-positive people who contract herpesvirus 8 eventually get Kaposi's sarcoma. Diagnosis is confirmed when a doctor biopsies the nodules.

Treatment modalities have not proved very successful. Often doctors use radiation or interferon to treat nodules that are painful or swollen. Lesions can be treated by cryotherapy. When these nodules spread widely and enter internal organs, a doctor can prescribe cancer drugs. Typically, treatment for AIDS-related Kaposi's sarcoma can relieve the pain of lesions, but no cure is available. Also, no one with this sarcoma should expect the treatment for Kaposi's to ensure a longer life.

Sometimes a doctor treats a person with fewer than 20 lesions with cryotherapy, surgical excision, or electrodesiccation. Use of one of these treatments can improve the appearance of the individual, potentially enhancing his sense of well-being and making him less likely to become homebound. In most cases, a patient with KS gets a single chemotherapy drug in the early stages of the cancer, and when it grows to an advanced stage, the physician tries chemotherapy drug combinations.

Disseminated Kaposi's sarcoma is characterized by presence of 25 or more lesions, appearance of 10 new lesions monthly, CD4 count below 200 cells/mm3, and spread of lesions to the lungs or stomach. At this advanced stage, a patient may benefit from systemic chemotherapy.

On the other hand, intralesional chemotherapy is the treatment of choice when there are a small number of lesions in the mouth. This form of chemotherapy, confined to the lesion (not a vein), does not infiltrate the person's entire system, affecting organs and tissues. Some Kaposi's sarcoma patients' tumors of the skin, anus, or mouth can be improved greatly by low-dose external irradiation—primarily for the lesions that are very visible. This may amount to one-session therapy or several treatments over a period of weeks. Some doctors prefer to use radiation because it produces less scarring than surgery does.

The major problem is that Kaposi's sarcoma lesions are usually widespread, and when one is minimized, another can pop up elsewhere. A relatively recent discovery by researchers is the finding that placing active molecules of some drugs into liposomes (protective globules made of fats) can make side effects less severe and make drugs more effective, causing them to settle into the lesions and act similarly to time-release treatment.

The Centers for Disease Control and Prevention found that AIDS patients who are treated with foscarnet (for any reason)—a medication that works against viruses such as the herpesvirus often found in KS lesions—usually are much less likely to develop Kaposi's sarcoma than are those who are not on this drug. Doctors who have tried using high doses of interferons also report improvements in patients with KS. Antiretroviral drugs, especially zidovudine (known as AZT), help, too. One study showed that patients who went into remission while taking antiretroviral drugs did not need to continue systemic chemotherapy for KS.

In *Science* (April 2001), Harvard researchers reported findings that suggest that cell-to-cell spread of the herpesvirus that leads to Kaposi's sarcoma can be stopped by blocking the action of one protein. This could lead to treatments for Kaposi's sarcoma, which is usually a very aggressive disease in AIDS patients. Investigators note that DNA from Kaposi's sarcoma–associated herpesvirus (KSHV) is found in most lesions related to KS. The study shows that a protein called latency-associated nuclear antigen (LANA) is also found in tumors infected with KSHV. Researchers found that LANA helps connect viral DNA to the infected cell's chromosomes during cell division, thereby smoothing the way for Kaposi's sarcoma–associated herpesvirus to enter new tumor cells. Hence, strategies that halt the process could possibly prevent and treat diseases the virus causes.

Kennedy–Cranston Amendment   The Kennedy–Cranston Amendment diluted the Helms Amendment, a controversial piece of legislation that nixed the idea of using federal funds to "promote or encourage, directly, homosexual sexual activities," and established a rule that all sex education materials had to put emphasis on sexual abstinence outside heterosexual marriage as well as nonuse of drugs. In 1988, it was replaced by the Kennedy-Cranston Amendment, a compromise that was advanced by Senators Edward Kennedy and Alan Cranston; it forbade using federal funds to promote or directly encourage IV drug abuse or homosexual or heterosexual activity.

kissing   Sometimes implicated in discussions of sexually transmitted diseases, deep kisses or French kisses actually have a very low risk of transmitting HIV. HIV in very small amounts has been found in saliva, but bleeding gums are the bigger problem because of the danger that contaminated blood will move from one partner's mouth to another's. Ordinary kisses that are virtual "pecks," however, do not pose a risk because no saliva or body fluid is exchanged. On the other hand, kissing of body parts that results in contact with vaginal secretions, semen, or fecal matter does carry the risk of contracting HIV. Also, one should not kiss an individual who has an infection such as mononucleosis, which can be transmitted by saliva.

Lactobacillus acidophilus   See ACIDOPHILUS.

lambskin condom   Condom whose use is not advisable for those seeking protection against sexually transmitted diseases because it does not provide such protection. This condom does, however, give some degree of protection against pregnancy.

laryngeal papilloma   A growth in the larynx (which contains the vocal cords) that is caused by a human papillomavirus strain. A mother who has genital warts when her child is born may possibly pass the virus to her baby; transmission may result in warts on the larynx or elsewhere. Laryngeal warts can be treated but can be very serious in children. The best approach is to treat the warts before birth so that they are not a factor during delivery. Even when an infected woman has a cesarean section, there is a risk of development of warts on her infant's larynx. It is important to note that mother-to-child transmission of human papillomavirus is very rare. Research indicates that the occurrence of laryngeal cancer is associated with certain strains of human papillomavirus.

laser surgery   The use of light beams with highly concentrated energies for various kinds of treatment. It can be used to operate on small areas of abnormality without damaging surrounding tissue. This approach is believed to have some advantages over traditional surgical procedures in that a laser light can be extremely precise, is noninvasive, and results in less swelling. The downside is that much of the success of laser surgery is dependent on the particular physician's skill, so it is extremely important to choose an experienced and talented doctor.

latency   A time during which a disease does not manifest itself in symptoms, although it has already been contracted. Herpes simplex virus is often triggered (and becomes symptomatic) during times of immune-system stressors and remains latent between outbreaks. HIV is often latent clinically in early years, so the infected individual thus does not have symptoms at that time.

latex allergy   An allergy that is a concern in respect to sexually transmitted diseases because condoms are made of latex, as are doctors' usual protective gloves. Sensitivity to latex can produce a wide range of reactions, from rashes to severe reactions (anaphylactic shock).

legal issues   It is important to note that in the realm of legal issues, those regarding authorization of medical treatment for young people present significant considerations. In Texas, for example, the legal definition of an adult is an individual who is age 18 or older, married, emancipated via court order if 16 or 17 years old, living apart from parents, or managing his or her own finances.

According to various state legal codes, a minor may consent to treatment in various situations, such as being on active duty with armed services or living apart from parents and managing her or his own finances. A minor can also legally consent to treatment for any infectious, contagious, or communicable disease that a physician is required by law to report; for hospital, medical, or surgical treatment if she is unmarried and pregnant; for drug addiction, dependency, or any condition directly related to drug use; and for hospital, medical, dental, psychological, or surgical treatment of his or her own biological child. A minor usually can consent to counseling that is related to sexual, physical, or emotional abuse; chemical addiction or dependency; and suicide prevention.

See Appendix V for a list of all states' rulings on minors' right to consent to HIV/STD services.

lentivirus   A family of retroviruses that includes human immunodeficiency virus (HIV). Escaping the body's natural defenses, lentiviruses can exist for long periods subclinically so that the person remains symptom-free. As a lentivirus, HIV is able to invade the brain and cause mental incapacity in some people who have HIV and AIDS.

lesbian health care   Human immunodeficiency virus (HIV) was initially viewed as a disease that was not transmitted woman to woman, but eventually it became clear that this disease could be spread from one lesbian (a woman who has sex with a woman) to another. Although lesbians' risk of contracting HIV in this manner is lower than in heterosexual activity, lesbians at higher risk are those who share needles and IV drug equipment, those who also have intercourse (anal or vaginal) with men who are bisexual, women with multiple partners, women who have sex with partners who use IV drugs or with hemophiliacs, women who received blood transfusions or blood products between the years 1979 and 1985, lesbians who have used semen for donor insemination from a donor of unknown risk status or high-risk status, and women who have used needles in unsafe ways for body piercing and tattooing.

Recommendations for lesbians that will reduce their probability of contracting HIV or other sexually transmitted diseases are the following: avoidance of contact that allows entry into the body of the other's vaginal fluids or blood via the mouth, anus, vagina, or a skin abrasion or cut; practicing of safe sex by using surgical gloves for penetration; vigilance in changing gloves between instances of anal and vaginal penetration; consistent use of latex or plastic barriers during oral sex and rimming; special caution used during times when either partner is having a menstrual period; avoidance of sharing of sex toys without thorough cleaning

between uses or using a new condom; avoidance of sadomasochistic activities that result in blood-letting; and avoidance of needle sharing.

lesion   A skin abnormality such as a bump, sore, or skin break.

leukoplakia   A condition in which white patches that cannot be scraped off appear on mucous membranes, typically of the mouth or vulva. These are generally considered precancerous and can become malignant.

Hairy leukoplakia is a viral lesion that primarily affects the lateral margins of the tongue. Both Epstein-Barr virus and human papillomavirus have been isolated from these furrowed lesions. As one of the hallmark signs of HIV, hairy leukoplakia alerts a health care provider that the individual being examined should be tested for HIV.

LGV   See LYMPHOGRANULOMA VENEREUM.

lifestyle   An umbrella term that encompasses a person's socioeconomic status, family particulars, sexual proclivity, and health, spiritual, personal, professional, and recreational priorities. Sexually transmitted diseases are most often seen in individuals whose lifestyle includes disuse (occasional or always) of safe-sex practices, numerous sexual partners, drug use, partners who have unknown or high-risk practices, and/or partners whose HIV and other STD status is unknown. Those who do contract sexually transmitted diseases often discover that their course of disease can be improved considerably by instituting and following a healthy lifestyle that features a good dietary regimen, an exercise program, and outlets for maintaining a sense of well-being.

lipodystrophy   A disturbance of fat metabolism or the distribution of fat in the body—a condition that may be found in people with HIV, many of whom suffer from facial atrophy. One of the newest treatments is the use of facial implantation in HIV patients who have lipodystrophy; polymethylmethacrylate (PMMA) implants have been shown to be safe and well tolerated. Also, these implants have had a beneficial effect on people's lives and well-being.

Marcio Serra, M.D., of CTA-AIDS/CREMERJ, Rio de Janeiro, Brazil, presented study results on July 11, 2002, during the XIV International AIDS Conference (AIDS 2002). The 184 people in the study were undergoing antiretroviral drug therapy for HIV. Results showed that PMMA implantation was easily done, had excellent cosmetic results, and lasted up to 36 months, compared to the lower and more varied levels of success in using facial implantation of collagen and polylactic acid to remedy lipodystrophy in HIV patients.

living will A document that records a person's wishes concerning whether artificial life support should be administered if he or she were in a condition of impending death. Not all states recognize living wills as legal documents.

living with herpes Information is power when it comes to dealing with genital herpes. After the initial shock of being diagnosed with herpes, people often find it helpful to arm themselves with knowledge. However, it is important to weigh the validity of sources one consults because, as is true of many diseases and conditions, far too many misconceptions and myths are disseminated.

The best course of action is talking to a physician and reading recently published books—those that are more likely to have up-to-date information. As far as the Internet goes, look for articles by physicians who are specialists in treating sexually transmitted diseases. For emotional support, many people with herpes have benefited from support groups and counselors.

A herpes-infected person needs to be aware of the legal repercussions of disease transmission. Disclosure of one's infection to all partners is generally considered to be the duty of a person with herpes. In some cases, individuals can be sued for transmitting the disease to a partner. Basically, there are three causes of action concerning the transmission of a sexually transmitted disease: misrepresentation (a person tells a new partner that he or she is

disease-free or not contagious, although he or she actually does not know whether he or she is shedding virus but does know that he or she has genital herpes), negligence (the infected partner's responsibility is to tell a partner that he or she is infected or to refrain from sexual activity), and battery (sexual contact that is intentional and harmful). However, it is difficult to prove in court that a certain person gave another genital herpes, because pinpointing of the exact time of transmission is problematic. There have been successful lawsuits in regard to transmission of herpes.

As far as health insurance goes, one must determine whether her or his health insurance carrier will consider herpes a "preexisting condition," because, if it is, that probably means that insurance claims in regard to treatment or care for herpes will not be covered.

living with HIV/AIDS A diagnosis of HIV or AIDS affects a person's body, mind, emotions, and relationships with others, and sometimes it even affects a job and legal and financial affairs. The course of HIV infection can vary, but it usually goes like this: an acute infection that is mononucleosis-like simply clears up in a few weeks. That is followed by a long period during which the HIV-infected individual feels good and is symptom-free. Next, the person has symptoms; finally, the disease progresses to full-blown AIDS, the markers of which are low numbers of the immune cells infected by HIV and/or opportunistic infections. The months or years an individual spends in each stage vary greatly, depending on mode of treatment, effectiveness of treatment, how early in the disease treatment was initiated, individual immune system and genetic characteristics, and the person's general health.

The effect of HIV on relationships also varies widely from person to person. Some HIV-infected individuals are fortunate enough to be surrounded by loving and supportive friends, family, and partners. Others are ravaged by isolation, worry, and feelings of helplessness and doom. Most people worry a great deal about how the disclosure of HIV infection will affect relationships with their children and their sexual partners. They are often concerned that an HIV diagnosis marks an end to their sexuality. Self-doubt may plague the individual who is going through the early days of coming to grips with an HIV diagnosis.

When HIV-infected parents tell their children that they have this disease, the youngsters usually need a great deal of support because they must deal with their own issues of feeling betrayed or abandoned and wondering who will care for them if the parent dies. Parents should consider the provisions they will make for their children in the event of death, so that this information can be shared.

The medical care of a person with HIV is a complicated picture, and there is a great deal of information to absorb. Still, the person with HIV should seek to be well informed and to know when a certain condition actually requires medical attention. Finding a doctor who specializes in taking care of HIV/AIDS patients is extremely helpful in that the patient will receive good advice and treatment, and a specialist stays abreast of all the latest developments in drug therapy, which are ever-changing and frequently upgraded. Dental care is another area in which a dentist who deals with HIV/AIDS patients should be an HIV-infected individual's first choice. These people usually have the compassion to approach dealing with saliva without making the patient feel like a pariah. Some dentists exhibit an overblown fear of contracting the disease, and this kind of dental office is not a pleasant place to be treated for the individual with HIV. Furthermore, HIV/AIDS specialist–dentists are good at treating the various diseases of the teeth and supporting structures that often plague people with this disease.

As for making a living, many who are HIV-positive find that staying in the workplace is usually best, especially when they have no symptoms, because maintaining a degree of normalcy helps greatly. Often the HIV-infected individual leaves a job when fatigue makes it impossible to continue.

To keep mental health problems at bay, people with HIV/AIDS can usually benefit from resources such as social workers, psychologists, and psychiatrists. AIDS-advocacy organizations can recommend good doctors.

In the years before progression of the disease to AIDS, few people have mental changes that are truly indicative of dementia. Being "at a loss for words" and having difficulty concentrating are very frightening to people with HIV, because they immediately associate these problems with HIV-associated dementia, which typically occurs only in the late stages of AIDS. A person who does have dementia experiences marked changes in attitude, usually characterized by extreme apathy, and changes in muscle control and mental acuity. Usually, days of sharpness alternate with days of slower mental processing of input. Also, an unsteady gait is a sign of HIV-associated dementia. The degree of impairment associated with dementia linked to AIDS varies widely: some people are affected in very minor ways, and others are hit severely.

Other aspects of living with HIV are taking a look at practical issues and attending to these while a patient still has the mental edge to do so. Knowing one's legal rights, understanding how to pay for medical care and how the government can help in this respect, and putting one's affairs in order all help a person with HIV feel more control over his or her fate and less helpless. A few of the many issues that need attention are understanding what insurance covers and what other options are available, how to assign power of attorney, and how to create a living will.

living with people with HIV   See HOME CARE in Appendix III.

low-risk sex   Those sexual practices that carry a low risk (but not zero risk) of contracting sexually transmitted diseases. Sexual intercourse with condoms falls into this category, as does mutual masturbation. However, the only route that has zero risk is abstinence (not having sex).

lymphadenopathy   The enlargement of lymph nodes (lymph glands). Infection or cancer can cause this condition of the lymph nodes. In some people, this is an early symptom of HIV infection. However, many medical conditions, such as infectious mononucleosis, also can cause swollen glands.

lymph nodes   Rounded masses of tissue composed of small groups of cells in the immune system that cluster in various body sites—such as the groin and under the arms. In infection or malignancy, lymph nodes can enlarge.

lymphogranuloma venereum   A sexually transmitted disease that is very rare in the United States but common in Asia, Africa, and South America. It is caused by a very virulent strain of *Chlamydia trachomatis.* Other types of the bacterium are causes of chlamydia infections. In the United States, lymphogranuloma venereum is often a result of an American having unprotected sex with an infected person in another country during travel.

The usual sign is a papule (a small bump), blister, or ulcer that appears in the genital area or on the cervix about a week to three weeks after exposure. Often the person does not even notice it. About a week or so later, painful enlarged lymph nodes develop on one side of the groin. At this time, the inflamed lymph nodes may rupture and drain pus or form chronic draining sinuses. The patient usually has fever, chills, and/or a rash. If there is anorectal node involvement, the person may have rectal strictures. This is one sexually transmitted disease in which men are more likely to have symptoms than are women.

A woman's cervix may be inflamed and infected. Oral sex with an infected person can result in mouth ulcers and lymph node enlargement in the neck. In some cases, rectal scarring can block stool passage.

A blood test checks for antibodies, and the doctor will probably screen for other sexually transmitted diseases. It is important to remember that HIV is transmitted more easily when someone has lymphogranuloma venereum because of the open sore in the genital area. Antibiotics such as doxycycline and erythromycin are used to treat lymphogranuloma venereum. The medication must be taken for 21 days, and sometimes rectal infection requires retreatment. A doctor may have to drain lymph nodes surgically. Any person who has had sex with an infected person within 30 days of becoming symptomatic should be treated with antibiotics, also, and tested for other sexually transmitted diseases. Condoms can be used to decrease risk of transmission of lymphogranuloma venereum. It is also spread from mother to child at birth.

major STDs   Major sexually transmitted diseases include chlamydia, gonorrhea, syphilis, genital herpes, genital warts, and HIV/AIDS.

malignancy   In cancer, the disease state in which cells grow in an unregulated way and can metastasize (spread) to other organs and parts of the body.

malnutrition   A condition in which an individual has a disordered state of nutrition—typically, a lack of food substances needed to sustain the body fully. Signs of malnutrition include sores in the corners of the mouth, bleeding gums, atrophy of the tongue, muscle soreness and lack of muscle tone, nonspecific vaginitis, corneal vascularization, skin rash, and thickening and pigmentation of skin. Researchers report that malnutrition is often a major problem in HIV because deficiencies set in early on and tend to influence the course of disease progression.

managed care   A health care system that manages health care delivery to control costs; this type of system relies on a primary care physician, who acts as gatekeeper, making decisions about when to refer patients to specialists. Those who want to sign up for a managed care program, usually one that was selected by an employer, should make themselves aware of the conditions concerning "preexisting" conditions and illnesses and determine whether the policy will cover any treatments that are needed for an existing sexually transmitted disease. In many instances, managed care programs have shown a reluctance to cover those patients they consider high-risk, such as people with HIV and AIDS. One of the major downsides of managed care is that those who administer the programs and make decisions are slow to accept various "new treatments" and even more reluctant to cover expenses for these. This may mean that HIV patients' access to treatment is limited even when their doctors want them to have access to expensive treatment modalities that could be beneficial and possibly life-extending. When the insured person is forced to pursue the matter through legal appeals, a court decision may be reached too late for someone who is fighting a terminal disease.

management of penicillin-allergic patients   In respect to sexually transmitted diseases, there are no proven good alternatives to penicillin available for treating neurosyphilis, congenital syphilis, or syphilis in pregnant women. Penicillin is also recommended for HIV-infected patients. However, in the United States, about 3 to 10 percent of the adult population, according to *Morbidity and Mortality Weekly Report* (January 23, 1998), have had responses such as upper airway obstruction, bronchospasm, and low blood pressure in reaction to penicillin therapy. If these patients receive penicillin again, they may have severe immediate reactions. Because anaphylactic reactions to penicillin can be fatal, health care providers are careful to avoid giving penicillin to those who are allergic to it, unless the sensitivity to penicillin has been removed by desensitization.

About 10 percent of those who report a history of severe allergic reactions to penicillin continue to be allergic; others, after some time has passed since their allergic reactions, may stop expressing penicillin-specific immunoglobulin E (IgE). Then they can be treated with penicillin. Studies show that skin testing with major and minor determinants can identify persons at high risk for penicillin reactions. Although these reagents are available in academia, the only ones available commercially are penicillin G and major determinant Pre-Pen. Experts estimate that testing with only the major determinant and penicillin G will identify 90 to 97 percent of patients with existing allergy. But skin testing without the minor determinants would still miss 3 to 10 percent of allergic patients, and serious or fatal reactions can occur among these minor-determinant-positive people. Hence, people should proceed with caution when the full battery of skin-test reagents is not available. Skin-test-positive people should be desensitized by means of a relatively safe procedure that is done orally or intravenously. Oral desensitization appears to be safer and easier. Desensitization should take place in a hospital setting in case an allergic reaction does occur, although this possibility is unlikely. The process takes about four hours and is followed by a dose of penicillin. Sexually transmitted disease programs should send patients to a referral center for desensitization.

mandatory reporting   A physician's legal obligation to inform health authorities when he or she diagnoses certain illnesses. In all of the United States, reporting of AIDS is required. State and national requirements vary as to which diseases must be reported.

See also NOTIFIABLE DISEASES.

mandatory testing   Any form of medical testing that is legally required. Some government agencies have mandatory testing policies for AIDS. Mandatory testing of pregnant women for certain sexually transmitted diseases has been widely recommended because treatment of the mother can often prevent transfer of the infection to the newborn.

manicure   The act or actions of nail styling or painting that involve cuticle trimming and shaping. Any cuts that occur during a manicure have the potential to provide an avenue for transfer of HIV infection from manicurist to client, or vice versa, because a person may be exposed to contaminated blood and thus have HIV infection transmitted. Infection is very unlikely by this route but is within the realm of possibility.

manmade HIV theory   A theory offered by Jakob Segal that HIV was created from a sheep virus (visna) and human T-cell leukemia virus (HTLV-1) by U.S. Army research labs in 1977 or 1978. Supposedly, the virus escaped accidentally after it was tested on prisoners. Robert Strecker has proposed another theory—that HIV was created from visna and bovine leukemia virus by the United States in the 1970s after about three decades of work on it. It was Strecker's theory that the virus was tested on African populations and then deliberately introduced into the United States gay population via the hepatitis B vaccination program. Evidence advanced to support this theory is that visna is very similar to HIV, and that although HIV is not similar to primate viruses, it can be formed by combining the genes of visna and bovine leukemia virus or human T cell lymphotropic virus. Supposedly, the government was working on biological warfare and wanted to manufacture an immune system–ravaging virus. An excerpt from congressional records is cited to support the premise (DOD Appropriations for 1970 Hearings, 91st Congress, Part 6, page 129):

> There are two things about the biological agent field I would like to mention. One is the possibility of technological surprise. Molecular biology is a field that is advancing very rapidly, and eminent biologists believe that within a period of 5 to 10 years it would be possible to produce a synthetic biological agent, an agent that does not exist and for which no natural immunity could have been acquired.
>
> Mr. Sikes: Are we doing any work in that field?
>
> Dr. MacArthur: We are not.
>
> Mr. Sikes: Why not? Lack of money or lack of interest?
>
> Dr. MacArthur: Certainly not lack of interest.

> MacArthur provides the following information:

The dramatic progress being made in . . . molecular biology led us to investigate the relevance of this field of science to biological warfare. A small group of experts . . . made these observations:

- All biological agents up to the present time are representatives of naturally occurring disease, and are thus known by scientists throughout the world. They are easily available to qualified scientists for research, either for offensive or defensive purposes.

- Within the next 5 to 10 years, it would probably be possible to make a new infective microorganism that could differ in certain important aspects from any known disease-causing organisms. Most important of these is that it might be refractory to the immunological and therapeutic processes upon which we depend to maintain our relative freedom from infectious disease.

MacArthur goes on to say that a research program to explore the feasibility of this could be done in about five years at a cost of $10 million. Strecker and Segal point to the fact that HIV appeared in the late '70s without a natural source, and that it could easily have been synthesized in a lab.

Dominating all of the many arguments is evidence overwhelmingly against these theories, which arose in the early '80s before simian immunodeficiency virus (SIV) was discovered and before the relevant viruses were sequenced. Genetic sequences show that HIV is much closer to SIV than HIV is to visna, BLV, HTLV, or any other known virus. HIV cannot be formed from splicing together parts of other known viruses. (See viral genetic sequences on the website http://www.ncbi.nlm.nih.gov in repository/aids.db.)

Other reasons the theories of Strecker and Segal do not hold up:

- The military testimony was only describing a future study to discover whether making a new agent would be feasible—not to produce this agent. They wanted an agent refractory to immunological processes—in other words, something that resists immunological processes. Testimony shows they were speaking of an agent

for which people lack a natural immunity—not one that destroys the immune system. That, further, would be much easier to produce than something such as HIV.

- Most scientists think that HIV evolved from SIV or a close relative. Also, HIV did not suddenly appear in the late '70s; it has been found in preserved blood samples from the '50s.

- Biotechnology was not sufficiently advanced in the '70s to produce something such as HIV, and many believe even today, that would be impossible. Since scientists do not even understand the details of HIV today, after years of research, it is unthinkable that HIV could have been purposely made in the '70s.

- At odds with the theory of the introduction of HIV by hepatitis B vaccinations is the finding that blood samples from the outset of the vaccination program have been tested and have shown that 6.6 percent of these people were already HIV-positive.

masturbation Self-gratification to achieve sexual pleasure or orgasm, which is usually done alone but can also be a part of couple's mutual pleasuring activities. If no partner has abrasions or skin lesions and thus there is no risk of blood or bodily fluid exposure, this amounts to relatively safe sex that carries a somewhat reduced possibility of contraction of a sexually transmitted disease. However, it is believed that genital warts can be spread via mutual masturbation, even in instances in which the warts cannot be seen.

Maternal HIV Consumer Information Project A program sponsored by the U.S. Health Care Financing Administration that offers a list of contacts in all states so that pregnant women with HIV can obtain information. This can be especially important for those who are seeking medication to prevent transmission of HIV infection to their offspring. The goal is to ensure that each state has a consumer information process to give women of childbearing age sufficient information to make informed decisions about reducing the risk of HIV transmission to their newborn infants.

For the list of state contacts' names and phone numbers, visit the website http://www.hcfa.gov/Medicaid/hiv/hivcipct.htm.

Medicaid   A program funded by the federal and state governments that pays for medical care for those Americans who cannot afford it. Disabled people are among those who qualify for Medicaid, including AIDS patients who have full-blown disease. Congress has considered extending Medicaid to HIV-positive people before symptoms of AIDS develop if these individuals have low incomes. The legislation was intended to enhance Medicaid benefits ordinarily available only when someone has AIDS or is disabled by AIDS. The Early Treatment for HIV Act was introduced by the House Democratic Leader Richard Gephardt, Representative Nancy Pelosi, and Senator Robert Torricelli. The bill would give states the option of expanding their Medicaid programs to provide coverage. Using a computer model to arrive at statistics, James Kahn of the AIDS Research Institute at the University of California, San Francisco, postulated that it appeared that more than 37,000 low-income people would enroll in the expanded Medicaid program over five years, and that this could result in about 15,000 fewer diagnoses of AIDS and 5,000 fewer AIDS deaths. Kahn also said that those five years of providing drugs and outpatient care would cost about $300 million.

Medicaid and its counterpart, Medicare, are the U.S. government's health insurance programs. Medicaid is federally supported and guided but state-run and administered. Medical benefits are made available via Medicaid to those citizens who have low incomes and meet eligibility requirements. Medicaid recipients are offered social services and a variety of inpatient and outpatient medical services. Welfare offices and Medicaid agencies provide information for those who want to apply for Medicaid.

According to information provided on the website of the Department of Health and Human Services, Medicaid is the largest single payer of direct medical services for persons living with AIDS.

Medicaid serves more than half of those living with AIDS and up to 90 percent of children with AIDS.

Estimates from the Health Care Financing Administration indicate that 116,000 Americans living with HIV were expected to be served by Medicaid in fiscal year 2001, and combined federal and state Medicaid expenditures for 2001 for this population were expected to be about $4.3 billion.

The following facts are from the Department of Health and Human Services:

- Most adults with HIV get Medicaid because they have low incomes, are disabled, and have limited assets. Others in families with dependent children are eligible for Medicaid when they meet standards for income and resources. In some states, people become eligible by virtue of their medical expenses alone. For the criteria for Medicaid, one can contact the state Medicaid agency.

- For pregnant women and babies, special income limits, which are higher than regular income limits for families and are designed to ensure prenatal care for pregnant women, have been set. To find out the state limits for pregnant women, check the Internet at http://www.hcfa.gov/hiv/subpg4.htm.

- In addition to providing eligible HIV-positive people with the full services indicated in the state plans, Medicaid can offer optional services. These can include prevention efforts, hospice care, and targeted case management.

- All states cover FDA-approved prescribed drugs, those used for prophylactic treatment of opportunistic infections and those administered for primary HIV disease. Zidovudine, known widely as AZT, is often provided to pregnant women and their infants.

- The HCFA's Maternal HIV Consumer Information Project spreads the word about the importance of women being tested for HIV, especially if they are of childbearing age. This is an effort designed to reduce the vertical transmission of HIV, from mother to infant during pregnancy, childbirth, or breast-feeding.

- Medicaid's Early and Periodic Screening, Diagnostic, and Treatment program and managed-care options offer health care for those with HIV and AIDS. EPSDT gives Medicaid-eligible people below age 21 access to services that are "medically reasonable" and necessary, whether or not they are covered under the particular state's Medicaid. Also, managed-care plans are offering persons living with AIDS (PLWAs) a chance to coordinate their health care through access to specialists, case management, home health services, social services, and implementation of new treatment protocols.

- In Washington, D.C., Massachusetts, and Maine, the HCFA has granted a demonstration waiver to extend Medicaid benefits to those living with HIV who are not disabled. The intention of this is to weigh the cost-effectiveness of extending Medicaid to them.

- In 16 states, people living with AIDS are given cost-effective alternatives to confinement to medical facilities and the options of home and community-based services waiver programs.

- The Ticket to Work and Work Incentives Improvement Act of 1999 gave states the right to expand Medicaid coverage of those with disabilities who wish to work by increasing the amount of income they can earn.

- In collaboration with the HCFA and other federal agencies, states work to make sure that those with HIV and AIDS are not discriminated against in seeking Medicaid and Medicare services.

For more information on Medicaid services, one can contact a particular state's HCFA regional office HIV/AIDS coordinator.

medical directive A means through which patients can express their desires and authorize the treatment they prefer for irreversible medical conditions. A written request in the form of a medical directive can be signed, along with a health care proxy, to assign a friend or relative the role of health care agent and decision maker. The medical directive has become a much-discussed option in the years since the outset of the HIV/AIDS epidemic.

See also LIVING WILL; NO CODE.

Medicare A U.S. government health insurance program. Medicare is designated for anyone 65 years old or older, anyone eligible for Social Security disability payments for at least two years, and anyone who has permanent kidney failure. This medical health insurance protection has no income requirements. The two programs involved are hospital insurance, Part A, and supplementary medical insurance, Part B. The benefits that are allowed vary. The Hospital Insurance Program enrolls all Americans 65 or older if they are entitled to benefits under the Old Age, Survivors, Disability and Health Insurance Program or the railroad retirement program, people below 65 who have been eligible for disability for more than two years, and insured workers (and their dependents) who require dialysis or kidney transplantation. The voluntary portion of Medicare is Part B, which covers physician charges and other individual provider services for all entitled to Part A who enroll and pay premiums. People who receive Social Security Disability Insurance benefits are automatically enrolled when the two-year waiting period ends. Others can apply at a local office of the Social Security Administration.

See also MEDICAID.

medication guidelines The specifics on how to use a drug, the dos and don'ts governing its use, and the foods and drugs that cannot be consumed or taken in combination with the drug. A doctor's instructions about medications should be followed carefully, and any variations from the treatment plan, even those as minor as vitamin or herb supplementation, should be discussed before they are used.

meditation The act of contemplation in an effort to achieve greater peacefulness and a heightened sense of well-being. This is often a segment of a person's overall mind, body, and health program or a means of spiritual grounding. Practiced regularly, this kind of exercise can relieve anxiety for some individuals who are dealing with the stress of coping with a sexually transmitted disease.

A typical routine for meditation involves the following: assume a comfortable position (sitting or lying down); close your eyes; take deep, slow breaths. Focus on the movement of your chest and abdomen as you breathe. Block out all intrusive thoughts and focus on saying the word *calm.* You can use an object or spot to stare at during the time that you are meditating. Think of your mind as actually emptying itself, banishing all tension and cares. Choose a scenario that you can bring to mind, one that reminds you of happy times and places—the day that your child gave you flowers she picked or a summer vacation spent on a beach when you felt carefree, basking in sun and surf. If a negative thought tries to intrude on your peacefulness, send it away. Any thoughts that upset you must not be replayed at this time. You want to learn how to shut off outside forces and quiet your mind.

membrane rafts   National Institute of Allergy and Infectious Diseases scientists at the National Institutes of Health have reported that HIV "rides" into human cells on membrane rafts. This discovery centers around the fact that HIV, which causes AIDS, must attach to cholesterol-rich regions of a cell's membrane in order to do its destructive work. Hence, the removal of cholesterol from cells showed researchers that HIV, in that particular state, lost much of its ability to wreak havoc (infect more cells and produce new virus). This raised an interesting possibility that is being studied further—that the cholesterol level–lowering drugs currently in widespread use may affect human beings in a way that is similar to that seen in lab studies. This idea was advanced by Eric O. Freed, Ph.D., NIAID investigator and senior author of a paper published in *Proceedings of the National Academy of Sciences* (November 20, 2001).

HIV has to navigate the cell membrane, which has both solid and fluid regions. Small, cholesterol-rich patches are referred to as rafts; their solidarity enables them to move as virtual rafts on water. Scientists contend that these rafts are in greatest evidence at points of cell-to-cell contact in the immune cells that HIV targets. What is needed, clearly, is a means of disrupting HIV's spread in order to incapacitate the virus in its flow into and from host cells. The HIV protein called gag has to attach to the cell membrane before new viruses can be spawned, and recent research shows that this attachment targets certain parts of the cell surface. Dr. Freed and his coauthor, Akira Ono, Ph.D., established that gag attaches to rafts; they created mutant gag forms and drew the conclusion that two pieces of the protein are necessary for attachment. That raised the question, What happens when HIV cannot get on rafts because it is kept off?

Freed and Ono used two compounds to deplete cholesterol from rafts; one could remove cholesterol rapidly from cell surfaces, and the other was an inhibitor of cholesterol synthesis. Used alone, each of these reduced greatly the ability of HIV to infect new cells. Researchers found that when the compounds together were applied to virus-producing cells, they almost totally abolished the ability of HIV to replicate—a powerful finding. This means that the gag-raft link is key to HIV replication, which must be interrupted in therapy of people with HIV.

Ono, A., and E. O. Freed. "Plasma Membrane Rafts Play a Critical Role in HIV-1 Assembly and Release," *Proceedings of the National Academy of Sciences* 98:13925–13930 (2001).

meningitis   An inflammation of the membranes around the brain and the spinal cord that can be caused by infection by almost any infectious agent, including the organisms responsible for syphilis, pneumonia, and tuberculosis. Meningitis can occur when bacteria from an infection in some part of the body travel via the bloodstream to the brain and spinal cord. Bacteria can also move directly to the spinal cord or brain from an ear, nose, or throat infection. There are also noninfectious causes of meningitis such as sensitivity reactions to certain medications. Acute bacterial meningitis can be caused by the bacteria *Pneumococcus* species, *Meningococcus* species, *Haemophilus influenzae, Listeria monocytogenes,* and by other organisms. Viral meningitis, which is typically milder than bacterial meningitis, can be caused by common intestinal viruses, mumps virus, herpesvirus, and others.

Cryptococcal meningitis is a fungal version that affects many people with AIDS. Usually it recedes after treatment with antifungal medicine, but often it recurs. Sometimes long-term antifungal drug therapy may be necessary for AIDS patients.

A person who has meningitis may have one or all of the following symptoms: fever, severe headache, stiff neck, loss of appetite, nausea, vomiting, and increased sensitivity to light and sound. Severe cases may include seizures. Sleepiness, confusion, and difficulty waking up should be cause for alarm, and the individual should be rushed to an emergency room as soon as possible. A baby with meningitis has different symptoms—usually these include lack of appetite, fever, irritability, constant crying, a bulging soft spot on the head, and extreme tiredness. A below-normal temperature in a baby is another possibility and a bad sign.

It is not unusual for early symptoms of meningitis to be mistaken for flu symptoms, and this can prove disastrous since prompt treatment of meningitis is critical. In most people, these symptoms appear very suddenly. With certain types of meningitis, the more time that passes before someone is treated, the more likely are permanent neurological damage and death.

Meningococcal meningitis is the most serious form. Viral meningitis can last 10 days or less. On the other hand, there are types of meningitis that are fatal, so anyone who has the symptoms described should see a doctor for medical evaluation of the problem. Diagnosis is based on physical examination, medical history, and diagnostic tests such as throat culture, CT scan, and the definitive test—analysis of cerebrospinal fluid, which is extracted by means of a spinal tap, also called lumbar puncture. This procedure often causes some discomfort during the fluid extraction and sometimes a headache afterward.

Bed rest, extra fluids, and analgesics are usually prescribed for viral meningitis. If a herpesvirus is the cause, an antiviral medication may be used. A person with bacterial meningitis, which is much more serious, is usually hospitalized for treatment and given intravenous antibiotics. Most patients who receive prompt medical treatment for meningitis do recover. The exceptions occur in instances when the disease moves with such speed that the person dies very soon after the outset, often within two days. Other bad outcomes are long-term neurologic problems caused by meningitis, such as brain damage, speech loss, blindness, or deafness, and other problems such as kidney failure.

Because some kinds of meningitis are contagious, good prevention measures are to avoid close contact with someone who is coughing and sneezing, avoid kissing or sharing utensils with someone who has the disease, try to avoid contracting upper respiratory infections and gastrointestinal infections, wash the hands thoroughly and often, and eat a healthy diet. This disease can spread fast in groups of people in close contact.

A pregnant woman is at increased risk for contracting the listeriosis bacteria, which may lead to meningitis. This can also put the fetus in jeopardy. One precaution a pregnant woman may want to take is to avoid eating cheeses that are made of unpasteurized milk and make sure all meat is thoroughly cooked (no pink in the middle).

Many children are vaccinated for pneumococcal meningitis, and there is also a meningococcal vaccine the CDC recommends for college students and travelers. The National Institute of Neurological Disorders and Stroke of the National Institutes of Health is doing research on meningitis, much of which is aimed at learning more about its causes, prevention, and treatments.

menstruation   A woman's monthly period; a flow of blood from the uterus that occurs as endometrium is shed when no fertilized egg implants in the uterus. An absence of the menstrual period can indicate pregnancy or a problem such as a hormone abnormality.

microsporidiosis   An intestinal infection that often occurs in people with AIDS and causes diarrhea and wasting. Two species of microspora cause microsporidiosis. The mode of transmission is not clear, but suspected means are unprotected sexual activity and consumption of food contaminated with microspora. No method of treatment tried thus far has worked well in treating patients with microsporidiosis.

minor STDs   The sexually transmitted diseases that are generally regarded as minor: chancroid, cytomegalovirus infection, molluscum contagiosum, pubic lice, scabies, HTLV-I and II, granuloma inguinale (donovanosis), lymphogranuloma venereum, and trichomoniasis.

molluscum contagiosum A common viral infection that often affects children and sexually active people, who pass it to other people. Usually the lesions it causes are benign, and the problem does not become chronic. Children almost always contract the infection through nonsexual contact. In adults, the virus is transmitted sexually, resulting in lesions on the genitals, lower abdomen, buttocks, or inner thighs.

Cause

Usually seen on the epithelium of the genitals or other skin areas, molluscum contagiosum is caused by a large DNA poxvirus. Transmission is typically via skin-to-skin contact, but it is also likely that a person can contract molluscum contagiosum from contact with inanimate objects such as clothing or towels. Further, a person can spread the infection on the body by touching a lesion and then touching a different part of the body.

Symptoms

Molluscum contagiosum results in skin lesions—painless, dimpled bumps that sometimes feel itchy or become irritated. These dimpled bumps show up as shiny, flesh-colored, domelike lesions with central umbilication (a "dent") and spread readily to extragenital sites, especially abdomen and thighs. Some people who contract molluscum contagiosum may have no obvious symptoms. Lesions in the genital region, upper thighs, or lower abdomen usually indicate that sexual activity was the means of transmission. In most of those with molluscum contagiosum, the bumps resolve spontaneously in a few months. (The time from infection to appearance of the lesions varies greatly from person to person; it can range from a week to a year or longer.)

In people who are HIV-infected, molluscum contagiosum is sometimes disfiguring and difficult to eliminate. When an individual with HIV has a low CD4+ cell count (below 200), these lesions may be many in number and have a tendency to spread. In some people, the lesions become extremely large when several merge. Some lesions disappear very quickly; others last for years.

Testing

Molluscum contagiosum is diagnosed by visual examination of the bumps. A papule incision shows a white waxy core. Although a doctor usually identifies this infection easily, a lesion may be biopsied to confirm diagnosis. Occasionally the physician lances a large lesion and expresses its virus contents to confirm diagnosis. A smear of contents reveals swollen epithelial cells. No blood test is used for diagnosis of molluscum contagiosum.

Treatment

Although these bumps usually resolve spontaneously, some people do not want to wait. For bumps that do not resolve spontaneously (or for people who do not want to wait for resolution), a doctor may use any one of several treatment options: liquid nitrogen, salicylic acid, curettage (surgical scraping of the lesions), 30 percent trichloroacetic acid, electrodesiccation, or cantharidin.

Prevention

Molluscum contagiosum can be transmitted to a sex partner by skin-to-skin contact, whether the person who is infected has symptoms or not. Therefore, maintaining a mutually monogamous relationship can help prevent infection with molluscum contagiosum.

monogamy The lifestyle of being married to only one person at a time, or the pattern of having a relationship (unmarried) with only one partner, who is also monogamous. The rise in sexually transmitted diseases in the United States has served as a reminder to those who are sexually active that in monogamous relationships both partners have lower risk of contracting diseases.

mood disorders A group of conditions characterized by a loss of the sense of control over one's moods and a resulting experience of distress. The two major mood disorders are major depressive disorder and bipolar disorder. Dysthymia and cyclothymia are also mood disorders. Mood disorders are commonly seen in people with HIV and AIDS. Some people have periods of depression from time to time; others have a more chronic version. Major depression is characterized by a period of at least two weeks of significantly low moods, feelings of overwhelming sadness, loss of interest in normal activities, and depression that (untreated) lasts six months to 18 months. Basically, the two traits that are benchmarks of a diagnosis of depression are anhedonia (lack of interest in things once enjoyed) and depressed mood state (sad, hopeless, teary). Furthermore, a person will have some of the following symptoms: sleep disturbances (excessive sleep, insomnia), weight loss or gain, agitation, extreme fatigue, feelings of worthlessness, suicidal thoughts, impaired ability to focus, or loss of libido.

Early treatment of depression can curb the duration and depth of the episode, and this is extremely important, because marked depression can lead to suicide. Medications commonly used to treat depression include fluoxetine (Prozac), sertraline (Zoloft), paroxetine (Paxil), escitalopram (Lexapro), and venlafaxine (Effexor XR). Bipolar disorder is a condition that features recurring cycles of depression and elation—lows and highs. This is also called manic–depressive disorder. The person who is in a manic state can make impulsive decisions that are unwise; also, a manic person may be wildly productive during up phases.

The depression of a bipolar person may be characterized by mood changes, sleep and appetite disturbances, persistent feelings of hopelessness, fatigue, difficulty in concentrating, and thoughts of suicide. When the person is in a manic phase, he or she may be talkative, have racing thoughts, and sleep little. This illness can be serious and debilitating. Some people have very severe bipolar disorder; in others the condition is very mild. There is no cure, and it often lasts a lifetime. However, it can be treated. If bipolar disorder is untreated, it often grows worse.

Although the cause of bipolar disorder remains unknown, it is believed that various genetic, environmental, and biological factors work together to trigger episodes. Differences in the chemical messengers in the brain from those in the normal brain have been noted in those with bipolar disorder.

In many cases, a person with bipolar disorder does not recognize the level of dysfunction caused by this problem, and it may be necessary for other people to recognize the signs and steer the person to professional evaluation and treatment. If you are a caregiver for a person with HIV or AIDS, or anyone else who appears to show the signs of bipolar disorder or depression, try to arrange for her or him to see a psychiatrist. The doctor can rule out other illnesses that produce similar symptoms and check whether the mood disorder is resulting from substance abuse or from a thyroid problem. Treatment for bipolar disorder usually involves psychotherapy and medication that evens out moods. The medications lithium and divalproex (Depakote) are commonly used to treat bipolar disorder. Electroconvulsive therapy (ECT) may be used when the person has suicidal tendencies or when medication does not work. Electrodes are taped to the person's head, and he or she is anesthetized or given a muscle relaxant, after which a small amount of electrical current is passed through the brain momentarily. A person with depression typically responds well after a few treatments.

Dysthymia is a persistent state of mild depression with symptoms less severe than those of major depression. People may experience frequent depressed moods, and this condition persists for years. The person feels hopeless and sad and has insomnia, poor appetite, and low energy. Treatment requires medication and therapy. In some cases, the dysthymic person's condition turns into major depression.

Cyclothymic disorder features mild mood changes, with times of mild depression and times of excitement. This disorder is notable for abrupt mood swings. The alternating episodes can last for years. It is treated in much the same manner used for bipolar disorder (although less aggressively because it is a less extreme problem).

morning-after pill   One of two different types of pills that have different purposes: the "emergency contraception" pill and the pill purported to prevent transmission of HIV after the fact.

The morning-after pill has spurred raging debate. The existence of a morning-after pill that prevents pregnancy remains shrouded in secrecy, and few

American women are even aware of it. Proponents believe that, if used properly, this pill could cut America's abortion rate in half. Emergency contraception consists of a high dose of the hormones found in birth control pills. When morning-after pills are taken within 72 hours of unprotected sex, pregnancy is prevented about 75 percent of the time. A woman can get a prescription for either of the two FDA-approved drugs, Preven and Plan B. Often, the morning-after pill is mistaken for a different drug—RU-486, which ends a pregnancy within weeks of conception. In contrast, emergency contraception is quicker, can prevent ovulation, or can prevent implantation of a fertilized egg.

Some physicians contend that emergency contraception pills should be made widely available. However, this idea is controversial. The American College of Obstetricians and Gynecologists has asked doctors nationwide to distribute information on emergency contraception when female patients have annual well-woman visits. The American Medical Association wants emergency contraceptives to become an over-the-counter product.

The effectiveness of the morning-after pill (actually, a drug regimen of pills) in preventing HIV infection after possible exposure to HIV has not been proved in research studies. However, doctors prescribe it, nonetheless, for patients who indulge in high-risk sex. At the same time, physicians are concerned that many people who are sexually active may mistakenly perceive using morning-after pills and condoms as a surefire way to prevent transmission of HIV, and this misconception may encourage promiscuity. It would be a disastrous outcome in that sex partners could contract diseases they believed they had been protected against, although they had not—since the verdict is still out on efficacy and safety.

The Centers for Disease Control and Prevention underscores that, in actuality, there is no such thing as a "morning-after pill" to prevent HIV infection. Multiple drugs are involved in postexposure antiretroviral therapy, and these must be taken for at least 30 days, several times a day. Too, there are no human data available on the effectiveness of postexposure therapy in reducing HIV infection after sexual or drug-related exposures. Some animal studies do suggest that there

could be benefits, but it remains unclear what this means for human beings. Important points are that animals are not exposed in the same way (different type of exposure through mucous membranes); are usually not exposed to the same virus (SIV is different from HIV); and metabolize drugs differently. Clearly, trying to prevent contraction of HIV by using postexposure antiretroviral therapy is unwise, particularly if it is used in place of safe sex.

Behavior that is believed to prevent HIV exposures includes abstinence, sex only with an uninfected partner, correct and consistent use of condoms, abstention from injection drug use, and use of clean equipment (for those who are IV drug users). Furthermore, antiretroviral therapy should not be used routinely, nor should it be used when a low risk of transmission exists or when people seek care more than 72 hours after exposure. Postexposure antiretroviral therapy—if it were indeed effective—would have to be started within an hour or two of exposure, and when started later than 24 to 36 hours after exposure would, in all likelihood, not be effective. This kind of drug therapy is extreme and can have severe side effects. Also, the cost is $600 to $1,000. Doctors should prescribe postexposure antiretroviral therapy only after informing patients of the experimental nature of this treatment and the possible risks associated with it. Also, it should be prescribed only after the patient has consulted an expert in the use of antiretroviral drugs.

Brown, Janelle. "High Noon for the Morning-After Pill," Salon. Available online. URL: http://archive.salon.com/mwt/feature/2001/06/20/pill.

mucopurulent Characterized by a combination of mucus and pus.

mucopurulent cervicitis Mucopurulent cervicitis (MPC) is identified by a purulent (pus-containing) or mucopurulent (mucus- and-pus-containing) discharge that is seen in the endocervical canal. Cervicitis is also suggested by easily induced cervical bleeding. Essentially, this common condition entails infections of the endocervix. No statistics are kept on mucopurulent cervicitis because it is not a reportable disease, but many women who are young and sexually active get these infections, including women who are pregnant, those who take oral birth control pills, and those who do not use any barrier method of protection against sexually transmitted diseases.

Cause

MPC can be caused by chlamydia and gonorrhea bacteria, by viruses such as herpesvirus, or by protozoa such as trichomonas. Often symptom-free, mucopurulent cervicitis can be found on physical examination and examination of discharge under a microscope. This disease is transmitted by sexual contact or contact with sex toys. Genital rubbing may sometimes transmit mucopurulent cervicitis.

Symptoms

An infected person can have yellow vaginal discharge, spotting with blood, redness of the cervix, pain with intercourse, and burning during urination. A doctor can diagnose mucopurulent cervicitis by observations during a patient's examination and by microscopic study of discharge. A doctor may have cultures done for specific bacteria and will try to determine whether the patient has pelvic inflammatory disease. Patients who have MPC should be tested for *Chlamydia trachomatis* and for *Neisseria gonorrhoeae*, but mucopurulent cervicitis is not a sensitive predictor of infection with these organisms because most women who have chlamydia or gonorrhea do not have MPC.

Treatment

MPC can persist even after several courses of treatment with antimicrobial therapy. If symptoms persist, women should return to the doctor for evaluation and abstain from intercourse even if prescribed therapy is complete. Partners of those being treated for MPC should be notified, examined, and treated for any sexually transmitted disease identified or suspected in the index patient.

The individual whose partner is diagnosed with mucopurulent cervicitis should be evaluated regardless of whether symptoms and evidence of infection exist. When a patient is treated for the infection that is underlying mucopurulent cervici-

tis, the cervicitis clears up in most cases. If the cause is bacterial, the patient is prescribed an antibiotic. When trichomonas or herpesvirus is the cause, the physician treats the infection. Extremely important in mucopurulent cervicitis is follow-up: a woman must make sure the problem has been resolved to ensure it does not escalate to pelvic inflammatory disease.

Prevention

An infected person can infect another during sexual contact. Condoms are not 100 percent effective in preventing any sexually transmitted disease. A person should not try to treat herself or take another person's medication. If a woman douches, that can also make diagnosis difficult in that it hides symptoms.

mucous membranes The mucus-secreting lining of some tissues of the body such as the vagina, mouth, nose, and eyes.

mucus Secreted by mucous membranes, a body secretion that has protective and lubricant action and is a carrier of enzymes.

Multicenter AIDS Cohort Study This is the largest continually followed group of HIV-infected or at-risk individuals in the world. The Multicenter AIDS Cohort Study (MACS) is sponsored by the National Institute of Allergy and Infectious Diseases (NIAID) and National Cancer Institute (NCI).

MACS research centers—funded by the NIAID—are located at the Johns Hopkins University, the University of Pittsburgh, Northwestern University, and the University of California at Los Angeles. The director of NIAID, Anthony S. Fauci, M.D., has stated that the study is "instrumental in advancing our understanding of the pathogenesis and natural history of HIV disease, and thus, has important implications for therapy." Since 1984, the MACS has enrolled 5,622, and there are now 1,705 active enrollees. Of enrollees, 2,779 are HIV-positive. Of the group of MACS volunteers, 1,585 have died of AIDS. As of March 2003, 1,781 participants have developed AIDS. For up-to-date information, see

"Dossier" on MACS at http://www.statepi.jhsph.edu/macs/dossier.

What has been especially beneficial is that the size and longevity of this study have enabled it to answer questions that would not be viable considerations for other investigations. Jack Killen, M.D., director of the Division of AIDS at NIAID, stated: "The MACS has amassed a wealth of clinical information and biological specimens. Together with the huge databases to which they are linked, these specimens provide the general scientific community with an invaluable research resource for multidisciplinary investigation."

When the project was proposed in the early 1980s, no one knew the cause of AIDS, and at that time, the disease mainly affected the gay community. NIAID, in hopes of pinpointing the cause, began a multicenter effort to enroll volunteers who were considered at risk for development of AIDS.

Soon after that, HIV was discovered, and its link to AIDS was revealed, thereby shifting the study's focus to progression of the disease (how and why) and prevention of HIV. At the outset, the MACS included clinical research centers at the institutions mentioned and at the University of California at Berkeley, but the latter left the MACS in 1988 to do its own NIAID-funded investigation, the San Francisco Men's Health Study.

Every six months, the MACS volunteers undergo evaluation. A visit includes an interviewer-administered questionnaire, physical exam, and collection of blood samples for analysis of the immune system and monitoring of HIV status. All quantitative information on sexual practice and use of illicit drugs is classified so that it is useful for analysis yet prevents disclosure of detailed private information.

As of December 12, 2001, data components included the following:

- The original cohort: the original 4,954 gay and bisexual men who had volunteered since the beginning of the study in 1984

- The new recruit cohort: recruitment was opened April 1987 through September 1991 to focus on minority and special target groups, such as part-

ners of the original cohort, and 668 new participants were recruited.

- The neuropsychological cohort: MACS centers began giving neuropsychological tests in 1987 to a subset of the original cohort.

Participants in the study are enthusiastic about the progress in HIV/AIDS research that has been fostered by MACS, which has played a critical role for many years. One of the earliest breakthroughs was in 1988, when John P. Phair, M.D., and his colleagues at Northwestern University reported that the risk of contracting *Pneumocystis carinii* pneumonia (PCP) increased greatly when an HIV-infected person's CD4+ T cell level dropped below 200 cells per cubic millimeter of blood. This finding paved the way for starting treatment to prevent PCP when a patient's T cell levels dropped below that number. In the year 1990, MACS had a switch in focus: whereas the scrutiny had been chiefly on clinical outcome questions, researchers moved into asking which features of the interaction between HIV and the person infected might explain variations in disease progression. MACS assembled virologists, immunologists, and epidemiologists to study this question.

Another landmark moment occurred in 1996, when John W. Mellors, M.D., and other MACS researchers at the University of Pittsburgh reported their finding that viral load was the single most important indicator of HIV disease progression. Before that, doctors had based treatment decisions on CD4+ T cell counts.

MACS data also enlarged knowledge concerning how differences in the genes that encode HIV coreceptors—the molecular handles where the virus attaches on immune system cells—make people HIV-resistant or affect progression of HIV once it is contracted. Analyses of cohort data have consistently contributed key information about opportunistic infections associated with AIDS, as well as the related cancers and neurological disorders.

Ongoing MACS research is studying how and why some patients have metabolic side effects to HAART and how drug resistance to HAART emerges. There is every reason to believe that MACS will contribute vital information to find the best treatment and, perhaps, a way to prevent HIV infection.

NIAID is a component of the National Institutes of Health (NIH). NIAID conducts and supports research aimed at preventing, diagnosing, and treating illnesses such as HIV and other sexually transmitted diseases, TB, malaria, asthma, and allergies.

multiple partners　A risk factor in all forms of sexually transmitted diseases involving a pattern of having multiple sex partners. One increases risk of being infected exponentially by involvement with various people and their own sets of exposures and existing sexually transmitted diseases.

mutation　A permanent change in the genetic material (DNA or RNA); this can lead to alterations in an organism's function. A mutation can be transmissible.

myalgia　Muscle pain, a frequent symptom of patients with human immunodeficiency virus (HIV). Although the term *myalgia* is most commonly used in the medical realm in relation to physical overuse of muscles, myalgia is also a problem of those with autoimmune disease and other medical conditions, such as flu.

When a person experiences generalized muscle pain, this can be a symptom of systemic illness, and typically the individual also feels ill and may have fever. Initially a person may want to try rest and over-the-counter medications, but it is advisable to call a doctor if the pain is persistent for several days, if fever is higher than 101°F, if a rash appears, or if the muscle pain is accompanied by new symptoms. Depending on the suspected cause of a person's myalgia, tests may be done, such as blood tests and a neuromuscular test (EMG; electromyography).

mycobacterium avium complex disease　Also known as MAC, this disease complex includes a group of germs that can infect those with HIV infection. Typically adults do not contract MAC disease until the T cell count is below 50 cells/mm^3. About 20 to 30 percent of AIDS patients contract MAC. Children are also vulner-

able to this disease. Usually they contract MAC sooner than adults—before the T cell count falls to 50 cells/mm^3.

It is believed that people with AIDS contract *Mycobacterium avium* complex disease via normal contact with food and water. MAC germs are found in most sources of drinking water, in soil, and in household dust. It is also seen in animals. MAC does not seem to be spread from individual to individual.

Symptoms of MAC, which infects the lungs or intestines, are fever, night sweats, weight loss, abdominal pain, diarrhea, and tiredness. Doctors can use lab tests to confirm that an individual has MAC.

Drugs that can reduce a person's risk of getting MAC disease are clarithromycin, azithromycin, and rifabutin. These medications are also used to treat MAC infection. A person who has had MAC disease should continue to take the medication to prevent another round of it.

myelosuppression　Bone marrow suppression that results in decreased production of red blood cells, white blood cells, and platelets. Some medications cause myelosuppression. For example, chemotherapy strongly affects both normal and cancerous tissues. Bone marrow is affected over a period of weeks until the patient being treated has a low dip in blood count, during which he or she is vulnerable to infection and becomes tired easily. Every patient's complete blood count must be checked before chemotherapy to ascertain whether values are abnormal. Any infection during this time can be fatal, so it is important for a patient and family or caregiver to monitor for fever, a new cough, a change in a cough, and an increase in weakness.

myopathy　Any disease of muscle. Myositis is an inflammation of muscle tissue with various causes including infections or an adverse reaction to a medication. A person with HIV often is subject to myopathy. Myopathies can be inherited or acquired. The individual who has myopathy usually has weakening and/or wasting of muscles in the upper parts of the arms and legs.

myths In the area of sexually transmitted diseases, as in most diseases, a number of myths and misconceptions exist. Examples are rumors that HIV can be transmitted by light kisses and hand holding and that a person can contract HIV if bitten by a mosquito that is carrying the blood of an HIV-infected individual.

name-based reporting At the outset of the AIDS epidemic, the medical community espoused the position that the victims of this disease should be identified so that their partners could be warned of their need for testing and so that the spread of the disease could be tracked. At the time victims had good reason to fear that disclosure of their HIV status could result in the loss of jobs, health insurance, friends, and family. While epidemiologists argued that name-based reporting was necessary, those on the other side of the controversy—the HIV/AIDS sufferers and their advocates—offered convincing rebuttals that putting a name on an HIV-positive report meant dooming that person to a loss of civil rights. Some states allowed anonymous reporting; others passed laws for name-based reporting. As time passed, the two opposing camps began to see each other's viewpoint. Even AIDS activist groups such as the National Association for People with AIDS contended that anonymous testing should be offered everywhere, but they became less militant in opposing name-based testing. Also, authorities at the CDC, who had once argued vehemently for compulsory reporting of those who tested positive for HIV, moved to a stance that anonymous testing is also needed for proper disease tracking and better dissemination of treatment. Many public health authorities concede that some people will not be tested if they think their name will be divulged, and that tendency would thwart the basic goal of public health—to stem the tide of disease spread.

The CDC has a toll-free HIV/AIDS hotline that uses a 50-state database to inform callers whether their state, city, or county requires name-based reporting. A CDC representative can also tell a caller where to have an anonymous test. The number is (800) 342-AIDS.

The Journal of the American Medical Association (JAMA) HIV/AIDS Resource Center online reports that some health care professionals fear that policies regarding confidential reporting by name to state health departments of those who are infected with HIV may cause some individuals to avoid HIV testing. However, in a study of six state health departments using analysis of data from the 12 months preceding the introduction of HIV reporting and the 12 months afterward, it was found that there was no significant decline in the total number of HIV tests provided at counseling and testing sites in the months after HIV reporting began, compared to reporting in any other state—except for those that were expected on the basis of existing trends before HIV reporting.

Increases occurred in Nebraska, Nevada, New Jersey, and Tennessee. Predicted decreases were in Louisiana and Michigan. Also, in all areas, the testing of at-risk heterosexuals actually increased in the year that followed implementation of HIV reporting. In men who have sex with men, declines in testing were seen in Louisiana and Tennessee after HIV reporting began, but testing increased for this group in Michigan, Nebraska, Nevada, and New Jersey.

Another issue is the adequacy of information. Some contend that because of the changed nature of the epidemic, particularly in respect to new therapies, AIDS case reports no longer offer enough information. There is a need for information on HIV-infected non-AIDS cases for prevention efforts, monitoring, planning, and allocation of resources. Previously, it was felt that AIDS-case reporting provided most of the information required to monitor and characterize the epidemic.

The Centers for Disease Control and Prevention has funded 65 project areas in health departments for HIV counseling and testing programs since 1985, and since 1990 most of these have sent the CDC the data they have collected on tests done. For each, information was collected on month and year test was done; sex, race, ethnicity; the testee's HIV risk exposure group (men who have sex with men, injection drug use, sex with a person infected with HIV or at risk for HIV); type of test site (freestanding, STD clinic, drug treatment center, family planning clinic, community health center, prison or jail, other); test result; and type of test (anonymous or confidential). The latter was added after 1992.

Basically, though, many states have been unable to establish HIV reporting policies because confidential reporting of HIV-infected people by name to health departments remains controversial. Some communities have opposed the practice. The American Civil Liberties Union has issued a position statement that "name reporting is a counterproductive public health measure that will cause individuals to avoid testing." An example of the public outcry that can result from opposition to name reporting is a Philadelphia hearing on Pennsylvania's plan to start an HIV reporting mechanism, which resulted in vociferous protests. Many activists attending the hearing aggressively opposed the name requirement. Offering an alternative, Anna Forbes advanced an idea that has made her nationally known, using "unique identifiers" (UIs) in place of names for HIV reporting. It is her belief that the use of UI systems will protect from stigmatization people with HIV/AIDS, drug users in recovery, women with termination of pregnancies, and those with mental illness. In this same context, Bruce Flannery of the Pennsylvania Coalition of AIDS Service Organizations described "a groundswell of opposition to reporting names." He explained: "Even in parts of the state where it's risky for people to publicly identify themselves as having the virus, people have been coming to these hearings and sacrificing their own privacy in order to plead with the state not to require names. Their major concern is that others with HIV, especially folks in high-risk populations, will stay away from testing and care, out of fear that their names will get out."

The long-range repercussions of reporting names concern many. David Fair, former director of the city's AIDS Activities Coordinating Office and of We the People Living with AIDS/HIV, takes the position that he does not trust the government with a list of HIV names, and he wonders whether someone in government may use the name of a person with HIV in some punitive manner.

National Electronic Telecommunications System for Surveillance The National Electronic Telecommunications System for Surveillance (NETSS) is a computerized public health surveillance information system that sends weekly data on cases of nationally notifiable diseases to the Centers for Disease Control and Prevention (CDC). A *notifiable disease* must be reported because regular, frequent, timely information is necessary to prevent and control it. The list of diseases varies over time and by state. Once a year, the CDC and the Council of State and Territorial Epidemiologists (CSTE) review and modify the list of nationally notifiable diseases. This list is available on the Internet at http://www.cdc.gov/epo/dphsi/phs.htm.

NETSS electronically transmits core surveillance data—date, county, age, sex, and race or ethnicity—and some disease-specific epidemiologic information for nationally notifiable diseases and for some nonnotifiable diseases as well. State and local health departments and CDC personnel work to make the demographic data as complete as possible, but there are cases in which complete information is not available for transmission. Factors that influence the thoroughness of the reports include type and severity of the illness, whether treatment is sought in a health care setting, diagnosis of an illness, availability of diagnostic services, disease-control measures in effect, the public's awareness of the disease, and the resources, priorities, and interests of the state and local health officials who are responsible for this kind of record keeping. Essentially, the completeness of the reporting differs from state to state and from one disease to another.

Personal identifiers (names and addresses) are never transmitted to the Centers for Disease Control and Prevention in reports of cases of notifiable diseases. The CDC and CSTE are required to keep the data confidential. Also, the CDC does not mandate state or territory participation. The reporting of nationally notifiable diseases is regulated by each state or territory.

The weekly reports of national morbidity data help public health managers and providers identify disease epidemics promptly and understand patterns of disease occurrence. This information enables them to monitor and investigate any changes they observe in demographics of disease—changes in age, sex, race or ethnicity, and geographic distribution. By means of NETSS, the CDC gets notifiable-disease reports from the 50 state health departments, New York City, the District of Columbia, and five U.S. territories. Health care providers who suspect or diagnose a case of a disease that is notifiable in their state initiate these reports. They send the case information by mail, telephone, or fax to the health department (local, county, or state). Clinical labs also report results.

NETSS is run by programmers and other support staff in the CDC's Surveillance Systems Branch, who are responsible for a variety of functions. Staffers develop, test, customize, install, and update computer software for health departments; develop and implement software to validate data sent to NETSS; identify problems (incomplete records, transmission errors, deviations); provide technical support; and convey specifications for record formats.

Anyone who wants to see current updates of data on notifiable diseases can check libraries (especially ones at medical schools and schools of public health) and read the CDC's weekly reports in *Morbidity and Mortality Weekly Report (MMWR)*. Final, corrected data are published in the annual *MMWR Summary of Notifiable Diseases, United States*. For *MMWRs* and data on case numbers, see http://www.cdc.gov. You can also check the CDC publication *National Vital Statistics Reports,* available online at http://www.cdc.gov.

National Institutes of Health Begun in 1887, the National Institutes of Health is now one of the world's foremost medical research centers, the federal focal point for medical research in the United States. The goal of the NIH is to uncover new knowledge that will improve the general health status of all. To work toward that mission,

the National Institutes of Health conducts research in its own laboratories; supports the research of nongovernment scientists in universities, medical schools, hospitals, and research institutions nationwide and abroad; helps train research investigators; and fosters communication of medical information. The goal of NIH research is to gain new information to help prevent, detect, diagnose, and treat disease and disability; research ranges from the rarest genetic disorder to the common cold.

The NIH is one of eight health agencies of the Public Health Services, which is part of the U.S. Department of Health and Human Services. Made up of 27 separate components, NIH has 75 buildings on more than 300 acres in Bethesda, Maryland. In 2001, the budget of NIH was $20.3 billion (in 1887, it was $300).

The impact of the NIH on the nation's health has been incredible. From 1977 to 1999, the mortality rate of heart disease dropped by 36 percent. In the same period, death rates from stroke dropped by 50 percent. Improved treatments and detection methods increased the relative five-year survival rate for those with cancer to 60 percent. Paralysis from spinal cord injury has been reduced greatly by rapid treatment with high doses of steroids. When treatment is given within the first eight hours after injury, it increases the likelihood of recovery of severely injured people who have lost sensation or mobility below the point of injury. Long-term treatment with anticlotting medicines has cut stroke risk by 80 percent from the common heart condition atrial fibrillation. New medications for schizophrenia can reduce or eliminate delusions and hallucinations in 80 percent of patients. Chances for survival increased for infants with respiratory distress syndrome. The 19 million Americans who suffer from depression can look forward to better lives thanks to effective medications and psychotherapy. Vaccines now protect against infectious diseases that once killed and disabled. Dental sealants have proved 100 percent effective in protecting chewing surfaces of children's molars and premolars, where most cavities occur. In 1990, NIH researchers performed the first trial of gene therapy in humans, with the result that scientists now are identifying functions of many genes and will eventually develop screening tools and gene therapies for cancers and other diseases. The NIH in the 21st century wants to discover better ways to prevent and treat cancer, heart disease, stroke, blindness, arthritis, diabetes, kidney diseases, Alzheimer's disease, mental illness, drug abuse and alcoholism, AIDS, and other diseases.

needle access   Improving access to clean needles and syringes is a huge thrust of HIV prevention efforts, because needle sharing is a major factor in the spread of HIV infection. Health care professionals seek to prevent illicit drug use, make treatment readily available to drug users, reduce the risk associated with continued drug use, and encourage the introduction or continuation of programs that improve knowledge about decontamination of injection equipment and provide access to sterile injection equipment to reduce spread of HIV and prevent new AIDS cases.

Consider this excerpt from a February 1997 letter to President Bill Clinton from the American Foundation for AIDS Research: The ethical imperative to provide sterile injection equipment to intravenous drug users is strongly supported by the nation's foremost bioethicists' consensus statement "On the Ethics of Denying Injection Drug Users Access to Sterile Injection Equipment."

- These principles inform our conclusion that the failure to fund needle exchange efforts, with the predictable loss of life that can be traced to HIV infections that might have been averted, is ethically unacceptable.

- We believe that a failure to lift the federal ban on funding of needle exchange programs represents a policy that will consign thousands of men, women, and children to early deaths. By every principle of medical ethics, this situation calls out for a change.

At the time, under the terms of Public Law 105-78, allocation of federal funds to support needle exchange programs was conditional on a determination by the secretary of health and human services that such programs reduce the transmission of HIV and do not encourage the use of illegal drugs. The act's restriction on federal funding, however,

was not lifted. The administration decided that local communities could implement their own programs with their own dollars to fund needle exchange programs. In a February 1997 report to Congress, Donna Shalala, Health and Human Services secretary, reported that a review of the findings of scientific research supported the belief that needle exchange programs could be an effective part of a comprehensive strategy to prevent HIV and other blood-borne infectious diseases "in communities that choose to include them." The next year she announced that a review of research indicated that needle exchange programs did not encourage the use of illegal drugs. While Congress has restricted using federal funds for needle exchange programs since 1989, lawmakers have authorized funding for research into the efficacy of needle exchange programs as a public health intervention to reduce HIV transmission and examine the impact of such programs on drug use.

needle exchanges   A program that allows intravenous drug users to exchange used needles and syringes for sterile ones. Some of these distribute needles. Others exchange needles and sell them. As of 2003, about 100 needle-exchange programs are in place in 40 communities in 28 states.

The goal of such programs is to reduce the spread of HIV by needle and paraphernalia sharing among IV drug users. Like many aspects of the HIV/AIDS spectrum, needle exchange programs have been subjects of much controversy. Proponents believe that the reduction in reuse of needles is a strong factor in prevention of further HIV spread by those who are IV drug users. Naysayers assert that setting up a needle exchange program simply means endorsing activity that is illegal and detrimental to society. Both government agencies and private organizations have set up these programs, with various formats. One clear advantage is that needle exchange programs make it possible for low-income drug users to get sterile equipment.

Reviews of scientific literature on needle exchange programs draw the conclusion that such programs can be an effective part of a community-based HIV prevention effort. Needle exchange programs also provide help that can link intravenous drug users to other important services such as risk reduction counseling, drug treatment, and support services.

Extensive research also underscores that needle exchange programs do not encourage illegal drug use and sometimes can reduce drug use because IV drug users are exposed to counseling and treatment. However, the U.S. Congress has continued to ban the use of federal funds for needle-exchange programs.

According to the Human Rights Campaign, a group working for equal rights for lesbians, gays, and the transgendered, many organizations that review research on needle exchange find that the evidence proves it is effective. These groups include the U.S. General Accounting Office, National Academy of Sciences, National Commission on AIDS, and the University of California, San Francisco. A study by Beth Israel Medical Center showed a two-thirds decrease in HIV infections in those who were participants in five needle-exchange programs in New York City.

needle sharing The act of one intravenous drug user sharing needles with another person or a group of people. In many cases, needle sharing refers to a drug addict's habit of reusing needles without sterilizing them even though they have been used by other individuals. These practices fly in the face of common knowledge that IV drug users can contract HIV by sharing their drug paraphernalia with others who may have the virus and have not disclosed the information. At the same time, it is believed that intravenous drug users can reduce their likelihood of contracting HIV by cleaning their drug paraphernalia carefully and by avoiding needle sharing. They are also encouraged to take advantage of needle exchange services, through which they can turn in used equipment for clean drug works.

needlestick The act of having skin pricked or punctured unintentionally with a hypodermic needle. Typically, this refers to the effect of this occurrence on a health care worker in a health care setting, so the term has come to suggest possible transmission of HIV. There is an element of risk

attached to a needlestick when the needle has been used for a patient who has HIV or AIDS.

nef A viral protein that is present in most human immunodeficiency virus strains; a person who has an HIV-1 strain that has a deletion of the nef gene tends to develop AIDS symptoms more slowly. When the nef gene is present, nef helps the human immunodeficiency virus overcome a person's immune defenses.

negotiated safety A type of unwritten "sexual contract" between the partners in a gay relationship that they can forgo using condoms because neither has HIV and they are monogamous. People who administer public health programs do not condone this practice because many believe the condom message applies to all—no flexibility for varied situations.

Some contend that the campaign for negotiated safety is based on assumptions that those involved can negotiate such difficult issues honestly, and then place absolute trust in each other. Many involved in education-and-prevention programs send a clear message that people should use a condom every time they have anal sex—with no exceptions.

Neisseria gonorrhoeae Gonorrhea is caused by the gram-negative diplococcus *Neisseria gonorrhoeae*.
See also GONORRHEA.

neonatal herpes The condition of an infant born with the herpesvirus as a result of the mother's transmission of genital herpes during childbirth. This is, however, a rather rare occurrence.

neuropathy See PERIPHERAL NEUROPATHY.

neurosyphilis Central nervous system disease can occur during any stage of syphilis. In primary and secondary syphilis, a lumbar puncture is not part of the routine evaluation unless a patient has clinical evidence of neurologic involvement with syphilis, such as ophthalmic or auditory symptoms, cranial nerve palsies, or signs of meningitis.

The early stages of a syphilis infection cause invasion of the nervous system by syphilis bacteria, and in about 3 to 7 percent of those whose syphilis is untreated, neurosyphilis develops. The time from infection to neurosyphilis development can be up to 20 years. Some individuals who have neurosyphilis do not have symptoms; others experience headaches, stiff necks, and fever caused by the inflamed lining of the brain. Other patients have seizures. If blood vessels are affected, the person with neurosyphilis may have stroke symptoms, with numbness, weakness, and/or visual problems. People who have neurosyphilis or syphilitic eye disease and who can take penicillin should be treated with aqueous crystalline penicillin for 10 to 14 days or, as an alternative regimen, procaine penicillin for 10 to 14 days. Durations of the recommended and alternative regimens for neurosyphilis are shorter than that of the regimen that would be used for late syphilis in the absence of neurosyphilis. All people who have syphilis should be tested for HIV.

newborn screening   Soon after a baby is born (usually on hospital-discharge day or within 48 hours of birth), his or her heel is pricked, and blood is taken for testing and dried on a piece of filter paper, which is then sent to the state health department for testing. The health department then contacts the family's doctor with the result. A baby is tested for eight different disorders, although guidelines vary in different states. Newborn screenings check for some or all of the following disorders: phenylketonuria (PKU), maple syrup urine disease, congenital hypothyroidism, congenital adrenal hyperplasia, galactosemia, homocystinuria, sickle cell disease, biotinidase deficiency, and hearing. Only New York routinely screens for human immunodeficiency virus (HIV). All states screen for some disorders, and private organizations offer screenings in addition to those done by state programs.

night sweats   Heavy sweating at night, which is usually a sign of disease, especially when a person also has fever. Two possible causes are non-Hodgkin's lymphoma and tuberculosis. Night sweats may also be indicative of a woman's onset of menopause. If the body is drenched in sweat the possibility of HIV infection is usually considered and investigated. A person who experiences night sweats should consult a health care provider for evaluation.

no code   A patient's instruction concerning lifesaving measures or life support when the individual is in dire straits as a result of a terminal condition or disease. A "no code" or "do not resuscitate" is a direction not to perform lifesaving measures. This direction is indicated on the patient's medical chart so that attending personnel will know what to do in case extreme measures are required to keep the individual alive.

nongonococcal urethritis   A urethral infection that is commonly sexually transmitted and is also called nonspecific urethritis.

See also NONSPECIFIC URETHRITIS.

non-Hodgkin's lymphoma   Lymphomas that encompass a wide variety of cancers that affect the lymphoid tissue and that have a wide range of aggressiveness, complications, and responsiveness to treatment. Although the cause is unknown, a factor that increases an individual's possibility of contracting this disease is an immunologic disorder. Non-Hodgkin's lymphoma is commonly seen in AIDS patients.

Possible symptoms include night sweats, enlarged lymph nodes, abdominal pain, fever, weight loss, bleeding, intestinal disturbances, and accumulation of fluid in the membranes lining the chest or abdominal cavities. Prognosis depends on which areas are affected and whether the disease has metastasized beyond the lymph nodes to other organs, such as the lungs, central nervous system, bone, or digestive tract.

Tests that may be used to diagnose non-Hodgkin's lymphoma are a peripheral blood smear, a complete blood count, and lymph node or bone marrow biopsy. The disease is then staged by some of the following: the doctor's examination of the patient, chest X ray, CT scan, lymphangiogram, laparotomy, liver biopsy, blood chemistry tests, MRI, and positron emission test (PET) scan.

Most critical in determining the progression of the disease and course of treatment is the state of the lymphoma cells and the rapidity with which the cancerous cells are growing. Non-Hodgkin's lymphoma (NHL) features uncontrolled proliferation of lymphocytes and appears in nodular or diffuse tumors. NHL is a kind of cancer that can be curable, but the patient who has a compromised immune system (such as someone who has HIV) usually does not respond to treatment as well as someone who has a healthy immune response. Another problem related to a non-Hodgkin's diagnosis is that some patients experience relapse, as the lymphoma arises again.

If a person is not having any symptoms, low-grade, or indolent, the disease is usually not treated aggressively. Within several years, the disease usually progresses and requires treatment. When it is time for treatment, the choices are chemotherapy, radiation, or both. Bone marrow transplantation is the treatment of choice for some people. For low-grade lymphoma, median survival rate is six to eight years. A patient who has high-grade lymphoma possibly may be cured, but the response to chemotherapy and/or radiation is ultimately the determining factor for longevity. The NHL patient must take extreme care to avoid people with colds and other infections when she or he is especially vulnerable in the weeks after chemotherapy.

nonhuman primate origins of HIV Scientists think that HIV-1 evolved from an immunodeficiency virus that was found in chimpanzees, simian immunodeficiency virus (or SIV cpz). Typically, viruses that infect one animal species, such as chimps, do not infect other species of animals, but this was apparently an exception; scientists are not sure exactly why this virus "jumped" from chimpanzees to people (called cross-species transmission). But the prevailing belief is that SIV cpz evolved into HIV-1 many decades ago, perhaps as early as the 1930s. HIV-2 is thought to have resulted from a cross-species transmission of an SIV from a sooty magabey monkey, according to the Centers for Disease Control and Prevention.

This has been a subject of much controversy. A statement from Kevin De Cock, M.D., director of the Division of HIV/AIDS Prevention, Surveillance and Epidemiology of the National Center for HIV, STD, and TB Prevention of the Centers for Disease Control and Prevention presented strong evidence that HIV-1 started in nonhuman primates, probably chimpanzees. University of Alabama at Birmingham researchers showed that they had pinpointed a new isolate of a retrovirus affecting a chimpanzee subspecies (*Pan troglodytes troglodytes*) and had established that this and other chimpanzee isolates are related to the different groups of HIV-1 that infect human beings. It is believed that HIV-1 launched human epidemic when the virus crossed from chimpanzees to humans through cross-species transmission. This finding led to greater understanding of HIV-1's evolution as well as providing insight into species-to-species transmission of viruses.

Because it is known that people have long hunted monkeys and apes for food, researchers conjecture that people could have been exposed to or infected with SIV or HIV during blood contact that occurred in preparing the meat. Then hunters may have spread HIV through sexual contact or rituals involving blood that happened to be contaminated, or even through injections and vaccinations with needles that had not been sterilized.

A 1959 blood sample showing HIV marks the early years of the virus. Researchers believed that comparing the virus's genome with that of later HIV strains could provide information on the evolution of the virus—and, perhaps, clues to how and when HIV jumped the species barrier from monkeys or chimps to humans.

When HIV was identified in 1983, researchers began to search for its origin. Problems grew from the fact of HIV's "starburst" phylogeny—the rapid genetic variation the virus had undergone since first infecting humans. Comparison of the ZR59 sequence in the 1959 blood sample containing HIV with current viruses in nonhuman primates might lead to the identification of common denominators that may pinpoint the primate that harbored the virus that first infected humans. The sample also helped researchers attempt to establish a timetable of HIV's evolution over the decades. The belief was that this knowledge might lead to an estimate of where the virus may be headed.

Researchers also wanted to know what kind of dynamics allowed HIV to explode later in the human population. Understanding HIV's origins may help to pave the way to development of a vaccine—a research endeavor that is hampered by the many strains with DNA sequences that vary from each other. It is hoped that a vaccine based on common features shared with HIV's early ancestors will prove more effective in battling the global AIDS epidemic than would vaccines based on cocktails of subtypes.

Another HIV origin theory was proposed by Leonard G. Horowitz, D.M.D., Walter Kyle, J.D., and Alan R. Cantwell, Jr., M.D., who believe that the simian immunodeficiency virus from the chimpanzee (SIV cpz)—generally regarded as the nonhuman primate virus most closely related to HIV-1 (or a closely related simian virus)—probably contaminated the experimental hepatitis B vaccines that were administered to gay men in New York City and to blacks in Central Africa during the 1970s. The AIDS authority Robert Gallo has theorized that HIV-1 evolved from a virus in African green monkeys that "jumped species" to infect the African human population. However, these authors reviewed the medical literature extensively and decided that HIV-1 evolved and jumped species as a result of human causes.

They point out that many people think HIV-2 and HIV-1 share the ancestor simian immunodeficiency virus from the African green monkey. Plus, they say, SIVmac—a macaque monkey virus lab contaminant—is identical to HIV-2. Because no macaques in the wild have been shown to have HIV-2, these researchers contend that humans with HIV-2 must have been infected via vaccines that were contaminated. In the years from 1972 to 1974, hepatitis B vaccine producers used chimps to grow hepatitis B virus that could not be grown in human or monkey cell cultures, and the MS-2 strain of hepatitis B was then used in the development of four subtypes of experimental hepatitis B vaccine. Horowitz, Kyle, and Cantwell assert that some vaccine researchers believed that a high percentage of their lab animals had been cross-contaminated with hepatitis B and other viruses. They also offer the hypothesis that the use of live viral vaccines in New York and Africa during the 1970s

could have resulted in AIDS virus progenitors such as HIV-2 and SIV cpz.

These researchers' inquiries about the original vaccines, which the FDA has in safekeeping, did not merit an answer because details of the vaccines were under the "classified for reasons of national security" umbrella. Further, they contend that their research supports their belief in a human, vaccine-induced AIDS origin. They believe that transmission of hybrid viruses from these contaminated animals and labs would also explain the fact that the first cases of AIDS in Africa occurred at the same time the epidemic began in New York as well as the initial incidence of AIDS primarily affecting white homosexual men in the United States and black heterosexual Africans. On the other hand, there is abundant evidence that supports the contention that HIV causes AIDS. First, before HIV, AIDS-type syndromes were unusual, whereas they have become common today, in those who have HIV. Examples are *Pneumocystis carinii* pneumonia (PCP), Kaposi's sarcoma (KS), and disseminated infection with the *Mycobacterium avium* complex (MAC). A 1967 survey reported that in the United States, the medical literature described only 107 cases of PCP and only 32 people with disseminated MAC disease. Yearly incidence of Kaposi's sarcoma in the United States was 0.021 per 100,000. By December 31, 1994, these statistics had changed radically: physicians reported to the CDC 127,626 patients with AIDS in the United States with diagnoses of PCP, 36,693 with KS, and 28,954 with disseminated MAC.

Another fact supporting the cause-effect relation of HIV and AIDS is that they are linked in time, place, and population group. Historically, AIDS-like illnesses have occurred on the heels of the appearance of HIV. In every place where AIDS has shown up, evidence of HIV infection has preceded it by a few years.

Also, many studies show that presence of HIV is the only factor that predicts development of AIDS. People of diverse backgrounds, sexual preferences, and lifestyles have all contracted AIDS, and their only common denominator is having HIV. Numerous serosurveys show that AIDS is common in populations in which many individuals have HIV antibodies. Conversely, populations with low seroprevalence of HIV antibodies rarely have cases of

AIDS. Severe immunosuppression and AIDS-defining illnesses are seen only in those who are HIV-infected; matched controls who lack HIV do not have these symptoms. A persistently low CD4+ T cell count is extremely rare in the absence of HIV infection or another cause of immunosuppression. Almost all of those with AIDS have antibodies of HIV. Testing methods enable researchers to find HIV in patients with AIDS with few exceptions.

According to Koch's postulates of disease causation, the agent that is infectious must exist in all cases of the disease; the agent must be isolated from the host's body; the agent must cause disease when injected into healthy hosts; and the same agent must be isolated from the newly diseased host. All four postulates have been fulfilled in three lab workers with no other risk factors in whom AIDS or severe immunosuppression developed after accidental exposure to concentrated, cloned HIV in the lab. In all three cases, HIV was isolated from the infected person, sequenced, and shown to be the infecting strain of virus. Two were infected in 1985; one was infected in 1991.

"Does HIV Cause AIDS?" *Journal of Acquired Immune Deficiency Syndrome* 2, no. 2 (1989).

Evans, A. S. "Causation and Disease: The Henle-Koch Postulates Revisited." *Yale Journal of Biology and Medicine* 49, no.2 (1976): 175–195.

"The Evidence That HIV Causes AIDS." Fact sheet, National Institute of Allergy and Infectious Diseases, National Institutes of Health.

Hahn, Beatrice H., and George M. Shaw. "AIDS as a Zoonosis: Scientific and Public Health Implications," *Science* 287, no. 5453 (2000): 607–714.

Hirsch, V. M., et al. "An African Primate Lentivirus (SIVsm) Closely Related to HIV-2," *Nature* 321, no. 24 (1989): 1621–1625.

"Oral Polio Vaccine and HIV/AIDS." CDC National Immunization Program. Available online. URL: http://www.cdc.gov/nip/vacsafe/concerns/aids/poliovac-hiv-aids.htm.

nonoxynol-9 A common spermicide that may increase the risk of STDs because of its propensity to damage epithelial tissues. Nonoxynol-9 is the active spermicide in most brands of contraceptive jellies, foams, tablets, and creams that are designed to be used alone or with diaphragms.

Nonoxynol-9 is also used in vaginal inserts, condoms, suppositories, and contraceptive film. In labs, nonoxynol-9 has been shown to kill chlamydia, HIV, and *Neisseria gonorrhoeae*, but in actual use, it can irritate tissues; tissue irritation is believed to increase infectivity of invading viral and bacterial organisms.

Many researchers and health care professionals have long believed that spermicides such as nonoxynol-9 can offer protection against transmission of sexually transmitted diseases. However, one report indicated that researchers had found that the common spermicide nonoxynol-9 irritated tissues of prostitutes who participated in a study and thus actually enhanced their probability of contracting HIV. Research at the NIH has spotlighted the possibility that using nonoxynol-9 with condoms and diaphragms may cause latex sensitization in men and women.

nonprogressor A person who has HIV but, for some reason, has not moved into the full-blown AIDS stage. Usually, the long-term nonprogressor is identified as a person with at least 10 years of seropositivity for HIV without symptoms or T cell depletion in the absence of therapy, according to Jay F. Dobkin, M.D., the medical director of Presbyterian AIDS Center in New York City and author of "New Insights into Nonprogressive HIV Infection" in *Infections in Medicine* (1998).

In large cohort studies, researchers have discovered that fewer than 10 percent of patients meet these criteria; those who do have proved to be a scientific curiosity. No one understands fully why some people get HIV and die within a few years, and others stay healthy for decades. Dobkin tells of a patient in his clinic who did not meet the criteria but had an even more telling trait—low-level or undetectable virus load. This is a key aspect of the nonprogressor phenotype, according to an article in the *New England Journal of Medicine* (1995). One general phenomenon in nonprogressors is that they have persistent immune responsiveness and preservation of lymph node integrity, although it has been hard to pinpoint a specific immune response that confers nonprogressor status. There is evidence that a person's genetic material accounts for some of the variability, and that age, too, may be a factor. Researchers have noted that an HIV-specific CD4+ helper response seems to persist in those who are nonprogressors but is lost early on in others.

On July 10, 2002, Keith Henry, M.D., reported on work by Dr. Brigette Autran's Paris group that identified a cohort of 70 long-term nonprogressors (CD4+ T cell counts greater than 600 for five years or more without therapy) and a control cohort of 50 HIV patients with disease progression. They concluded that long-term nonprogressors are unusual patients and data is needed as to what would protect newly infected patients from progression versus what may protect long-term nonprogressors.

Henry, Keith. "Immune Responses in Long-Term Nonprogressors." The Body Website. Available online. URL: http://www.thebody.com. Downloaded July 10, 2001.

nonsexual HPV transmission   The transmission of genital warts or human papillomavirus (HPV) by means other than sexual activity. This can occur by way of surgical gloves or by mother-to-infant transmission, but both routes of transmission are extremely rare.

nonspecific urethritis   Inflammation of the urethra in men. Also known as nongonococcal urethritis, this is commonly sexually transmitted and not gonorrhea-related. The cause may be *Chlamydia trachomatis, Ureaplasma urealyticum,* or *Trichomonas vaginalis.* In rare instances, it is caused by herpes simplex virus or other viruses or bacteria. Often, men with nonspecific urethritis do not have symptoms; if they do occur a few weeks after infection, they usually take the form of painful urination, penis discharge, and an irritated-feeling penis. Often this disease arises in men who perform anal sex and become infected with stool bacteria in the urethra. In most cases, the use of condoms prevents development of nonspecific urethritis.

Testing includes a urethral swab that is examined for white blood cells. Usually nonspecific urethritis is treated with antibiotics. Partners must be evaluated and treated even if they are symptom-free and show no signs of infection. Until treatment is completed and symptoms cease in all partners, sexual activity should not be resumed.

nonvenereal genital lesions   Genital lesions that are not sexually transmitted. These include lichen planus, candidiasis, psoriasis, tinea cruris, Reiter's disease, erythrasma, contact dermatitis, herpes zoster, pearly penile papules, and seborrheic keratosis, according to the *Update in Sexually Transmitted Diseases 2001.*

Norwegian scabies   A very severe form of scabies that manifests itself in an extreme infestation of mites. This disease appears in people who have severe systemic disease, retardation, senility, and immunosuppression.

The difference between Norwegian scabies and regular scabies is the number of mites found on the infected individual. Regular scabies usually causes a person to host about 10 to 15 mites at a time; a patient who has Norwegian scabies has thousands to millions. As a result, the skin problem is much more severe, creating thick crusts on various parts of the body. Interestingly, the type of mite is the same in both varieties of scabies. The host is the difference because the person who contracts Norwegian scabies almost always has an immune system that is compromised. Underscoring this point is the fact that when a person who has a normally functioning immune system contracts scabies from someone with the Norwegian type, the former experiences only a typical case of ordinary scabies—not the extreme Norwegian presentation.

Sarcoptes scabiei cannot jump or fly, so a person contracts the infection by direct contact with someone who is infected or by contact with infected items: linens, furniture, clothing, and so on. A health care worker who touches anything in the room of a patient with Norwegian scabies is likely to get the infection unless he or she wears gloves.

Time from infection to symptoms is brief for Norwegian scabies—only about 10 to 14 days—whereas regular scabies usually causes symptoms in about four to six weeks. For Norwegian scabies, the treatment is topical ectoparasiticide cream

(Permethrin) followed by application of 6 percent sulfur in petrolatum. The treatment takes several weeks.

nosocomially acquired HIV HIV infection that is acquired in a hospital or health care setting. The means of transmission would be a needlestick in which a health care worker is infected by the blood of a person with HIV or by touching (ungloved) the blood, feces, or other body fluids of an HIV-positive patient who has an open lesion.

notifiable disease A disease that must be reported to health authorities. By law, doctors have a list of diseases they are required to report. Nationally notifiable sexually transmitted diseases change from year to year. As of 2002, the nationally notifiable infectious diseases included the following: acquired immunodeficiency syndrome (AIDS), anthrax, botulism, brucellosis, chancroid, *Chlamydia trachomatis* genital infections, cholera, coccidioidomycosis, cryptosporidiosis, cyclosporiasis, diphtheria, ehrlichiosis, arboviral encephalitis (California serogroup viral, Eastern equine, Powassan, Saint Louis, Western equine, West Nile), enterohemorrhagic *Escherichia coli*, HIV infection, legionellosis, listeriosis, Lyme disease, malaria, measles, meningococcal disease, mumps, pertussis, plague, paralytic poliomyelitis, psittacosis, Q fever, rabies (animal and human), Rocky Mountain spotted fever, rubella (congenital syndrome), salmonellosis, shigellosis, invasive group A streptococcal disease, streptococcal toxic shock syndrome, *Streptococcus pneumoniae* (drug-resistant, invasive disease), syphilis, neurosyphilis, congenital syphilis, syphilitic stillbirth, giardiasis, gonorrhea, *Haemophilus influenzae* (invasive disease), Hansen disease (leprosy), Hantavirus pulmonary syndrome, hemolytic uremic syndrome (postdiarrheal), viral hepatitis (acute), hepatitis A (acute), hepatitis B (acute), hepatitis B virus perinatal infection, hepatitis C (non-A, non-B, acute), tetanus, toxic-shock syndrome, trichinosis, tuberculosis, tularemia, typhoid fever, varicella (deaths only), and yellow fever.

nukes The nickname for nucleoside analogs used in the drug treatment of HIV. They inhibit the reverse transcriptase of HIV. These are called nucleoside reverse transcriptase inhibitors (NRTIs) or "nukes."

Nureyev, Rudolf When the famous ballet star Rudolf Nureyev died on January 6, 1993, rumors flew around the world that his friends said he had succumbed to AIDS. But his physician had told the media that the cause of death was "a cardiac complication, following a grievous illness." This spurred a controversy in that many found Nureyev's desire to conceal the true cause of death cowardly. A week later, his physician told a French newspaper that Nureyev had indeed died of AIDS. He also stated that the ballet great had lived for about 13 years with the virus. He had not gone public because a number of countries, including the United States, refused entry to people who were HIV-positive. Nureyev died of a rare case of pericarditis caused by cytomegalovirus.

nutrition The process of nourishing one's body or the processes by which a human being takes in food and utilizes it. *Nutrition* refers to the complete intake and use of food, which includes ingesting, digesting, absorbing, and metabolizing, making the body function. Someone who is malnourished is not well equipped to fight off infections. Good nutrition is extremely important to maintaining the health of individuals with sexually transmitted diseases. Some people with HIV also use megavitamin supplementation in hopes of boosting their immune systems. However, no established evidence confirms that food supplements do help a person with HIV.

One of many dietary regimens that have had a number of proponents in HIV (and cancer) circles is the macrobiotic diet, known for its emphasis on the consumption primarily of vegetables and grains. However, some dietitians criticize this plan as deficient in needed nutrients and claim that it cannot enhance one's overall health. In most cases, physicians encourage those people who are dealing with a sexually transmitted disease to follow a dietary regimen that is nutritious and features plenty of healthy choices, including protein, vegetables, grains, fruits, and sufficient water. This is favored over any plan that is based on dietary extremes. A consultation with a registered dietitian to set up a food regimen may help an STD-infected individual get on the right track and understand the role that correct diet can play in the healing process.

occupational exposure Exposure to sexually transmitted disease that occurs during the normal course of one's occupation. An example would be a sex worker's heightened chance of contracting diseases as a result of overexposure to high-risk activities and individuals, or a health care worker's heightened exposure to blood that may be contaminated with HIV.

ocular herpes A herpes infection of the eye that is caused by transfer of the infection from an infected part of the body to the eye. A person with a herpes infection of the eye should consult an ophthalmologist (eye doctor) immediately.

OI See OPPORTUNISTIC INFECTION.

oncogenic potential The likelihood of a disease to cause tumors.

oral–anal sex A form of sexual activity viewed by health care experts as extremely high-risk because a partner can come in contact with feces, which may transmit a sexually transmitted disease. The act of performing oral–anal sex puts one individual's mouth in contact with the anus of the other partner, thus enhancing the likelihood of transmission of disease.

oral–genital sex Cunnilingus, oral sex performed on a woman's clitoris and other sexual organs; fellatio is oral sex performed on a man's penis. Either can transmit HIV, but the one more likely to transmit HIV is fellatio, because an HIV-positive man's semen contains more HIV than does an HIV-infected woman's vaginal secretions.

See also ORAL SEX.

oral mucosal lesions Lesions or sores in the mouth caused by several sexually transmitted diseases. These can be infectious and can be transmitted to a sex partner by means of oral sex. Gonorrhea and chlamydia can cause a throat to be sore and red. Symptoms of oral herpes are bumps, blisters, or ulcers on the lips, roof of the mouth, or gums and throat. One can contract herpes type 2 in the mouth by performing oral sex on someone who has genital type 2 herpes. However, typically type 2 herpes in the mouth does not result in symptoms. A person who performs oral sex on a partner with syphilis may acquire syphilis infection; the initial manifestation is a painless ulcer on the tongue, gums, or throat. Anyone who has a yeast infection in the mouth (white patches, redness, soreness) should seek HIV testing.

It is also important to note that many other physical conditions besides sexually transmitted diseases can cause mouth sores and ulcers. These include Crohn's disease, ulcerative colitis, and some autoimmune conditions. The most common oral ulcers that are not sexually transmitted are called aphthous ulcers—the painful small ulcers that sometimes occur on the sides of the mouth or the inside of the lips, last about a week, and then disappear spontaneously. The cause of these is unknown, but they are not herpes lesions, as is often mistakenly believed. A sore in the mouth that does not heal is characteristic of oral cancer; these lesions often occur under the tongue.

See also GENITAL HERPES.

oral papillomas Benign growths that appear on the skin or mucous membranes of the oral cavity (mouth) and protrude above the surrounding tissue. A wart is a papilloma. In respect to sexually transmitted diseases, oral papillomas are seen in the context of the disease genital warts (which has been transmitted to the mouth of a partner via oral sex) and HIV/AIDS. Warts in the mouth are common in patients who are treated in HIV/AIDS clinics.

oral sex The act of giving sexual gratification to a partner via one's mouth on the other's genitals. The sexually transmitted diseases that can be passed on by performing oral sex are HIV, genital warts, syphilis, gonorrhea, herpes, chlamydia, lymphogranuloma venereum, and nongonococcal urethritis.

The risk of transmission with oral sex is heightened if a person has cuts or sores in the mouth or throat; if the partner ejaculates in his or her mouth; or if the partner has pre-existing sexually transmitted disease. To prevent infection in the act of having oral sex with a male partner, it is important to use a latex condom on the penis or a plastic condom if one partner has an allergy to latex. Condoms reduce risk greatly. The individual who is having oral sex with a female partner should use a latex barrier such as a dental dam or cut-open condom (it should form a square between the mouth of the person performing oral sex and the other's vagina). In the case of HIV, evidence suggests that the risk is lower for oral sex than for unprotected anal or vaginal sex. The virus can be transmitted via blood, semen, preseminal fluid, and vaginal fluid.

Researchers who reported on the most definitive study to date on the link between oral sex and HIV transmission found evidence that "a significant percentage" of new HIV infections in some groups of men who have sex with men are due to oral sex. This is noteworthy when one considers that many people tend to view this mode of transmission as almost nonexistent. However, at the 7th Conference on Retroviruses and Opportunistic Infections (2000), the Centers for Disease Control and Prevention reported that 7.8 percent of a group of HIV-infected men were infected via oral sex. This study looked at risk

behavior for 102 gay and bisexual men who had been recently infected with HIV and found that the only risk behavior eight of the men practiced was oral sex. Although it is true that, overall, oral sex is less likely to transmit HIV than are other forms of sexual activity, repeated exposures can pose a more formidable risk. Also of note is that before this study, it was hard to discover whether an individual had been infected through oral sex because few engage in that sexual activity exclusively, and it was also impossible to zero in on time of infection.

oral signs Signs of a sexually transmitted disease that are in evidence in the mouth area. The chancre (painless ulcer) of primary syphilis can occur in the mouth or on the lips. In secondary syphilis, mucous patches can occur in the mouth. Oral signs of HIV include oral hairy leukoplakia and thrush.

See also HIV; LEUKOPLAKIA.

orgasm The peak of sexual excitement that culminates in ejaculation in men and vaginal contractions in women.

orifice An opening. Body orifices include the mouth, anus, and vagina.

ostracism The act of excluding someone from a group, often by agreement. In cases of sexually transmitted diseases, it is not unusual for an individual with a disease to be held at arm's length by prospective sexual partners. For this reason, deceiving potential partners is not an unusual practice among some people who have sexually transmitted diseases that have not been cured or cannot be cured.

outercourse Referred to as sex play without intercourse, certain methods listed by Planned Parenthood that allow people to "have sex" without sperm having a chance to join an egg. These include masturbation (alone or with a partner), erotic massage, and body rubbing. These methods are effective in preventing transmission of HIV and other sexually transmitted diseases unless partners exchange body fluids via oral or anal intercourse or come in contact with infectious lesions.

ovary The female sex organ that releases eggs from menarche (the start of menstruation) to menopause (the end of menstruation). The ovary also makes estrogen and progesterone.

over-the-counter drug A medication that is available without a doctor's authorization or prescription.

painful intercourse Pain during intercourse does not automatically signal that a person has a sexually transmitted disease. Genital herpes sores can cause pain, or a woman may feel pain during penetration by her partner's penis if she has a vaginal infection (trichomonas or a yeast infection, for example). When deep penetration is causing a woman to experience pain, that may mean that there is an infection of the cervix or pelvic organs—chlamydia, gonorrhea, pelvic inflammatory disease, or mucopurulent cervicitis. Causes of painful intercourse that are unrelated to sexually transmitted disease include endometriosis, vaginal muscle spasms, and a condition resulting from being postmenopausal (thinned tissue resulting from estrogen loss).

pandemic A worldwide epidemic that affects a very high proportion of the global population. A pandemic disease affects most of the people in a country or countries.

Papanicolaou smear In a Pap smear, also referred to as a cervical smear, a doctor scrapes from the surface of the cervix and just inside its opening a specimen of cellular material (usually during a woman's yearly well-woman examination) and sends the specimen to a lab for analysis. It is examined microscopically for signs of cancer or precancerous changes in the cells. In the spectrum of sexually transmitted diseases, human papillomavirus, the virus that causes genital warts, can cause abnormal Pap smear results that merit further investigation. In some cases, the abnormal Pap smear finding is the woman's first indication that she has contracted genital warts and thus warns her that she needs further evaluation and possible treatment.

The Pap test is named after the physician George Papanicolaou, who introduced this technique in 1949. Although this important innovation has served to reduce the incidence of cervical cancer, researchers have continued their study of cervical disease causes. By the 1970s, much evidence suggested that cervical abnormalities had a close link to sexual activity and perhaps to certain STDs. Ten years later, scientists had narrowed their search to human papillomavirus (HPV). Some types of HPV lead to genital warts or cervical abnormalities, and some of the signs that show up in a Pap test result signal HPV.

Although the Pap smear remains significant in screening, researchers now can identify the DNA of many HPV types, and new diagnostic tests can help to confirm the presence of the HPV types that are linked to cervical disease. A major HPV DNA test approved by the FDA, Hybrid Capture II, accurately detects up to 13 high-risk HPV types and some low-risk ones.

According to the SexHealth Web Site (October 1, 2001, "Is the Pap Smear Obsolete?"), HPV typing is not yet routine in gynecologic care. The Hybrid Capture test is approved by the FDA for those women whose Pap smear results are "of unknown significance." This test does not necessarily require an extra office visit because Pap tests done with a new collection system called ThinPrep result in a sample that can also be used for HPV typing tests. It is important for women to know that having Pap smears does not eliminate the need for the tests that diagnose sexually transmitted diseases more effectively. A study of 278 women in the Netherlands published in the *Journal of Pathology* showed that HPV testing using Digene's Hybrid Capture II HPV DNA Test was more effective than a Pap smear test in indicating which of the women with borderline Pap smear results were truly at risk for cervical cancer. The Digene HPV Test was 96.3 percent sensitive in pinpointing women who had moderate- to high-grade cervical disease, whereas the Pap smear had 56 percent sensitivity. This underscores the important role in cervical cancer detection that HPV testing can play. (Source: www.docguide.com, "Human Papillomavirus Testing Highly Valuable in Cervical Cancer Screening.")

In the article "HPV Screening Plus Pap Tests Every Two Years Found Better, More Cost-Effective than Pap Tests Alone" (Elda Hauschildt, *Journal of the American Medical Association,* 2002; 287: 2372–2381), researchers go on record as saying that "screening women for human papillomavirus (HPV) plus Pap tests biennially from age 20 can save additional years of life at a reasonable cost, compared to Pap tests alone." The combination of biennial HPV and Pap tests served to avert the greatest number of invasive cervical cancer cases and deaths.

Pap smear report   After a Pap smear is done, the sample is sent to a lab for examination. The report is sent to the patient's doctor, who informs the woman of the result, the Pap smear report. It may be normal or may highlight that the cervix showed cellular changes that are precancerous or indicative of cervical cancer. Cervical intraepithelial neoplasia 1 (CIN 1) is mild dysplasia; CIN 2 is moderate dysplasia; CIN 3 indicates that the woman has severe dysplasia or carcinoma in situ (preinvasive cancer). If a woman does receive a Pap smear report that points to some kind of abnormality, her doctor discusses with her what the results mean and whether any further testing or treatment is necessary.

papule   A small, discrete skin bump.

parent–adolescent communication   Most parents in the United States are acutely aware that teen pregnancies and sexually transmitted diseases are major problems among youth and that they need to be able to communicate good information concerning sexuality to their adolescent children.

But in a study reported in *Adolescence* (1998), the parents interviewed claimed that they not only felt uncomfortable discussing sex with their kids, but also felt they lacked information. The researchers reviewed 26 articles in the popular press that appeared from 1984 to 1993, all of which offered advice on how parents could effectively convey this kind of information. They discovered that these articles were flawed in that they addressed white readerships and mothers in traditional families; plus, there was little advice given on difficult issues such as AIDS and contraception. Findings suggest that the popular press could be an informational vehicle for disseminating sex information to young people and their parents, but the tips and guidelines published must be appropriate for a very broad audience.

partner counseling   Verbal advice from a doctor or counseling professional aimed at a couple who are sex partners. Sexually transmitted diseases have become a huge part of the public health picture, and it is important that sex partners seek counseling when one of the couple has difficulty understanding or accepting the existence of a sexually transmitted disease. Sometimes a health care professional's urging is necessary to persuade the other partner to seek treatment or use safe-sex methods; in such cases, partner counseling can be extremely valuable. Prevention and educational counseling are most effective when provided non-judgmentally and in a way that is appropriate to the couple's culture, language, sexual orientation, age, and developmental level.

partner notification   See RIGHT TO KNOW.

partner selection   Choice of a sexual partner. For anyone who is sexually active, the question of partner selection is always a critical one, but particularly in a period when sexually transmitted diseases are running rampant in the United States as well as worldwide. Key to this issue is understanding that one cannot detect whether a person actually has a sexually transmitted disease by looking at him or her. A person can be impeccably groomed, extremely articulate, and perfectly dressed and yet have HIV. Thus, good communication in the arena of sexual activity is critical. Furthermore, many people try to deceive potential sex partners because they fear that their diseased state will be a roadblock to sex. This points up the importance of avoiding a promiscuous approach to dating in favor of seeking meaningful relationships in which sexuality is but one ingredient of a satisfying bond—and the partners know each other and feel some sense of responsibility for safeguarding each other's health.

pathogen   A microorganism that causes a disease.

patterns of condom use   In the early days of the AIDS epidemic, there was a rush to the use of condoms as the knowledge that one could die from this sexually transmitted disease sent people scurrying to stores and health agencies for preventive options. In recent years, however, a new and frightening complacency has made the use of condoms much sketchier in that many sexually active people are less afraid of HIV/AIDS because HAART has extended the lives of many Americans who are HIV-positive. The irony is that a very positive outcome—increased longevity—has had a very negative effect: a more lax attitude to taking precautions when having sex.

In 1999, the CDC issued a report reiterating its stand that condoms are a good means of protection from STDs. The CDC news release stated that lab studies show that latex condoms are effective barriers to HIV and other STDs, and several studies show compelling evidence that these are extremely effective in protecting against HIV when used for every sexual act. The findings are from studies of discordant couples (couples in whom one member is infected with an STD and the other is not); in a two-year study of discordant couples in Europe, among 124 who used latex condoms consistently, none of the uninfected persons became infected. However, of 121 couples using condoms inconsistently, 12 (or 10 percent) of the uninfected partners became infected. Another study showed that in a group of 134 discordant couples not using condoms at all or using them haphazardly, 16 partners became infected.

In a study of condom use among adolescents (*Pediatrics,* June 2001), it was found that sexual activity and pregnancy rate decreased slightly among adolescents in the 1990s, reversing trends of the two previous decades, and condom use among adolescents increased significantly. This decrease is attributed to the success of adolescent-framed prevention campaigns. At the same time, though, rates of acquisition of STDs and HIV in adolescents remain extremely high, underscoring the need for continued education efforts and showing that higher use of condoms can decrease but never eliminate the acquisition of STDs and HIV as well as unwanted pregnancies. No evidence exists that condom education programs increase teen sexual activity.

Researchers report mixed findings on the effectiveness of condom use in preventing the spread of sexually transmitted diseases. It appears that condoms are effective against transmission of HIV and gonorrhea in men, but less effective in women and in prevention of other sexually transmitted diseases, including genital herpes, chlamydia, and syphilis; basically, the jury is still out. In response, the Physicians Consortium accused the CDC of overstating the effectiveness of condoms in respect to preventing STD transmission. In rebuttal to the Physicians Consortium's blast, the CDC retorted that the new report does not discount condom use as ineffective, but rather states that they only found sufficient evidence to support the finding that condoms work well in preventing transmission of HIV and gonorrhea. The CDC still takes the stand that male latex condoms, used correctly and consistently, are highly effective in protecting people who are sexually active against HIV and can reduce the risk of contracting other sexually transmitted diseases.

Many in health care note that the findings are varied: studies alternately show that condoms provide poor protection against STDs, or moderate protection, or good protection. Many health care providers note what they have long known—that condoms offer little or no protection against the transmission of genital warts—yet this remains a fact that is not widely known or disseminated to the public.

Physicians now face a unique situation in which recommending condoms is still a good idea because of the benefits they do offer. At the same time, they cannot tell patients that condoms will protect them fully against syphilis, chlamydia, and herpes since the evidence does not support that assertion.

A report in *Journal of the American Medical Association* (June 27, 2001) indicated that even inconsistent condom use appeared to offer significant protection of women in a study of genital herpes in discordant couples. Women who used condoms during at least 25 percent of their sexual encounters had just 8 percent of the type 2 genital herpes risk of women who used condoms less often. The researcher Anna Walk, M.D., M.P.H., of the University of Washington, adds that although they have not yet analyzed and published the data for men, there is no reason to think that condoms do not work for men and endorses using condoms for herpes prevention across the board.

pediatric AIDS A case of pediatric AIDS, as defined by the CDC, is a child who has had (1) a reliably diagnosed disease that is at least moderately indicative of underlying cellular immunodeficiency, and (2) no known cause of this immunodeficiency or any other reduced resistance associated with that disease. The diseases that are indicative are the same ones that define AIDS in adults except for congenital infections such as toxoplasmosis or herpes simplex in the month after birth, or cytomegalovirus in the six months after birth. There were 543 pediatric HIV cases reported to the Centers for Disease Control and Prevention in the year 2001 in the United States in children younger than 13—a dramatic increase from 224 in 2000. Most pediatric AIDS cases in recent years have been acquired by mother-to-child, or perinatal, transmission, according to the Centers for Disease Control and Prevention. Through December 2001, 9,074 children younger than 13 had AIDS, and of these, 58 percent (5,257) had died. During 2001, 175 new cases of AIDS in children were reported, 150 of whom had gotten AIDS via perinatal exposure. In 2002, worldwide about 2,000 children younger than 15 became infected with HIV *every day,* and 3.2 million children younger than 15 were living with HIV/AIDS.

During the early 1990s, before perinatal preventive treatments were available to American pregnant women, about 1,000 to 2,000 infants were born with HIV every year in the United States. The dramatic decline in perinatal HIV transmission is a result of the success of U.S. public health service recommendations made in 1994 and 1995 for routine counseling and voluntary testing of all pregnant women for HIV; for use of zidovudine (AZT) by pregnant women with HIV during their pregnancy and delivery; and for drug therapy for newborns.

From 1992 to 1997, perinatally acquired AIDS cases in the United States dropped by 66 percent. Among women who participated in the CDC's Perinatal AIDS Collaborative Transmission Study, AZT use increased after Public Health Service guidelines were published; the rate of perinatal transmission went from 21 percent to 11 percent. Included in this study were women from New York City, Newark, Baltimore, and Atlanta. Experts predict that without U.S. perinatal care interventions (HIV counseling, testing, and AZT treatment for infected mothers and children), many more lives would be lost, and a 24 percent mother-to-infant transmission rate would result in the births of an estimated 1,750 HIV-infected infants every year in the United States (with lifetime medical costs of about $282 million). Every year, perinatal prevention efforts in the United States cost about $67.6 million; they prevent approximately 656 HIV infections and preclude the need for $105.6 million in medical care costs.

Since about 91 percent of AIDS cases in U.S. children result from mother-to-infant HIV transmission (during pregnancy, labor, and delivery or through breast-feeding), it is clear that the rate of pediatric AIDS cases can be dramatically reduced by preventing infection in women and promoting early prenatal care with HIV counseling and testing. Because statistics show that women who use illegal drugs during pregnancy are the least likely to seek and get prenatal care, many organizations are attempting to increase efforts at all levels to enlarge HIV prevention activities and substance abuse programs and to help pregnant women get the care they need.

The rate of disease progression in an infant with HIV/AIDS bears a direct correlation to the severity of the disease when the mother gives birth, according to the European Collaborative Study (1992). Most infants born to seropositive mothers have HIV antibodies that are detectable—a state that may last for as long as 15 months. However, in most cases, this does not point to actual HIV infection. Rather, it indicates that antibodies have crossed the placenta. The European Collaborative Study (10 European centers) of mothers, most of whom had histories of intravenous drug use, found that AIDS or immune deficiency had developed in none of the 343 children who no longer had maternally transferred HIV antibodies, but of the 64 who were HIV-infected (and retained their HIV antibody response), 30 percent had AIDS in six months, and by age one 17 percent had died.

pelvic inflammatory disease (PID)   Infection of the fallopian tubes, which carry eggs from the ovary to the womb, and of other internal reproductive organs in women. Not counting AIDS, pelvic inflammatory disease is the most common and serious complication of sexually transmitted diseases among women. This infection of the upper genital tract can affect the uterus, ovaries, fallopian tubes, and other related structures. Untreated PID can lead to serious consequences, such as infertility, ectopic pregnancy, chronic pelvic pain, and abscess formation.

Cause

When disease-causing organisms migrate up from the urethra and cervix to the upper genital tract, pelvic inflammatory disease sometimes develops. Various organisms can cause PID; the most common are gonorrhea and chlamydial infections. There is also a role played by bacteria that are normally present in the vagina and cervix. *Neisseria gonorrhoeae* causes PID by traveling to the fallopian tubes and causing the sloughing of some cells and invasion of others. It is believed that within and under these cells, the organism multiplies, then spreads the infection to other organs, leading to more inflammation and scarring.

Researchers think that *Chlamydia trachomatis* and other bacteria act similarly. However, it remains unclear how bacteria that normally exist in the vagina gain entrance to the upper genital tract. Perhaps the cervical mucus plug and secretions help prevent microorganisms from spreading to the upper genital tract—a form of protection that is probably less effective during ovulation and menses. Another contention is that the organism that causes gonorrhea has greater access during menses if the menstrual blood flows backward from the uterus to the fallopian tubes, moving the organisms along. In some women who have gonorrhea and chlamydia, symptomatic PID develops.

Symptoms

Symptoms of pelvic inflammatory disease vary from nonexistent to severe. Women who do experience symptoms usually report lower abdominal pain. Other signs are fever, a foul-smelling vaginal discharge, discomfort during sexual intercourse, painful urination, pain in the right upper abdomen, and irregular menstrual bleeding.

It is interesting to note that most women who are diagnosed with tubal infertility do not report ever having had PID symptoms. That is because PID may cause only mild symptoms or none at all, even while it is doing serious damage to the woman's reproductive organs. This finding underscores the sometimes silent nature of this malady, in which an organism invades the tubes and scars them, thus blocking eggs from normal passage into the uterus.

A tubal pregnancy, wherein a fertilized egg does not pass into the uterus to grow, is about six to 10 times more likely when a woman has had PID. When pelvic inflammatory disease is untreated, some women have long-term pelvic pain.

When PID is caused by chlamydial infection, there usually are few symptoms, if any. However, it can damage the reproductive organs, regardless of the absence of symptoms. According to the Centers for Disease Control and Prevention, chlamydia, if untreated, can lead to pelvic inflammatory disease in up to 40 percent of cases.

PID is a serious infection of the reproductive organs that affects about 1 million women in the United States every year. Half of the cases are attributed to chlamydial infections, many of which occur symptom-free.

Diagnosis

Pelvic inflammatory disease can be hard to diagnose when the symptoms are subtle. A diagnosis is based on clinical findings. When the patient reports lower abdominal pain, the doctor performs a physical exam; if she also has fever, abnormal discharge (cervical or vaginal), and evidence of cervical chlamydial or gonorrhea infection, the doctor is likely to arrive at a diagnosis of PID.

If more information is needed before initiating treatment, the doctor may order an ultrasound or laparoscopy, which can help ascertain whether it is pelvic inflammatory disease or another disorder that has similar symptoms. Via laparoscopy—a surgical procedure in which a tiny flexible tube with a lighted end is inserted through a small incision below the navel—the doctor can view the internal abdominal and pelvic organs. At the same time, she or he can take specimens for cultures or microscopic studies if necessary. A pelvic ultrasound is helpful in diagnosing PID because an ultrasound can view the pelvic area to see whether the fallopian tubes are enlarged or an abscess is present.

Treatment

Antibiotics can cure PID, and prompt treatment can prevent severe damage to pelvic organs. However, antibiotic treatment cannot reverse existing damage. A doctor usually prescribes at least two antibiotics that effectively wipe out a wide range of infectious agents. Mode of delivery is by mouth or by vein.

Before the infection is cured, the symptoms may disappear. If a patient becomes symptom-free, she should nevertheless complete the course of the medication to cure the infection. A patient should return to the doctor about three days after starting treatment to make sure the antibiotics are working. About a fourth of those with suspected pelvic inflammatory disease have to be hospitalized, particularly those who are very ill with high fever, HIV-infected, are pregnant, or cannot use oral medications (because of nausea and vomiting) and need intravenous administration of drugs in a hospital setting.

If symptoms persist, or if an abscess cannot be eliminated, surgery may be necessary. Complica-

tions of PID—chronic pelvic pain and scarring—are hard to treat, but sometimes surgery improves the condition. If a woman has pelvic inflammatory disease, her sex partners also need treatment to prevent reinfection.

Complications

If a woman is treated early for pelvic inflammatory disease, complications can be prevented in most cases. Women who have recurrent episodes of PID are most likely to suffer the scarring of the tubes that spins off into infertility, tubal pregnancy, and/or chronic pelvic discomfort.

When pelvic inflammatory disease is not treated, permanent damage to the female reproductive organs can occur. Infection-causing bacteria can silently invade the fallopian tubes, causing normal tissue to turn into scar tissue. Scar tissue prevents normal movement of eggs into the uterus. If the scar tissue totally blocks fallopian tubes, an egg cannot be fertilized by sperm or move to the uterus to develop into a fetus. The most severe result of PID is this scarring of the fallopian tubes, because the blockage prevents fertilization from taking place in the woman's body, thus rendering many women infertile (unable to conceive). A woman is infertile if her tubes are totally blocked, and even partially blocked or slightly damaged fallopian tubes can cause infertility. Of women with PID, approximately one of five becomes infertile, and multiple episodes of PID heighten a woman's likelihood of becoming infertile.

There are also cases in which scarring interferes with the passage of a fertilized egg down into the uterus, causing the egg to implant in the fallopian tube. This is called an ectopic, or tubal, pregnancy. Not only does this threaten the mother's life; it also results in loss of the fetus.

Furthermore, an infant exposed to *C. trachomatis* in the birth canal may contract an eye infection (conjunctivitis) and/or pneumonia. If an infant is infected, eye discharge and swollen lids typically appear within the first 10 days of life. A severe cough and congestion, caused by pneumonia, develop within three to six weeks of birth. (Doctors treat both conditions with antibiotics.) Since the risks to the baby's health are great, it is not uncommon for doctors to recommend routine testing of pregnant women for chlamydia.

At Risk for PID

The following are at highest risk for PID:

- Women who have sexually transmitted diseases, especially gonorrhea and chlamydia. A prior episode of pelvic inflammatory disease heightens risk of another episode because the body's defenses are usually damaged during the initial bout of infection.
- Sexually active women younger than 25.
- Women who have many sex partners or have a sex partner who has multiple partners.
- Women who douche.
- Women who have an intrauterine device (IUD) may have a slightly increased risk compared to women who use other contraceptives or no contraceptives at all. Mutual monogamy is encouraged for those women who use an IUD to decrease the risk of PID.

Sexually active teens have a greater chance of development of PID than do older women. Further, an episode of pelvic inflammatory disease makes a woman more likely to have another one.

Prevention

Women can take a proactive approach to making sure that they do not contract PID; if they have PID, they can seek early treatment to ensure that the condition does not prevent them from having children. The main cause of PID is an untreated sexually transmitted disease, so women can protect themselves from PID by taking action to make sure they do not contract sexually transmitted diseases and by being treated early if they do.

The following are good precautions:

- Check with your doctor if you have any suspicion that you may have a sexually transmitted disease. Do not have sex, and go to see a doctor immediately. Watch for any genital symptoms: rash, discharge with odor, sore(s), burning with urination, or bleeding between menstrual cycles.
- Seek prompt treatment to prevent development of PID.

- Correctly and consistently use male latex condoms to prevent transmission of STDs. This means using them during every sex act.
- Avoid douching. Regular douching once or twice a month appears to make a woman more likely to contract PID than does a woman who douches less often or not at all.
- Have a screening test for sexually transmitted diseases.
- If you are not abstinent, limit sexual contact to one partner, and do not have sex with anyone who has genital sores. (This is not to suggest, however, that all sexually transmitted diseases can be seen—often they cannot).

Research

Studies on the effects of antibiotics, hormones, and immune-system boosters are under way with the goal of discovering ways to prevent infertility and other PID complications. Also in development are topical microbicides and vaccines to prevent gonorrhea and chlamydial infection. Researchers are also working on tests that are quick and easily used for diagnosis of chlamydia and gonorrhea.

penis pain   External genital discomfort or itchiness, irritation inside the penis, or pain during urination, which require medical evaluation and treatment. Such symptoms may be mild or severe; they may come and go; it is possible that a discharge may accompany the discomfort. Usually a male mistakenly attributes such problems to other causes, but, in most cases, the cause is one of the following: chlamydia, nongonoccal urethritis, gonorrhea, urinary tract infection, urethral warts, prostate infection, or genital herpes. (See separate entries on these conditions.)

periodontal disease   Usually considered synonymous with gum disease, a disorder that actually encompasses bone, periodontal membrane, and gums. Caused by the action of plaque on the teeth adjacent to these tissues, periodontal disease in its early form is called gingivitis. In more severe stages, it is periodontitis, wherein bone loss and gaps between teeth and gums can occur. People with poor oral hygiene often have periodontal disease, but it is also a major problem for those who have compromised immune systems, such as individuals who have HIV or AIDS.

peripheral neuropathy A complication associated with HIV and AIDS, a painful sensory nerve disorder. Although not a disease, peripheral neuropathy is a manifestation of a number of conditions that can cause damage to peripheral nerves.

A person's peripheral nervous system includes all the nerves that are not in the central nervous system (CNS), which consists of the brain and spinal cord. The central nervous system uses the peripheral nervous system to work in concert with the rest of the body. Damage to the nerves of the peripheral system disrupts the flow of communication back to the CNS and from the CNS to other parts of the body. Peripheral neuropathy may indicate damage to a single nerve, a nerve group, or many nerves. There are times when the cause cannot be determined. Other body structures may be compressing a nerve or nerves; surgery may cause some nerve damage; and maintaining a cramped position for extended periods can result in the injury of a nerve. Systemic causes of neuropathy include hereditary conditions, metabolic disorders, medical conditions that damage nerve tissue, and disorders that affect blood supply to nerve cells and that affect the connective tissues of nerves.

Some of the medical conditions that are associated with neuropathy are AIDS, HIV, syphilis, Guillain-Barré syndrome, botulism, Colorado tick fever, diphtheria, leprosy, rheumatoid arthritis, amyloidosis, lupus, sarcoidosis, dietary deficiencies, Charcot-Marie-Tooth disease, Friedreich's ataxia, diabetes, alcoholism, uremia, multiple myeloma, lymphoma, leukemia, lung cancer, and various infectious or inflammatory conditions. Also associated with neuropathy are exposure to toxins, use of certain drugs, prolonged exposure to cold, and decreased oxygen and blood flow.

Symptoms depend on whether sensory or motor nerve fibers are affected. If the sensory fibers are damaged, a person can experience changes in sensation, including decreased or lack of feeling or pain. These sensation changes generally start in the feet or hands, then move toward the body's center. Damage to motor fibers blocks impulses to an area and causes impairment of movement of the area supplied by the nerve. Deficient nerve stimulation to a muscle group translates to weakness or reduced control of movement. Muscle atrophy (wasting) can result from the lack of nerve stimulation.

The cause must be found and treated. Treatment involves removal, if possible, of the agent causing the problem, as in toxic neuropathy caused by alcoholism, and treatment of any associated systemic illness. Sometimes steroids are prescribed.

Numerous treatment modalities may be considered for their appropriateness, from nutritional supplements to physical therapy. Safety measures need to be emphasized for those who are having movement and sensation difficulties. For the pain of neuropathy, a person may need to use over-the-counter analgesics or prescription pain medications. For stabbing pain, a doctor may prescribe tricyclic antidepressants or anticonvulsants.

A new treatment for peripheral neuropathy is the lidocaine patch, which was reported at the 14th International AIDS Conference (July 2002). According to "AIDS 2002: Lidocaine Patch Treats HIV-Associated Peripheral Neuropathy" (www.docguide.com), a pilot study has shown that this treatment can provide symptomatic relief for some HIV patients. The patches were worn by 10 patients, who used them 12 of every 24 hours for four weeks. Reduction in the intensity and sharpness of pain, how "hot" the pain felt, and how bad the surface discomfort felt were reported. It appeared that the patch did improve the subjects' ability to work, sleep, and walk because the peripheral neuropathy was less of a factor.

persistent generalized lymphadenopathy Abnormal enlargement of the lymph nodes, which creates a chronic problem that lasts for more than a month in at least two separate areas (not including the groin). This condition is commonly seen in early HIV infection.

person living with AIDS An individual whose HIV infection has progressed to full-blown AIDS.

pet ownership   In people who are ill, a practice that is believed to be a significant stress reducer. The daily chores involved and the unconditional acceptance both can help an individual with HIV/AIDS, for example, have a better quality of life and achieve a state of relaxation. In later stages, however, a person living with AIDS may need help in caring for a pet, as the disease becomes more debilitating and makes her or him less mobile.

phallus   Another name for the penis.

pharyngeal gonorrhea   Gonorrhea infection that has infected the throat, usually as a result of oral sex with a gonorrhea-infected partner.

physician selection   The choice by a person who has a sexually transmitted disease of a treating physician who can help to ease the difficulty of dealing with an unpleasant diagnosis through good rapport. A family physician, urologist, gynecologist, or internal medicine doctor can take a matter-of-fact approach to discussing the problem and outline the options for treatment and/or cure. In the case of HIV patients, it is important to have a doctor who is experienced in HIV/AIDS medicine directing drug therapy.

PID   See PELVIC INFLAMMATORY DISEASE.

piercing   The penetration of skin by a pointed instrument. Body piercing can be a means of contracting HIV or hepatitis if the personnel in the piercing facility reuse needles and other equipment that may have remnants of blood from previous customers. The piercer should use a new, disposable needle for each person.

"ping-pong" infection   Transmission of a sexually transmitted disease back and forth between sex partners.

planned sex   Preparing oneself to have sex, in order to enjoy a feeling of being in charge of one's life, which is always a good thing. The old saying "Planned sex is bad sex" has been proved untrue

time and again. Some people argue against the use of condoms because "they take away the spontaneity" of the sexual encounter, but, in fact, in a loving context both partners should be concerned about each other's health and well-being. Having sex with someone who has no interest in whether you contract a disease is definitely a bad idea.

One huge advantage of planning sex is that both partners can feel more relaxed and less anxious about the possible health outcome. Furthermore, a sex partner who is actually a person worth having sex with is someone interested in concerns that a partner may express. No one should fall for the "If you loved me, you'd do it for me" logic. Being swept away in the "magic of the moment" is considerably less exciting if a partner realistically thinks about the scary possibilities that are inherent in unprotected sex. Remember, people living real lives are not bullet-proof TV characters; it is possible to get pregnant, and it is possible to get a sexually transmitted disease. It is also possible to prepare and plan sexual activity that is fulfilling and relatively safe.

PLWA   The abbreviation of PERSON LIVING WITH AIDS.

***Pneumocystis carinii* pneumonia**   *Pneumocystis carinii* is a fungus whose importance as a human pathogen in the United States increased dramatically after the onset of the AIDS epidemic. PCP is the most common severe infection that affects those with HIV, and it can be fatal. Advances in understanding *Pneumocystis carinii* pneumonia (PCP) have reduced the associated morbidity and mortality rates. The mode of transmission in humans is not known, though it is likely that PCP is spread in the air.

Cause

This is a form of pneumonia that is caused by infection with *Pneumocystis carinii*. Also referred to as PCP, this severe illness often affects adults and children with HIV and AIDS. The infection also occurs in other people with compromised immune systems and in premature or ill infants. Among children with AIDS in the United States, PCP is the most common serious infection. Most people who are infected with this fungus do not get pneumonia because they have a normal immune system that can combat it. PCP is not sexually transmitted, according to the CDC.

Symptoms and Diagnosis

Pneumocystis carinii causes clinically apparent pneumonia virtually exclusively in immunosuppressed patients. Typically, an infected adult has fever, shortness of breath, nonproductive cough, difficulty in breathing, and substernal tightness. Symptoms in children are fever, cough, and breathing difficulty. It is important for those who care for such children to seek medical help as soon as possible, because a child with PCP can die unless treatment is begun immediately. The doctor can diagnose PCP via lab tests of fluid or tissue from the lungs. For adults, too, prompt medical treatment is very important.

Treatment

Usually the best medicine for treating PCP is trimethoprim-sulfamethoxazole (TMP-SMX). It is also sold under the brand names Bactrim, Septra, or Cotrim. People with very severe PCP are usually treated in a hospital with IV medicine, and as they improve, they can then take pills for the PCP.

Prevention

The latest findings suggest that it is safe for HIV-positive people who are taking HAART drugs and have CD4 cell counts of 200 cells/mm3 or higher to stop taking drugs to prevent *Pneumocystis carinii* pneumonia. According to a study reported in *The New England Journal of Medicine*, researchers think that combination antiretroviral therapy induces a clinically significant restoration of immunity against *P. carinii*. But researchers warn that patients who have already been exposed to the infection still have a risk of PCP; thus, they must continue prophylaxis. The best drug for prevention is TMP-SMX. A person with HIV should have regular blood tests to check the strength of his or her immune system; if the CD4 cell count falls below 200 cells/mm3, the doctor can prescribe TMP-SMX. Other conditions for which a doctor may consider TMP-SMX necessary are temperature above 100°F for two or more weeks or coexisting fungal infection in the mouth or throat (a

problem known as thrush). The downside of using TMP-SMX is that it may cause slight sickness or rash. If this occurs, the patient should ask the doctor whether to continue taking it.

Children whose mothers have HIV can take antiviral medications to prevent PCP. Starting this medicine when infants are four to six weeks old is recommended for all newborns of HIV-infected mothers. If the doctor discovers that the infant does not have HIV, the medication can be discontinued. A child with HIV should take TMP-SMX until age one. Because a child who has *Pneumocystis carinii* pneumonia can contract it again, it is important that an HIV-infected child be treated even after a PCP infection in order to prevent contracting it a second time.

Note: A pneumonia vaccine does not protect a person against PCP because the vaccine is only designed to prevent pneumococcal infections. Someone who has had PCP can get it again. According to the CDC, taking TMP-SMX can prevent second infections with PCP.

After checking with his or her doctor, a person who has HIV and is taking medications to control HIV may be able to stop taking medicine to prevent PCP if these conditions apply: this individual has never had PCP; his or her CD4 cell count stays above 200 for three to six months; and blood tests show a low or undetectable viral load.

pneumonia An inflammation of the lung that is caused by various pathogens, but most commonly by bacteria. Symptoms are cough, fever, shortness of breath, and chest pain. The most common form of pneumonia is bronchopneumonia, thus named because it starts around the bronchi and bronchioles. *Streptococcus pneumoniae*, the most common bacterial cause, results in lobar pneumonia, which affects whole lobes of either or both lungs. Pus can fill the air sacs and thus exclude air.

Some other common bacterial pathogens are *Haemophilus influenzae*, *Staphylococcus aureus*, *Mycoplasma pneumoniae*, and *Chlamydia pneumoniae*. Antibiotics are used to treat bacterial pneumonia. Sometimes people require hospitalization for treatment of pneumonia.

polio vaccine and HIV/AIDS   One of many controversies related to the HIV/AIDS epidemic was kicked off in 1992 by a *Rolling Stone* article that spawned the rumor that AIDS may have been caused by an experimental oral polio vaccine that was used in the 1950s. In 1999, *The River* by Edward Hooper supported this idea. This movement, of course, spurred an investigation of the renegade theory, which overturned the experimental oral polio vaccine/HIV link theory as "very unlikely," in view of the evidence of HIV traits and origins, the production of the polio vaccine in question, and the lack of HIV/AIDS cases in some areas where the experimental vaccine was given.

The human immunodeficiency virus, which causes AIDS, is passed from person to person by sexual contact and by blood-to-blood and vertical transmission (mother to infant) when pregnant HIV-positive women are not treated. In most people who have HIV, AIDS develops; HIV-1 and HIV-2 can both cause AIDS, but there have been only a few HIV-2 cases in the United States. When an HIV-infected individual can no longer fight off illness because HIV has weakened the immune system, AIDS is the result. As for polio vaccines, the two types are inactivated, or "killed," polio vaccine (IPV), given as a shot, and live (attenuated or weakened) oral polio vaccine (OPV), a liquid that is swallowed. IPV is made with dead polio virus that is grown in a lab on a monkey kidney cell culture and then killed with formaldehyde (or other chemicals that harm the virus). OPV is made with live polio virus weakened so that it cannot cause disease. Polio virus for making OPV is also grown in a lab on monkey kidney cell culture—then chemicals are used to weaken it, and it is frozen and diluted so that it can be used as a vaccine. The history of polio vaccines dates back to the 1950s, when they were developed and tested. Jonas Salk introduced the first one that was widely used as a polio vaccine as a shot in 1954. His shot was replaced by Albert Sabin's OPV, placed on sugar cubes and eaten. In 1957, Dr. Hilary Koprowski introduced an oral polio vaccine that people swallowed. In testing procedures, early vaccines were used on monkeys, chimpanzees, guinea pigs, mice, and rabbits.

Monkeys were most commonly used to grow polio virus for early vaccines.

Scientists believe that HIV-1 evolved from an immunodeficiency virus found in chimpanzees—simian immunodeficiency virus. But what about the fact that viruses that infect one species usually do not infect other species of animals?

Scientists are not sure why or how simian immunodeficiency virus "jumped" from chimps to people, but the evolution from simian immunodeficiency virus to HIV is thought to have occurred a number of decades ago. The belief is that some people who were hunting monkeys or apes for food had contact with the animals' blood while preparing the meat, and then these hunters spread HIV through sexual contact with other humans, or through rituals that involved contact with contaminated blood, or through use of nonsterile needles for injections or vaccinations.

All of this leads back to the article in *Rolling Stone* and the 1999 book suggesting that the oral polio vaccine Dr. Koprowski originated introduced HIV-1 into people's bodies. Most HIV/AIDS experts do not believe this theory. By the time his vaccine was being used, HIV-1 had already formed (in the 1930s, originally). Plus, there is the compelling fact that it is hard to contract HIV by ingesting it, especially in tiny amounts (a couple of drops in a vaccine). Early cases of AIDS occurred in Africa only, and not in the European countries given Koprowski's vaccine—Poland, Switzerland, Croatia. Furthermore, some of this vaccine that had been stored in a lab has been tested in recent years and found free of HIV or similar viruses.

The Koprowski vaccine was used from 1957 to 1959. In recent years, there has been a switch from Dr. Albert Sabin's oral polio vaccine to use of the inactivated polio vaccine. All vaccines are now carefully monitored and tested by the Centers for Disease Control and Prevention, the U.S. Food and Drug Administration, the National Institutes of Health, and other federal agencies. No one should be able to contract HIV from the vaccines used today, which all go through extensive testing in labs and animals and three phases of testing in human volunteer groups. All tissues and cells that are used to grow and produce any vaccine must be tested and cleared of any virus, including HIV.

Even after the FDA and CDC clear a vaccine and license it, they continue to monitor it for continued safety.

Health care workers and others can report any negative reactions that they observe after vaccinations to the Vaccine Adverse Event Reporting System ((800) 822-7967).

In 2002, researchers told the Institute of Medicine that simian virus (SV40) is in humans and plays a role in causing cancer, including in those who got virus-contaminated polio vaccines (in the 1950s and 1960s). An SV40 strain found in non-Hodgkin's lymphoma matched the one in 1950s vaccine samples. Other researchers disagree.

Highfield, Roger. "AIDS Link with Polio Vaccine Finally Rejected," *Daily Telegraph,* April 26, 2001.
"Oral Polio Vaccine and HIV/AIDS," CDC National Immunization Program. Available online. URL: http://www.cdc.gov/nip/vacsafe/concerns/aids/polio-vac-hiv-aids.htm.
"Study: HIV Not Tied to Polio Vaccine," MSNBC. Available online. URL: www.msnbc.com. Downloaded January 15, 2002.

power of attorney   A legal arrangement that gives an assigned individual the right to sign checks, give medical consent, and conduct other business for a person with a terminal illness such as HIV or AIDS. A durable power of attorney can be exercised in the event that the ill person becomes mentally incapacitated or unconscious. In most states, this power can be assigned to anyone older than 18 years old. The basic plan is that this person will then have the right to sign on the person's behalf if that becomes necessary. The goal is to prevent legal, financial, and medical matters from being left in limbo. In some states, if this designation is not assigned to a specific person, a family member is named to serve as a surrogate.

Durable power of attorney can begin at two times: when an individual decides he or she wants it to go into effect or when the ill person becomes incompetent. The "incompetent" state comes into play when someone is no longer able to make informed decisions based on the information provided. Two physicians' agreement is required to declare incompetence in a patient.

Durable power of attorney can be revoked; if it is never revoked, it continues until the person who assigned it dies.

In the context of handling this matter for people with HIV/AIDS, assigning power of attorney can be accomplished simply by contacting a local AIDS organization for forms and free legal aid. Forms are also available through state agencies and hospitals. Basically, the two kinds of durable power of attorney are one for health care decisions and one for financial decisions. A person who has durable power of attorney concerning finances does not automatically have the right to give medical consent.

In filling out legal forms, the person who has a terminal disease designates the jobs he or she wants to be taken care of by the person with durable power of attorney. The HIV-positive person can opt to assign medical and financial power to the same person or to different people.

The person who is chosen to make health care decisions via durable power of attorney can decide to authorize or withhold treatment and life support measures. Also, the legal document can give or deny this agent the right to admit the ill person to a psychiatric facility, the right to authorize psychiatric medications and treatments, and the right to decide about nursing home placement. Special instructions can also be included in the document. Those who do assign someone durable power of attorney for health care may want to update it occasionally because laws regarding durable power of attorney are subject to frequent change.

pregnancy   The period during which a woman carries a developing fetus. From conception to childbirth, pregnancy lasts about 266 days. Women with sexually transmitted diseases sometimes require medications during pregnancy in order to ensure that their infants are not infected with the diseases. The doctor who is supervising the pregnancy should be informed of all pertinent health information concerning the mother, and that includes any sexually transmitted diseases or recent exposures to STDs (even though the pregnant woman may not have tested positive thus far).

pregnancy in HIV-positive women   See HIV.

prevention messages   Public service announcements and publications for which the U.S. government has spent millions of dollars in an effort to spread prevention and education messages concerning sexually transmitted diseases. The goal is to convey to sexually active people that they need to make certain behavior changes if they are currently at risk for acquiring or transmitting STDs.

The person who is starting a new sexual relationship needs to make sure that both partners are tested for sexually transmitted diseases, including HIV. This important step should be taken even if the new partner is absolutely certain he or she does not have an STD. (Remember that thousands of Americans who have STDs today are not aware of it and have never been diagnosed or treated.) When partners do not have testing before having sex, or if someone has sex with someone whose STD status has not been determined or knows the person has an existing sexually transmitted disease, safe sex is imperative. Both partners should make sure that a new condom is used for each separate act of intercourse.

An STD prevention message for IV drug users amounts to advice to any individual who injects drugs not to use drug paraphernalia that have been used by another person—no syringe, no needle. Using clean needles is critical. If a person insists on continuing to use equipment that other drug users have used, water-and-bleach cleaning of equipment is better than nothing, although it does not sterilize the equipment. This is no insurance that HIV will not be transmitted, but it should reduce the rate of HIV transmission in those sharing needles, according to the 1998 *Guidelines for Treatment of Sexually Transmitted Diseases* of the U.S. Department of Health and Human Services of the Centers for Disease Control and Prevention. Ideally, those who are drug users will seek help in a drug-treatment program.

Another proactive move that a person can take before engaging in sex with a partner who could have an STD is preexposure vaccination. Hepatitis B vaccination is a good idea for anyone being evaluated for STDs, according to the Centers for Disease Control and Prevention; hepatitis A vaccination is recommended for homosexual men, bisexual men, and those who use illegal drugs.

The most important prevention message is this: avoiding sexual contact with other people is the only surefire way to prevent getting a sexually transmitted disease. Also, for the sexually active, observing the following precautions can help to reduce the likelihood of contracting a sexually transmitted disease:

- Have a mutually monogamous sexual relationship with an uninfected partner.

- Use a male condom correctly and consistently with sex partners.

- Use clean needles if you are involved in injecting IV drugs.

- Use safe-sex practices in order to prevent contracting STDs. That will decrease your susceptibility to HIV infection and reduce the infectiousness of those who are already HIV-infected.

- Become sexually active later rather than earlier. It is clear that the younger a person is when she or he has sex for the first time, the more likely he or she is to contract an STD. Risk of acquiring sexually transmitted diseases also increases with multiple partners.

- Have regular checkups for STDs, especially if having sex with a new partner.

- Become well educated about common STD symptoms.

- Avoid sex during menstruation. Women are probably more susceptible to infection with an STD at that time. HIV-infected women are also more infectious at this time.

- Avoid anal intercourse. (If this is practiced, it should be done with a male condom.)

- Avoid douching, which removes some of the vagina's normal bacteria, thus heightening the risk of sexually associated problems such as bacterial vaginosis and yeast infections.

primary brain lymphoma   Lymphoma that originates in the brain. Lymphoma is a cancer of the lymphatic system. Often, people with AIDS have lymphomas that are non-Hodgkin's lymphomas, which tend to be very serious and occur in unusual anatomical sites, such as the brain. Because those with HIV have a compromised immune system, they have much higher rates of lymphomas than the general population.

privacy   Keeping a diagnosis secret from others, if a person wants to, is based on an individual's right to keep medical records private. On April 14, 2003, the first federal privacy standards to protect patients' medical records and other health information took effect. These standards give patients access to their own medical records and more control over how their health information is disclosed. The regulation covers health plans, health care clearinghouses, and health care providers who electronically conduct such transactions as enrollment, billing, and eligibility verification. Certain small health plans have an extra year to comply, but most health insurers, pharmacies, doctors, and other health care providers had to meet the April 14, 2003, deadline. (See http://www.hhs.gov/ocr.hipaa.)

Basically, the new regulations ensure a national minimum of privacy protections for patients by limiting the ways that health plans, pharmacies, hospitals, and other entities can use personal medical information.

The new standards also require that health plans and providers adopt policies and train their personnel on how to properly follow procedures.

For civil violations of the new standards, the Office for Civil Rights may impose penalities up to $100 per violation, up to $25,000 a year, for each requirement or prohibition violated. Criminal penalities apply for actions such as knowingly obtaining protected health information in violation of the law. Penalties range up to $50,000 and one year in prison for certain offenses; up to $100,000 and up to five years in prison for offenses committed under false pretenses; and up to $250,000 and up to 10 years in prison for offenses committed with intent to sell, transfer, or use protected health information for commercial or personal gain, or malicious harm.

See also RIGHT TO KNOW.

proctitis   An inflammation of the rectum that is characterized by diarrhea, bleeding, and unproductive straining to have a bowel movement. This occurs in ulcerative colitis and sometimes in Crohn's disease and can also result from other conditions. An unusual cause is lymphogranuloma venereum.

proctocolitis   Inflammation of the rectum and colon that is usually associated with ulcerative colitis.

prodrome   The stage of early symptoms that signal an infection or outbreak. For example, genital herpes outbreaks are often preceded by prodromal symptoms.

See also GENITAL HERPES.

profiles of behavior   Epidemiological researchers often study various groups of people to determine what sorts of lifestyles appear to contribute to the spread of certain diseases. In the case of sexually transmitted diseases, profiles of behavior can spotlight groups whose needs should be addressed insofar as disseminating information on transmission, treatment, and prevention of STDs.

prophylactic   Something that is used to prevent acquiring a disease; a condom is an example.

prophylaxis   A means that a person undertakes in order to prevent disease and preserve health. An example would be an HIV-positive person's use of the medication trimethoprim-sulfamethoxazole (TMP-SMX) (Bactrim) to prevent *Pneumocystic carinii* pneumonia.

prostatitis   An inflammation of the prostate gland.

Causes

By far, the most common type of prostatitis is nonbacterial. The others—chronic and acute bacterial prostatitis—stem from bacteria. Inflammation of the prostate gland as a result of infection is common in men 50 and younger.

Symptoms

A man who has nonbacterial prostatitis has pain (perineal, suprapubic, or low back) and urinary symptoms (frequent irritation, difficulty in urinating). Chronic prostatitis often causes recurrent urinary tract infections, low back pain, urination problems, pain after ejaculation, penile pain, and/or testicular discomfort. Subtle symptoms also can accompany the chronic variety.

Someone with acute bacterial prostatitis usually experiences fever and chills with urinary tract infection (or obstruction) symptoms, such as frequent urination or difficulty urinating. A person who has acute prostatitis may experience low back pain, perineal pain, joint pain, and malaise and will probably feel very ill.

Testing

Diagnosis of prostatitis is a matter of excluding possibilities because prostate cancer, benign prostatic enlargement, and prostatitis can coexist and symptoms may overlap. In the case of chronic prostatitis, the urinalysis and culture findings generally indicate a low-grade bacteriuria (*Escherichia coli* or other member of the gram-negative Enterobacteriaceae, *Enterococcus faecalis, Staphylococcus aureus,* or coagulase-negative staphylococcus). Prostatic secretions of a person with chronic prostatitis may show more than 10 to 15 WBCs per high-power field. Chronic nonbacterial prostatitis yields sterile cultures—no bacteria or uropathogens. Microscopic examination shows 10 to 15 WBCs per high-power field, which points to the presence of inflammation. With acute prostatitis, the prostate is enlarged, indurated, and very tender. If acute prostatitis arises during a hospital stay, it may be associated with the use of a Foley catheter (to empty urine from the bladder) and may be the result of *Pseudomonas* species, enterococci, or *S. aureus.* Imaging may be necessary, if a person is extremely ill, to rule out an abscess, which may require surgery.

Traditionally, nonbacterial prostatitis has been characterized by the absence of significant numbers of bacteria from prostatic fluid—the fluid reveals microscopic purulence. Recently reclassified as chronic abacterial (type III) prostatitis, this is responsible for more than 90 percent of all prostatitis cases. Unfortunately, diagnostic tests for chronic abacterial prostatitis are not definitive. There is not enough evidence of the accuracy of the gold standard four-glass test, long used to classify prostatitis as infectious, inflammatory, or noninflammatory. Furthermore, studies that have examined currently used treatment methods are considered flawed, and not one has been done in the United States. The treatments reviewed were finasteride and other alpha-blockers, antiinflammatory medications, antibiotics, thermotherapy, and various agents. Researchers in a review reported in August 2001 that routinely giving antibiotics or alpha-blockers to men with chronic abacterial prostatitis is not justified. However, some evidence supports using the two-glass test, and some small studies have shown that symptoms and quality of life of patients with prostatitis were improved by transrectal microwave hyperthermy. Also, some abacterial prostatitis patients find relief from pelvic pain via antioxidants (tomato extract, selenium, lycopene). In the largest prostate cancer prevention study to date, the National Cancer Institute's Selenium and Vitamin E Cancer Prevention Trial (SELECT) will study the effectiveness of these supplements in 32,400 men over a period of 12 years. Each man's participation is seven to 12 years. The final results will not be computed until the end of the 12-year period. Enrollment lasts from 2001 through 2006. (See http://www.crab.org/select.)

Treatment

If the acute prostatitis is caused by sexually transmitted bacteria, treatment for infections such as chlamydia, gonorrhea, and nongonococcal urethritis is initiated. (See the separate entries on these conditions.) If STD-caused urethritis is treated promptly, there is less possibility that it will progress to a prostate infection. Acute prostatitis caused by an STD does not usually result in chronic infection.

Usually, for acute bacterial prostatitis, a doctor prescribes a 10- to 14-day regimen of antibiotics. If the person is very ill, however, hospitalization may be necessary in order to ensure bed rest and supply adequate rehydration, intravenous antibiotics, pain relief medication, stool softeners, and medications for fever. If a person is suffering from chronic prostatitis, it may be very difficult to eliminate the problem, and the typical antibiotic course is four to six weeks.

For chronic nonbacterial prostatitis, a doctor treats with several weeks of antibiotics (because of the uncertainty of the cause of the prostatitis). To ease irritation, the patient may try nonsteroidal anti-inflammatories, muscle relaxers, warm sitz baths, normal sexual activity, and regular mild exercise, and should avoid spicy foods, caffeine, and alcohol. Some people believe that this kind of infection can be eradicated by repeated instances of ejaculation via masturbation, but this idea has not been proved. Partners of a man who has prostatitis caused by an STD should be treated as sexual contacts.

psychiatric disorders   Mental abnormality. There are a number of psychiatric disorders that are associated with sexually transmitted diseases. Doctors note that some people are so devastated by hearing the news of a sexually transmitted disease diagnosis that they require counseling, whereas others seem to accept it relatively well. Much depends on the basic temperament of the individual, his or her medical history up to that point, and the particular disease (naturally, those that are incurable affect the individual more drastically). Suicide attempts are not unusual among those who have just received HIV-positive test results.

Depression and anxiety are common problems of those dealing with an STD diagnosis. A pivotal factor for such individuals is finding help and support in treating the psychosocial and psychiatric complications that can go hand in hand with having an STD. Even psychiatric complications of AIDS, such as delirium, mania, psychosis, organic brain disease, depression, and panic disorder can be treated.

Often, as someone becomes more ill with HIV/AIDS, he or she is more likely to experience a form of psychiatric distress, which can stem from central nervous system disease, complications from medications, and/or spiritual and emotional dysfunction. It is important that those who care for HIV/AIDS patients be able to separate normal anxiety states from signs of serious psychiatric disorder that require a doctor's care. Patients experiencing depression, for example, must be warned not to self-medicate without consulting their treating physician, who can monitor drug interactions. Monitoring is especially critical for a person who is undergoing HAART. Also, caregivers should not let their own feelings prevent them from providing the help needed. (For instance, a caregiver may well think, "I would be feeling depressed if I were HIV-positive, too, so this reaction is natural.") An HIV patient who is having many bouts of disturbed sleep, malaise, tearfulness, and constant fatigue may need counseling or medication for depression. One should also remember that chronic pain can be a cause of

depression and anxiety, and in HIV, frequent headaches and extremity pain are not unusual.

One serious complication of HIV is delirium, which can be the result of central nervous system opportunistic infections, medication side effects, and systemic illness. Most of the time, people with delirium need to be treated in an intensive care unit because they must be monitored carefully. In those who have HIV, delirium is often the result of drug (recreational or prescribed) withdrawal, low oxygen concentration in the blood, electrolyte disorders, low blood sugar level, or low blood pressure.

AIDS-associated mania usually stems from organic HIV-associated brain disease. Mania can also arise from the anxiety of dealing with a chronic illness. Unfortunately, the gold standard for treating mania—lithium—is considered too high-risk for use by an AIDS patient, who may be dehydrated and experiencing vomiting and diarrhea. Often doctors prescribe perphenazine (Trilafon) with or without lorazepam (Ativan) to stabilize the condition, followed by valproate or carbamazepine.

Signs of psychosis in HIV patients are hallucinations, delusions, and paranoid delusions, which are usually treated with midpotency neuroleptic medicines such as Trilafon. Psychiatric consultation is recommended.

HIV-associated organic brain disease can lie at the base of any of the psychiatric syndromes mentioned. High-dose AZT therapy can reverse impairment in some people who have cognitive impairment only, but if both mood and cognitive signs are in evidence, dextroamphetamine sulfate (dexedrine) or methylphenidate hydrochloride (Ritalin) may be required.

Patients who have organic brain disease are less responsive to caregivers and less functional, conditions that sometimes result in distancing. However, these patients still need empathy and warmth, and counseling can help caregivers get through this difficulty. The patient who is cognitively impaired can be cared for at home, where he or she may well experience less anxiety in the familiar setting.

Chronic anxiety can also be debilitating to some people going through drug withdrawal and/or living with HIV/AIDS or herpes. The person experiencing chronic anxiety may have difficulty in concentrating, feel exhausted and agitated, and have trouble sleeping. Some people experience very frightening panic attacks. It is important to treat panic and anxiety aggressively, and there are a number of medications that work well. Behavior modification therapy can help, too.

Another mental health problem is seen in certain HIV-negative people with high-risk lifestyles, who become obsessed with whether their next HIV test will have a positive result.

puberty The period during one's life when sex organs mature. In girls the menstrual period begins and breasts and pubic hair develop; in boys scrotal, testicular, and penis growth begins; pubic hair grows; and secondary sex characteristics, including chest hair and deepening voice, develop. After puberty, the reproductive organs become functional; this means a girl can become pregnant, and a boy who has reached puberty is capable of impregnating her with his sperm. The pituitary hormones of the body stimulate the testes (in males) and ovaries (in females), touching off an increase in sex hormones that brings about the physical changes of puberty. The age at which an individual reaches puberty can range from nine to 15.

pubic lice Extremely tiny insects that infest the pubic hair and survive by feeding on human blood—and thus are external parasites of humans.

Cause
Pubic lice (pediculosis pubis) is caused by blood-sucking lice (*Phthirus pubis*) that feed off human blood. They infest pubic, perianal, or thigh hair and occasionally axillary (armpit) hair or even eyelashes. These are usually spread by sexual contact, although, in rare cases, people have contracted pubic lice from infested bedding and clothing. Most people discover they have pubic lice when the insects cause itching in the pubic area. Scratching often spreads the infestation. For this reason, the person with pubic lice should try to avoid touching the infected area.

Symptoms and Diagnosis
Pubic lice cause itching. Often they are visible to the naked eye. Nits (tiny white eggs of lice) that are cemented to the base of hair are examined microscopically to confirm diagnosis. Pubic lice are the size of a pinhead and look brownish red because they contain blood.

Treatment
Most people use over-the-counter lotions and shampoos to kill pubic lice. Doctors can also provide prescriptions such as permethrin (Elimite) or lindane (Kwell) lotion. Permethrin is more commonly used. A second treatment is done seven to 10 days after the first in order to kill newly hatched lice. Pubic lice die within 24 hours of being separated from the human body. Because the eggs may live up to six days, it is important to apply the second treatment.

Pregnant women definitely should not use a product with lindane. If the lotion or cream is being used on a child, it is important to follow a doctor's instructions for its use. Apply the lotion as directed in order to eradicate all eggs. For any itching that remains after the lice are gone, some people use calamine lotion.

For treating eyelashes, a person should thickly apply a prescription petrolatum twice a day for seven to 10 days.

Sex partners, family, and anyone else who has close contact with a person who has pubic lice should be treated. Clothing and bedding must be washed in very hot water and dried at a high setting.

quality health care Most people agree, in relation to sexually transmitted diseases, quality medical care is that which addresses all aspects of a sexually transmitted disease, from treatment to management of anxiety to use of precautions for partner protection and prevention to follow-up. Open and candid communication with health care providers can help to elicit information and instructions as needed. Although most doctors are not likely to impose their sexual morals or standards by giving patients unsolicited advice, they are definitely interested in preventing the spread of sexually transmitted diseases and in answering people's questions about safe-sex options, modes of transmission of sexually transmitted diseases, testing, and treatment.

quality of life Degree of satisfaction with one's life, usually used in the context of a person living with a disease. The individual who is living with a particular sexually transmitted disease is obviously in the best position to evaluate his or her own quality of life. In some cases, though, it becomes clear that this person needs assistance, and at such times, social services workers and counselors can help to improve the outlook of someone who must deal with an STD diagnosis. Certainly, it can be overwhelming to discover that one has a disease that may result in unexpected medical care expenses, partner notification, and social ostracism. Thus, the goal for caregivers is to help each patient attain the highest level of quality of life that is possible when living with a sexually transmitted disease.

quarantine A period during which a person is kept in isolation to prevent the spread of a disease that is contagious. Quarantine periods are of different lengths, depending on the disease. In regard to sexually transmitted diseases, the quarantine comes into play in the realm of artificial insemination, for example.

According to a March 1998 *Lancet* report detailed on Doctor's Guide Web Site, a woman in Germany contracted HIV after artificial insemination. The sperm donor had tested HIV-negative at the time of insemination but on retesting three months later tested positive. The recipient and the donor had HIV with identical viral sequences. Germany is a country that has no regulation requiring a three-month quarantine of sperm before its use. Researchers warn doctors against using fresh sperm for artificial insemination and remind the medical community that artificial insemination should be looked at as a potential source of HIV-1 infection.

In respect to ideas about containment of a bioterrorist-disseminated disease, U.S. researchers report that quarantine may not be the answer. However, "if the disease is contagious, the specific mechanism of transmission must drive disease-containment strategy." What this would mean is that those who have clinical or lab evidence of a contagious disease would be isolated from those who do not. Even so, the isolation could be restricted to body fluid or skin contact—not full physical contact with all who are healthy, and this is determined, of course, by the illness under consideration. Rather than using quarantine, it is more likely that measures recommended to prevent disease spread would be along the lines of rapid vaccination or treatment, use of disposable masks, short-term voluntary restrictions on public meetings, and closing of mass public transportation.

Hauschildt, Elsa. "Bioterrorism Containment Depends on Disease's Communicable Level," *JAMA* 286 (2001): 2711–2717.
"IVF Clinics 'Shun' HIV Patients." AVERT. Available online. URL: www.avert.org. Downloaded on February 12, 2001.

Rapid Ethnographic Community Assessment Process The process, also known as RECAP, developed through the Innovations in Syphilis Prevention (ISP) initiative, with the goals of determining point of access for those at risk for syphilis, figuring out effective prevention messages and strategies, and tailoring screening efforts for this disease.

rapid HIV test According to the Centers for Disease Control and Prevention, a screening that produces quick results, typically in about five to 30 minutes. This is much faster than the commonly used HIV oral fluid enzyme immunoassay screening test (EIA), for which results are not known for one to two weeks.

The FDA has licensed only one rapid HIV test, and its availability may vary by locality. The rapid test is considered as accurate as the EIA. Both look for the presence of antibodies to HIV. Results of all screening tests, including the EIA and the reactive rapid HIV test, require confirmation before a diagnosis of infection can be made.

rectal pain and discharge Discomfort that occurs in the rectum (the terminal part of the intestine ending at the anus) or fluid release (discharge) from the rectum can have various causes. A person who has an infection in the anal and rectal area may experience severe symptoms (pain and discharge) or be symptom-free.

Unprotected anal sex carries a risk of infection with sexually transmitted diseases in women and men. Chancres (of syphilis) are typically painless unless they become infected by bacteria. Chancroid can cause painful anal (and genital) ulcers. Donovanosis can cause anal scarring that results in rectal pain. Rectal pain, bleeding, and discharge can occur after having anal sex with a person infected with gonorrhea or chlamydia. A person can become infected with herpes through anal sex and have painful herpetic lesions in the anal area.

Certain intestinal infections can be contracted through unprotected anal sex with someone who is infected.

It is also important to note that a person may commonly experience rectal pain as a result of warts, Crohn's disease, ulcerative colitis, and hemorrhoids (dilated blood vessels in the anal area that result from straining during a bowel movement, pregnancy, or the extra strain of childbirth). Hemorrhoid symptoms can recede spontaneously or with certain treatment measures but often recur.

For more on each sexually transmitted disease, see the individual entries on chancroid, donovanosis, gonorrhea, chlamydia, lymphogranuloma venereum, syphilis.

recurrent infection A repeated episode of an illness after its first occurrence, which may appear in some sexually transmitted diseases. This can mean that a person is at risk of contracting the disease a second, third, or fourth time. In other words, having the disease once does not prevent reinfection. An example is *Pneumocystis carinii* pneumonia, which commonly recurs in people with AIDS who are not taking prophylactic medication.

reporting and confidentiality A person who may have been exposed to HIV can go to an anonymous testing site and be tested anonymously (the identifying information is not linked to the HIV test result) or can choose to be tested confidentially (the test result is linked to the identifying information such as patient and provider names—often the method used by medical clinics). In states that require HIV case reporting, the health care providers in confidential medical or testing sites must report HIV-infected persons to public health authorities.

Of course, not all people who have HIV are tested, and for those who are, the actual testing occurs at different stages of HIV infection. The HIV test can produce a negative result in a newly infected person. This means that HIV surveillance data provide a minimal estimate of the number of HIV-infected persons in the United States and most clearly reflect those who have had HIV infection diagnosed in medical clinics and other settings that offer confidential HIV diagnosis. This figure would include those found to be HIV-infected who know they are at risk and thus seek testing; those who are offered testing, such as pregnant women and people who go to sexually transmitted disease clinics; those for whom testing is required (blood donors and military recruits); and those who have HIV testing because they have symptoms of HIV-related diseases. According to Centers for Disease Control and Prevention estimates, in 1996, about two-thirds of all infected people in the United States were diagnosed as HIV-positive in such settings. Also, it is important to note that HIV surveillance data may not represent those who remain untested, those who test at anonymous sites, and those who use home collection kits, but the popularity of anonymous testing is important in promoting knowledge of HIV status among at-risk populations, and offers a chance for counseling in order to reduce high-risk behavior and provide voluntary referrals to medical services. Surveyed individuals who had undergone HIV testing reported that their reasons for delays in being tested were fear of having HIV infection diagnosed or belief that they were not likely to have been infected with HIV. Fear of "reporting to the government" may have contributed to delays in seeking testing for 11 percent of heterosexuals, 18 percent of IV drug users, and 22 percent of gay men.

Listing name-based reporting as a primary reason for not being tested for HIV were 1 percent of heterosexuals, 1 percent of IV drug users, and 4 percent of gay men. Concern about name-based reporting of HIV status to the government was a factor in not being tested for HIV in 13 percent of heterosexuals, 18 percent of IV drug users, and 28 percent of gay men.

These findings in studies by researchers at the University of California at San Francisco and participating health departments, supported by the CDC, suggest that name-based reporting policies may well deter a small number of people who practice high-risk sex or drug-use behavior from seeking HIV testing and thus underscore the need for strict adherence to confidentiality safeguards of public health testing and surveillance data. Also, the survey substantiated a widely held belief: consistently high numbers of respondents who knew that anonymous testing was available planned to be tested in the future.

Sampling the use of alternatives to confidential name-based reporting for HIV surveillance, several states tried using numeric or alphanumeric codes to report cases of HIV or low CD4 counts (a marker of immunosuppression in HIV-infected people). Other states tried to do case surveillance without name identifiers by using codes designated for nonsurveillance purposes. The Centers for Disease Control and Prevention reported that the states recommended that the CDC evaluate additional coded identifiers and help document and disseminate their results. Several subsequent studies could not find a code system that worked as well as name-based methods. Texas switched to name-based HIV case surveillance on the basis of published evaluations, and several states (Maryland, Illinois, Maine, Massachusetts) as well as Puerto Rico all implemented HIV reporting using four different coded identifiers.

Also, a review of state confidentiality laws in 1994 documented that all states and many localities have legal safeguards for confidentiality of government-held data on HIV status. Most states have specific statutory protections for public health data related to HIV infection and other sexually transmitted diseases. But these protections vary, and the CDC is in favor of strengthening privacy protections of public health data. For maintaining the confidentiality of those in whom HIV has been diagnosed by public or private health care providers, the CDC recommends stronger standards for enhancing the confidentiality of HIV and AIDS surveillance data.

In 2000, a report that spotlighted a drastic shift in standard HIV reporting practice in the United States surfaced. The Centers for Disease Control and Prevention, mainstream medical journals, and many state legislatures are supporting state-level proposals requiring public health officials to adopt name reporting—monitoring HIV by name, not by number. The shift from the practice of confidential and anonymous HIV reporting represents the belief of many that the "duty to warn" should take precedence over the long-held professional advocacy of confidentiality.

research   U.S. medical research is continually under way in hopes of finding new and better ways to treat sexually transmitted diseases and to create vaccines that will stop the upswing in the spread of many types of sexually transmitted diseases. Research is directed to investigating genital herpes, genital warts, HIV, and other diseases that are prevalent in the U.S. population and worldwide.

Sexually transmitted diseases ravage society at great cost to everyone, and the physical and emotional suffering of millions is unmeasurable. The National Institute of Allergy and Infectious Diseases (NIAID) conducts and supports numerous research efforts that are designed to improve prevention measures and find better avenues of diagnosing and treating STDs. Furthermore, the NIAID supports several university-based sexually transmitted disease research centers. In recent years, NIAID research has unveiled new tests for faster and more accurate diagnosis of STDs. New drug treatments are being studied by NIAID research scientists—a key effort in the war against STDs in view of the fact that some sexually transmitted diseases are developing resistance to currently used drugs.

Researchers are developing and testing vaccines and assessing their efficacy in preventing AIDS, chlamydial infection, genital herpes, and gonorrhea. An example of research in the area of STDs is documented in Centers for Disease Control and Prevention reports (May 9, 2002) showing that recent studies reveal that frequent use of the spermicide contraceptive nonoxynol-9 (N-9) can be a hazard to one's health because it can cause genital lesions in the vagina, which may actually enhance tissue receptiveness to HIV transmission. This means a person may increase risk for HIV transmission by using N-9. Also, N-9 can damage the rectum's lining, thus allowing entry of HIV and other STDs. Guidelines on treating STDs for 2002 cautioned that spermicides, especially those containing N-9, should not be used during anal intercourse.

The level of N-9 that is used as a condom lubricant is much lower than what is deemed harmful, but health care experts still do not recommend using condoms lubricated with N-9 spermicide because of their short shelf life, their higher cost, and their association with urinary tract infections in females. On the other hand, CDC representatives also announced that people who have on hand any unexpired condoms with N-9 can use these, anyway, since the protection a condom provides still outweighs N-9's potential risk. (To see the 2002 guidelines, visit http://www.cdc.gov/std.)

resistance to antiretroviral therapy   Some strains of HIV develop resistance to antiretroviral therapy, making it necessary for a patient's multidrug regimen to be changed, eliminating the drug that is no longer effective. In fact, HIV drug therapy often fails because of the appearance of multidrug-resistant virus. Two possible reasons for the creation of drug resistance in response to therapy are that resistant virus may preexist at low frequencies in drug-naive patients and is thus rapidly selected when it is in the presence of drugs, or that resistant virus may be absent at the start of therapy and be generated during therapy. Some contend that treatment failure is probably caused by the preexistence of resistant mutants, but it may also be attributed to a patient's failure to adhere properly to the drug regimen, and, therefore, the virus evolves resistance to each of the drugs used while the patient is on therapy if only a subset of the prescribed drugs is taken for certain periods. At the same time, though, it is important to note that drug resistance also occurs in patients who faithfully follow the drug regimen.

In people in North America newly infected with HIV, the prevalence of transmitted resistance to antiretroviral drugs is estimated at 1 to 11 percent. Researchers did five years of retrospective analysis of susceptibility to antiretroviral drugs before treatment and drug-resistant mutations in HIV in plasma samples of 377 subjects with primary infection. These people had not yet received treatment and represented 10 cities in North America (1995–2000). A study reported in *The New England Journal of Medicine* (August 8, 2002) concluded that over the five years, there was a significant increase in transmitted drug resistance; the proportion of new HIV infections that involve drug-resistant virus is increasing in North America; initial antiretroviral therapy is more likely to fail in patients who are infected with drug-resistant virus; and testing for drug resistance before therapy is now recommended even for those who are recently infected with HIV.

Little, Susan J., et al. "Antiretroviral Drug Resistance Among Patients Recently Infected with HIV," *New England Journal of Medicine* 347, no. 6 (August 8, 2002): 385–394.

responsible sexual behavior The use of safe-sex practices, which includes using latex condoms consistently and using new condoms with every sex act; having no sexual relations with people of undetermined STD status; avoiding all forms of sexual behavior, including oral sex, in which one has contact with blood, feces, or other bodily fluids; and maintaining good overall health. Behaving responsibly in sexual activities can reduce the likelihood of contracting a sexually transmitted disease in an era when high-risk behavior has made STDs a huge threat to the health of sexually active people.

rest and relaxation Allocation of time for sufficient rest and relaxation as a part of a healthy-living regimen, which is important for the person who is living with a sexually transmitted disease. Fatigue and stress can affect one's immune system, making the individual more susceptible to contracting other diseases.

retinitis An inflammation of the eye's retina that leads to loss of vision in some people with AIDS. This results from cytomegalovirus and is referred to as cytomegalovirus retinitis.

retrovirus A type of virus that stores genetic information on an RNA molecule rather than the more common DNA. HIV is a retrovirus. A retrovirus uses the enzyme reverse transcriptase to synthesize viral DNA, which is then integrated into the infected cell's DNA.

right to know The right of a person to know the STD status of a sex partner. From the beginning of the AIDS crisis, doctors have known that respecting the privacy of those with HIV is important because of the clear potential for discrimination. The advent of the HIV/AIDS epidemic created legal and ethical obligations for health care providers and sexually active individuals.

When many instances of bias were broadcast widely, people with HIV and AIDS moved quickly to ensure that their HIV/AIDS status would be held confidential and to establish protections for this confidentiality. At the same time, the entire matter was complicated by the fact that most people agreed that there was a compelling second issue—the duty to inform those who may be exposed to HIV because they are sex partners of HIV-infected individuals or because they share IV drug needles and paraphernalia with someone who is HIV-positive. Insisting on one's "right to know" is understandable, considering the enormous risk associated with exposure to HIV. People want to know whether their sex partners or IV-drug partners have HIV; they assert that it is unfair for someone to expose them to such a danger without their prior knowledge or consent. At the same time, U.S. courts have found doctors liable for failure to inform persons of the risk of HIV infection, so this means physicians are faced with the perplexing quandary of maintaining patient confidentiality and revealing confidential information to those at risk of contracting HIV (partners).

Most U.S. jurisdictions leave no doubt that physicians are obligated legally to inform a patient of a positive HIV test result. Also, many courts declare that one has a "duty to warn" all known sexual and needle-sharing partners. Decades ago, the California Supreme Court found in *Tarasoff v. the Regents of California* that doctors have a legal duty to inform known third parties of significant risks posed by their patients.

It is clear that the privacy principle is being tested as many U.S. agencies and groups claim that they have a right to know. For example, those who risk exposure to a patient's HIV-infected blood (doctors, nurses, police officers, prison guards) believe they have a right to be informed. This has led to the changing of some U.S. laws on confidentiality, granting a need-to-know right to such groups. Most agree, however, that the strongest claim to a right to know is that of people who are conducting ongoing sexual or needle-sharing relationships. Many believe that, in these cases, the law should give health care providers a power to disclose if they think it is necessary because of a significant risk of transmission. First, however, health care professionals should ask the patient to disclose HIV status to his or her sex partner(s), who can proceed with the relationship (or not) on an informed basis.

rimming   A term sometimes used to describe oral-anal sexual contact.

risk control   In relation to sexually transmitted disease, only with abstinence (no involvement in sexual activity) can a person be absolutely sure of controlling the risk of sexually contracting HIV and other STDs. Other than that, though, sexually active people can control their risk of infection to some degree by avoiding the main modes of transmission of HIV: sexual contact with genital secretions that may be infected, transfusion, or IV-drug infection with blood that may be infected with HIV. Also, it is important to remember that a pregnant woman who has HIV can transmit HIV to her child during childbirth or breast-feeding; treatment, however, can prevent transmission in many cases.

risky behavior   According to a report on trends in STDs, researchers underscore the fact that the key high-risk behavior in HIV transmission is unprotected anal and vaginal intercourse; oral-genital sexual contact is viewed as somewhat less risky. For other STDs, the degree of risk of different types of sexual behavior is not clear and may depend on the particular STD. (See individual entries on sexually transmitted diseases in this book). However, it is clear that any sexual contact without barrier protection increases a person's risk for contracting a sexually transmitted disease. Examples of other factors that affect probability of exposure, promote transmission, or provide a context that may act as a trigger for risk behavior are sex with multiple partners, sex without condoms, early sexual activity, excessive use of alcohol and substances that impair judgment, sex with partners who have multiple partners, and sex for money.

Ryan White Comprehensive AIDS Resource Emergency Act of 1990   On August 18, 1990, the U.S. Congress passed Public Law 101-381, the Ryan White Comprehensive AIDS Resource Emergency (CARE) Act. It was enacted in response to reports from major U.S. metropolitan areas that were experiencing severe hardship due to the cost of care of many Americans living with AIDS who lacked health insurance or had insufficient coverage.

The act supported development of systems of care that respond to local needs and resources. It is named for the Indiana teen Ryan White, whose struggle with AIDS and against AIDS bias helped to educate Americans about the needs of AIDS sufferers. He died at age 19 on April 8, 1990, a few months before Congress passed the act. In the years since 1991, CARE Act programs have served about 500,000 people with HIV and AIDS each year. The fiscal year 2002 appropriation was $1.91 billion.

This federal program devised to improve care for those with HIV/AIDS and their families was amended and reauthorized in 1996 and again in 2000 for a five-year period. As part of the federal budget, it is administered by the Health Resources and Services Administration (part of the U.S. Department of Health and Human Services). The titles and Part F of the act, administered by the HIV/AIDS Bureau of HRSA, are as follows: Title I, grants for outpatient health care and support services for eligible metropolitan areas based on case rates; Title II, grants to states for health care and services for people with HIV/AIDS; Title III, support to primary care providers through local health departments, homeless programs, community and migrant health centers, family planning centers, and hemophilia centers; Title IV, health care and support services for children, adolescents, women, and families via community-based care systems; Part F, Special Projects of National Significance, which are competitively awarded grants to encourage the development of models of HIV/AIDS care that are innovative and focus on hard-to-reach populations.

SAFE (Serostatus Approach to Fighting the HIV/AIDS Epidemic)   A program of the Centers for Disease Control and Prevention, Serostatus Approach to Fighting the HIV/AIDS Epidemic, or SAFE, springs from the CDC's tradition of supporting interventions to prevent HIV infection in high-risk individuals. Because many experts believe that a person with HIV needs to begin highly active antiretroviral therapy (HAART) as soon as possible to achieve better and longer-lasting results, it is important to spread information that makes people more likely to seek testing and treatment early. The CDC programs include the following:

• Conducting operational research for development and testing of innovative approaches, such as rapid testing, public service announcements to promote HIV testing, and counseling and testing in both nontraditional and private practice health care settings.

• Disseminating information on counseling, testing, and referral services.

• Building capacity and giving assistance, including assessing community readiness for more HIV testing, supporting community groups in communities of color, and holding workshops on HIV counseling and testing.

• Setting up projects that promote knowledge of serostatus and prevention and care for those living with HIV.

• Promoting knowledge of serostatus for those in high-risk groups through communication (multimedia) and mobilizing of private-sector involvement (Partnership Council and Leadership Action Alliances).

safe sex   The term for the actions of a sexually active person who takes certain precautions to prevent exposure to sexually transmitted diseases—in particular, HIV. A person who is practicing sex with moderate risk avoids contact with semen and vaginal fluids and uses a new latex condom correctly during each instance of sexual activity (vaginal, anal, and oral) for the full duration of the sexual activity. Deep kissing is considered a moderate-risk activity. Forms of low-risk sex include self-masturbation, mutual masturbation, and dry kissing. *Safe sex* became a household term after the first few years of the HIV/AIDS epidemic, when local, state, and national groups launched large-scale efforts to educate the U.S. population about the importance of using protection during sexual activity to reduce the probability of contracting the lethal human immunodeficiency virus.

scabies   A skin infestation that is fairly common throughout the general population, scabies is highly contagious and can be spread via sexual contact. It also can be transmitted by contact with skin or infested sheets, towels, or even furniture.

Cause

Scabies is caused by infestation by the mite *Sarcoptes scabiei*. What confuses matters is that the skin reaction may not occur until a month or more after infestation. During this time, the person may pass the disease unknowingly to a sex partner or someone with whom he or she has close contact.

Symptoms

Scabies causes intense itching, which is usually worse during the night. Small red bumps or lines appear on parts of the body where the female scabies mite has burrowed into the skin to lay eggs.

Typical sites of scabies lesions are between the fingers and on wrists, elbows, abdomen, and genitals.

Sometimes, scabies can be confused with other skin irritations, such as poison ivy or eczema. To make a diagnosis, a physician can take a scraping of the irritated area and examine it under a microscope to look for the presence of a mite.

Treatment

Ectoparasiticide cream (Permethrin) or scabicide lindane lotion can be used to treat scabies. Sex partners and family members of the affected individual should be treated, too. The lotion is applied at bedtime to all skin below the neck and then washed off in eight to 12 hours. Permethrin can be repeated in seven days if necessary. Itching resolves in two to three weeks. Some patients use a sulfur preparation to treat scabies, which works but has an objectionable smell and leaves a lingering skin irritation. For relief from itching, a patient may want to use a hydrocortisone cream. Pregnant women and young children should not use lindane.

Twenty-four hours after treatment with medicated lotion, the person who has scabies is no longer contagious. It is important, however, to make sure all mites have been eliminated from bedding and clothing by washing with hot water.

See also NORWEGIAN SCABIES.

school-based prevention Part of the overall grand scheme of prevention programs aimed at decreasing the spread of sexually transmitted diseases, school-based efforts are critical because school is often the site where sex-related information is spread among young people and thus becomes a key portal for sexual activity that can involve great risks in the era of rampantly spreading STDs. Also, it is estimated that half of the new HIV infections in the United States—about 40,000 every year—occur in people younger than 25. This means that prevention activities and interventions must begin well before young adulthood. To address this need, the Centers for Disease Control and Prevention has created school-based HIV prevention programs. Although the CDC itself does not determine the content of these programs, it does highlight curricula that have been effective in reducing health risks in young people and offers resources to ensure that interventions and training are available. The CDC recommends that specific content of prevention programs be determined by local communities so that they will be in line with parental and community values.

screening Testing that can be done to evaluate for the presence of sexually transmitted diseases or other medical conditions in an individual. Various types of tests are used to determine whether an individual has contracted a sexually transmitted disease. Outside the context of STDs, there are numerous forms of medical screenings, including the mammogram, which screens for breast cancer; colonoscopy, which screens for colon cancer; and the Pap smear, which screens for cervical cancer.

self-talk A method used to encourage oneself; negative self-talk is banished, and the individual repeats positive and proactive affirmations. This practice can be helpful to people who have sexually transmitted diseases, in that positive thinking can provide a greater sense of empowerment over the disease and over one's eventual fate in regard to the disease.

semen A milky fluid that a male ejaculates from his penis during sexual climax, or orgasm. Besides sperm, it contains fluids from the testicles, prostate, and seminal vesicles. Each ejaculate may contain up to 500 million sperm. Fertilization, required for pregnancy, is the fusion of a spermatozoon and an ovum (egg).

semen with blood Presence of blood in the semen, which is usually the result of a ruptured blood vessel and which is not serious and may follow masturbation or ejaculation during sexual activity. This requires no treatment, but a man who sees blood in his semen must seek medical evaluation as soon as possible in case the cause is more serious. A doctor needs to rule out possible malignancy and infection. A prostate infection and infections in the urethra can cause blood in the semen. Another possible cause is prostate cancer, which only rarely causes blood in the semen.

seroconcordance   In the context of HIV/AIDS, a couple's HIV status. A couple can be HIV seroconcordant (both are either HIV positive or HIV negative), or a couple can be HIV serodiscordant (the two partners' serostatuses are different).

seroconversion   The process of developing antibodies to infection. Seroconversion time is the period required for detectable antibodies to develop once an infection has occurred. Typically, the body takes a few days or weeks to react to a foreign substance such as a virus and develop antibodies to it. In the case of HIV, antibodies may not appear (thus a person may not test positive for HIV) for a minimum of several months. That is why repeat testing is recommended for people who believe they may have been exposed to HIV.

serologic test   A blood test that can detect a disease such as herpes by looking for antibodies in the blood or serum. Blood tests can be done even when no symptoms are apparent or after symptoms are gone.

The antibodies that are detected by serologic tests are substances produced by the immune system to help fight infection. If antibodies are discovered in the blood, they indicate that a person has been exposed to or infected with the disease in question.

To get a more accurate herpes blood test result, a person should ask for a type-specific assay, which can distinguish HSV-2 from HSV-1. There are many kits available in the marketplace that do not make this distinction. Remember, too, that after a person is exposed to herpes, herpes antibodies may not show up in the blood for anywhere from two weeks to three months. (Once a person does have antibodies, they remain in the body for a lifetime.)

sex toy   A toy that is used for sexual stimulation or gratification with or without a partner. Examples are vibrators and dildos.

sexual accommodation   The act of accommodating one's partner via participation in sexual activities that gratify the other individual.

sexual assault and sexual abuse   Sexual assault is any form of nonconsensual and unwanted sexual conduct, attack, rape, or activity perpetrated by means of force or a threat of force or violence or coercion if the victim does not cooperate. Rape in marriage is included.

Sexual abuse is sexual activity (inappropriate acts) involving a betrayal of trust by an adult perpetrator with a minor or unwilling party; this may include a single instance or activity over a long period. Traditionally, when children are sexually abused, it is a case of incest (sexual activity with a relative) or pedophilia (sexual activity with a sexual predator who preys on children). Sexual abuse is most commonly perpetrated by someone who has authority or power over a child—a family member, teacher, church or club authority figure, and so on.

The U.S. Department of Health and Human Services issues recommendations for treating people who have been sexually assaulted or abused, limited to the identification and treatment of sexually transmitted diseases commonly seen in sexual assault and abuse cases. (Documentation of findings and collection of nonmicrobiologic specimens for forensic purposes and the management of potential pregnancy or physical and psychological trauma are not included.) Among sexually active adults, identifying STDs after an assault is usually more important for the psychological and medical management of the patient than for legal purposes, because the infection could have been acquired before the assault.

The diseases most often diagnosed in women who have been sexually assaulted are trichomoniasis, bacterial vaginosis, chlamydia, and gonorrhea. Because these are STDs that are rampant in the sexually active population, their presence after an assault cannot be definitively declared "acquired during assault." Of special concern in such situations are chlamydia and gonorrhea in women because of the possibility of ascending infection (pelvic inflammatory disease and its potential complications such as infertility). In addition, if a person is exposed to hepatitis B virus during an assault, postexposure administration of hepatitis B vaccine and hepatitis B immune globulin can prevent infection.

After sexual assault, the initial examination should include the following procedures:

- Cultures for *Neisseria gonorrhoeae* and *Chlamydia trachomatis* are made from specimens collected from any sites of penetration or attempted penetration.

- If chlamydia culture is not available, a substitute such as a nucleic acid amplification test is acceptable. If a nonculture test is used, a positive test result should be verified with another test. EIA and direct fluorescent antibody are not good alternatives because of their potential to produce false-negative results.

- Wet mount and culture of a vaginal swab specimen for *Trichomonas vaginalis* infection are made. The wet mount should also be checked for bacterial vaginosis and yeast infection.

- A serum sample is collected for immediate evaluation for HIV, hepatitis B, and syphilis.

Those who have been sexually assaulted should have follow-up examinations to detect new infections acquired during or after assault, to complete hepatitis B immunization (if indicated), and to complete counseling and treatment for other STDs. Two weeks after assault, an exam for sexually transmitted diseases should be done again. This is important because infectious agents acquired during assault may not have produced enough concentrations of organism to test positive at the initial examination, so it is critical to perform culture, wet mount, and other tests at a two-week follow-up visit, unless prophylactic treatment was already provided. Serologic tests for syphilis and HIV should be done again at these intervals: Six, 12, and 24 weeks after assault (if results initially were negative).

Many health care experts recommend routine preventive therapy after a sexual assault. Most people probably benefit from prophylaxis because follow-up for sexual assault victims is difficult, and

they may be reassured by treatment or prophylaxis for possible infection. The following prophylactic regimen is recommended:

- Postexposure hepatitis B vaccine and hepatitis B immune globulin should protect against hepatitis B virus. Hepatitis B vaccine should be given to victims of sexual assault at the time of the initial exam. Follow-up doses of vaccine should be administered one to two and four to six months after first dose.

- An empiric antimicrobial regimen for chlamydia, gonorrhea, trichomonas, and bacterial vaginosis should be given.

Other considerations are that patients should be counseled about symptoms of STDs and the need for immediate examination if these occur, and abstinence from sexual intercourse until STD prophylactic treatment is completed should be emphasized.

The risk for acquiring HIV through sexual assault is low, although HIV-antibody seroconversion has been reported among those whose only risk factor was sexual assault or abuse. The likelihood of getting HIV during a single act of intercourse depends on type of activity (oral, vaginal, or anal); presence of oral, vaginal, or anal trauma; site of victim's exposure to attacker's ejaculate; viral load in his ejaculate; and the presence of a preexisting STD in the victim.

The probability of HIV transmission may also be affected by postexposure therapy for HIV with antiretroviral agents. Postexposure therapy with zidovudine is associated with reduced risk for HIV infection, according to the results of a study of health care workers who had percutaneous exposures to HIV-infected blood. Because of these results and the effectiveness of antiretroviral agents, postexposure therapy has been recommended for health care workers who have percutaneous exposures to HIV. But whether these findings apply to other HIV-exposure situations such as sexual assault remains a question.

In children, finding sexually transmissible agents after the neonatal period is indicative of sexual abuse. Exceptions are the following:

- Rectal or genital infection with chlamydia that has resulted from perinatally acquired infection (it can last for up to three years)

- Genital warts, bacterial vaginosis, and genital mycoplasmas, which have been seen in children who have been abused but also in those who have not

- Hepatitis B virus (HBV) transmitted to children through household exposure to persons with chronic HBV

If the child has no apparent risk factor for infection and has an STD, the possibility of sexual abuse should be investigated. When the only evidence of sexual abuse is the isolation of an organism or the detection of antibodies to a sexually transmissible agent, findings should be confirmed and implications scrutinized. The determination of whether sexual abuse has occurred should be made by people who are experts in evaluating abused and assaulted children.

Evaluation for sexually transmitted infections in abused children must be done in a manner that minimizes further pain and trauma. Situations that have a high risk for STDs and a strong need for testing are the following:

- The offender has a sexually transmitted disease or is at high risk for STDs.

- The child shows symptoms of an STD.

- The community has a high prevalence of STDs.

- Evidence of genital or oral penetration or ejaculation exists.

- Other people in the child's household have sexually transmitted diseases

Obtaining specimens for STD testing is delicate in children. This must be done so that the child is not further traumatized physically and psychologically. Ideally, the person doing the examination and collecting of specimens should be someone with experience and training in dealing with abused and assaulted children. Also, the child needs a follow-up visit two weeks after the sexual exposure for another examination and a second collection of specimens. To make sure there has been time for development of antibodies, the child should have a third follow-up 12 weeks after the sexual event. The following are the tests and exams that are recommended:

- Visual inspection (genital, perianal, oral areas) for genital warts and ulcerative lesions

- Cultures for gonorrhea collected from the pharynx and anus in boys and girls, the vagina in girls, and the urethra in boys

- Cultures for chlamydia from specimens collected from the anus in both boys and girls and from the vagina in girls

- Culture and wet mount of a vaginal swab specimen for *Trichomonas vaginalis* (presence of clue cells in the wet mount or a sign such as a positive whiff test finding suggest bacterial vaginosis in girls with vaginal discharge)

- Collection of a serum sample to be tested immediately, preserved for later analysis, and used as a baseline for comparison in follow-up tests

In the exam 12 weeks after the last sexual exposure, there will have been time for antibodies to infectious agents to develop (if baseline test results were negative). A child's risk for sexually transmitted diseases from sexual abuse is undetermined. Presumptive treatment is not recommended in most cases because it appears that young girls are at lower risk for ascending infection than adolescent or adult women.

Every state and U.S. territory requires reporting of child abuse. State requirements vary.

sexual communication Emphasis on talking to one's sex partners about existing sexually transmitted diseases, use of condoms, realistic protection expectations, and so on, as a proactive means of maintaining overall health. Active sexual communication is recommended in order to promote greater "global" protection of sexually active individuals.

sexual ethics A code of sexual behavior that requires ethical treatment of partners, including safe sex and protection of others from transmission of sexually transmitted diseases.

sexual intercourse Intercourse between a male and a female in which the penis is inserted into the vagina; or intercourse between individuals that calls for genital contact that does not involve insertion of the penis into the vagina. This is also referred to as coitus. Usually sexual intercourse involves penetration by the penis.

sexuality One's sexual self, or the ability to respond to and experience sexual feelings and act as a sexual being. The era of HIV/AIDS and other sexually transmitted diseases has given rise to many conflicting feelings and messages about sexuality. It is clear from reports from the Centers for Disease Control and Prevention National AIDS Hotline that adolescents in the United States often have trouble finding accurate information about sexuality in a safe and anonymous way. Every year the hotline gets hundreds of thousands of condom-related calls, many from adolescents who are seeking reliable information on proper use of condoms.

sexually transmitted disease A disease that is transmitted by sexual contact. Once called "venereal diseases," sexually transmitted diseases (STDs) are among the most common infectious diseases today in the United States. There are more than 20 STDs, according to *Journal of the American Medical Association (JAMA)* Women's Health Sexually Transmitted Disease Information Center.

In today's era of widespread dissemination of these diseases, sexually active people definitely need a good understanding of STDs, how they are spread, their symptoms, and more. It is extremely important for people to know that many sexually transmitted diseases do not have symptoms at the outset, and sometimes—in fact, often—a partner may not even be aware that he or she has a disease. To complicate matters even more, safe sex (using a latex condom) is not a surefire solution, because some STDs can be contracted even when condoms are used. (See entries on individual STDs in this book.) This points to the obvious conclusion—that the only way a person can be sure of not contracting a sexually transmitted disease is to abstain from having sex and any sexual conduct, and that includes oral sex.

Although two-thirds of those who have STDs are younger than 25, it is not unusual for older people to contract these diseases, especially considering the trend toward multiple sex partners, which increases one's risk of getting an STD.

In some cases, a woman can become infertile as the result of an untreated STD. Or she may have a tubal (ectopic) pregnancy, which can sometimes lead to death. The STD human papillomavirus infection can give a person genital warts, but it can also lead to cervical cancer. Further, some STDs can be passed from a pregnant woman to her fetus or to her baby when she gives birth. In some cases, the infant can be cured, but other times, the child may contract HIV or a permanent disability or even die.

The Centers for Disease Control and Prevention emphasizes that a great deal of scientific evidence suggests that the presence of sexually transmitted disease(s) in an individual enhances his or her likelihood of both transmitting and getting HIV.

STDs probably increase a person's susceptibility to HIV infection in two ways: genital ulcers (syphilis, herpes, chancroid) cause breaks in the genital tract lining or skin, which can create portals of entry for HIV. Second, nonulcerative STDs (chlamydia, gonorrhea, trichomoniasis) increase the concentration of cells in genital secretions that can serve as HIV targets (CD4+ cells).

Also, studies underscore that when HIV-positive people have other sexually transmitted diseases, they are more likely to have HIV in their genital secretions, meaning that they are more infectious. As an example, consider the fact that men infected with both gonorrhea and HIV are more than twice as likely to shed HIV in genital secretions as those who have HIV alone. And the median concentration of HIV in semen can be 10 times higher in men who have both HIV and gonorrhea than in men who are only HIV-infected.

Thus, it is clear that STD treatment can help to reduce a person's ability to transmit HIV and also reduces the spread of HIV in communities.

It has been seen that continuous interventions to improve access to treatment are more effective in reducing HIV transmission than interventions that are intermittent, such as periodic mass treatments.

Second, sexually transmitted disease treatment is most effective in reducing HIV transmission where STD rates are high and the heterosexual HIV epidemic is young. Third, treatment of symptomatic sexually transmitted diseases appears to be especially important.

The upshot of this is that strong and comprehensive efforts to prevent, test, and treat STDs can go a long way toward preventing the spread of HIV sexually. Also, STD trends provide researchers with insights so that they can determine where the HIV epidemic may grow and try to address this trend with appropriate interventions.

Major STDs that sexually active people must be aware of include HIV/AIDS, chlamydia, genital herpes, genital warts, gonorrhea, and syphilis. Other disorders that can be sexually transmitted include scabies, pubic lice, trichomoniasis, and cytomegalovirus.

To prevent an STD, a person can avoid all forms of sexual activity (abstinence) or practice safe sex to reduce the likelihood of contracting an STD. Some risk-reduction suggestions are the following:

- Be monogamous (have one partner).
- Use a male condom with each sex activity.
- If you have HIV, try to make sure you do not get another STD.
- Reduce your chance of contracting HIV by avoiding the transmission of any sexually transmitted disease.
- Postpone sexual activity as long as possible. The younger you are when you begin, the more likely you are to contract an STD.
- Limit your number of lifetime sex partners.
- Have regular screenings for sexually transmitted diseases.
- Make sure you know common STD symptoms.
- Remember that you cannot rely on a "visual test." A person's appearance tells you nothing about whether she or he has an STD in most cases.
- Avoid anal intercourse.
- Do not douche.
- Avoid having sex during menstruation, because you are more susceptible to infection.

If you do discover that you have an STD, follow these steps:

- Be sure to seek treatment as soon as possible. In addition to preventing complications and transmission of the disease to other partner(s), a pregnant woman can reduce the risk of transmission to her infant.
- If you plan to breast-feed, discuss this option with your gynecologist.
- Inform sex partners of your STD and advise them of treatment options.
- Do not have sex while you are undergoing treatment for a sexually transmitted disease.
- Follow your doctor's suggestions, and take all of your medication. Later, have a follow-up test to make sure the infection is gone.

sex without penetration   Sexual activity between partners that does not involve the penetration of an orifice of the body. In the realm of sexually transmitted diseases, sex without penetration is often an appealing choice when one partner or both do not want to risk pregnancy or transmission of a disease. However, sexually transmitted diseases also can be transmitted by sex play that does not involve penetration, such as oral sex.

sex worker   A person who works in an industry that sells sex as a service—the prostitution of individuals, male or female. The term is also applied more loosely to include strippers, actors in porn films, and the like.

shingles   Shingles, or herpes zoster, usually begins with pain along the distribution of a nerve—typically, in the face, abdomen, or chest. Occasionally someone also has fever, chills, and headache. A person may experience itching, tingling, or severe discomfort along the nerve distribution about three to five days before the development of skin lesions—red skin with clustered blisters. The skin eruption is localized to one side of the body. These lesions, which pop up for several days to three weeks, resemble chickenpox lesions but are grouped rather than singletons. Within several weeks, they contain pus and crust over; by the time they are crusting, they do not contain virus.

The person with shingles feels better in a few weeks, but the area of the nerve may continue to be painful for months (and in rare cases, for years). This is called postherpetic neuralgia. The virus that causes herpes zoster can also cause chickenpox in children.

Basically, the varicella-zoster virus is known to be associated with both shingles (zoster) and chickenpox (varicella). What is peculiar about varicella-zoster is that even after a child has chickenpox and recovers from it in a couple of weeks, the virus becomes dormant in sensory ganglia, and it may reactivate decades later, when it produces shingles or herpes zoster.

Two possible complications of shingles are postherpetic neuralgia and bacterial infection. The latter can be a major problem because the person may have superficial gangrene, resulting in scars. If a person has zoster in the eyes, a bad infection may cause corneal opacification or secondary bacterial infection.

Shingles can be diagnosed by clinical examination and lab analysis. Occasionally differentiating between herpes zoster and herpes simplex can be difficult. Lab testing can accurately diagnose herpes zoster.

To treat shingles, the doctor prescribes an antiviral medication such as acyclovir, valacyclovir, or famciclovir. Oral famciclovir effectively treats herpes zoster and decreases duration of postherpetic neuralgia.

In people with HIV or AIDS, herpes zoster is relatively common. Also, in about half of elderly people shingles is likely to develop. A study is being conducted with a new formulation of chickenpox vaccine to see whether vaccinating people older than 55 can reduce the frequency or severity of shingles.

skin conditions Any irregularity or abnormality of the skin. Skin conditions that occur in people who have sexually transmitted diseases include the following:

- HIV/AIDS: Weeks after infection, one may have a diffuse rash. Later the HIV-infected individual may suffer from Kaposi's sarcoma, dry skin, molluscum contagiosum, herpes simplex, shingles, genital warts, and hairy leukoplakia.
- Gonorrhea: There may be skin lesions on the arms or legs that appear to be sores filled with pus or blood and that are set amid reddened skin.
- Hepatitis B: Chronic hepatitis B can cause a skin disorder called polyarteritis nodosa.
- Pubic lice: The skin may be irritated by the lice attached to the skin in the genital area. Where lice attach, there may be a small bit of bleeding.
- Molluscum contagiosum: Often mistaken for warts, molluscum skin lesions are white, waxy bumps that are painless and have dimpled centers.
- Syphilis: The first symptom is a chancre, a painless sore. In second-stage syphilis, a person may have a rash that appears all over the body, including the palms of the hands and soles of the feet. There may be bumps in the genital area that resemble warts.
- Chancroid: There can be one or several painful ulcers.
- Donovanosis (granuloma inguinale): This causes genital ulcers that enlarge and form beefy red sores.
- Genital herpes: Lesions are painful blisters or ulcers. Sometimes initially there are red itchy bumps.
- Genital warts: Bumps that are flat or cauliflowerlike and usually harder than the surrounding skin.
- Scabies: Scabies forms itchy bumps and lines.
- Yeast infections: These can cause a rash on the penis or a red, scaly genital rash that itches.

Social Security Administration disability benefits
An American who is disabled or too ill to have a job may be eligible to receive disability payments from the Social Security Administration at any age. Health problems the Social Security Administration lists as serious enough to merit disability payments are HIV or AIDS, heart disease, chronic arthritis, multiple personality disorder, mental retardation, schizophrenia, cancer, emphysema, stroke, paraly-

sis, kidney failure, loss of a limb, or visual impairment (loss of some or all vision).

It is the Social Security office in the state in which a person resides that actually makes the final determination as to whether someone qualifies for payments. Sometimes medical problems other than those listed merit payments. An attorney can file claims for the individual who is ill, and this is usually the best course of action because the filing procedure and subsequent steps can be complex.

social services The variety of community and public services that are made available (at no cost or low cost) to those who have sexually transmitted diseases, as well as people with other health problems. Services can include counseling, testing, treatment, and support groups.

socioeconomic impact The way a disease affects a person socially and economically. The socioeconomic impact of sexually transmitted diseases is absolutely mind-boggling, particularly when one considers the billions devoted to research, treatment, and testing for HIV/AIDS patients. Sexually transmitted diseases can take a toll on an individual's personal finances, and they also are a major force in allocation of governmental funds for efforts ranging from prevention and education and intervention to treatment and counseling and outreach projects on all levels—local, state, national, and international.

specialists in HIV When a person receives an HIV-positive diagnosis, it is important to seek counseling and treatment as soon as possible; typically, the individual is advised to find a medical specialist who treats HIV patients routinely. These health care providers are usually the most up-to-date on the ever-changing highly active antiretroviral therapy (HAART) drugs and can provide the latest advice on self-care and ways to enhance health and live an active, high-quality life.

sperm The short form of the word *spermatozoa* (plural), the sex cells from a man that can fertilize an egg (ovum), resulting in pregnancy. Sperm is contained in the semen that a man ejaculates when he has an orgasm.

spermatorrhea Abnormally frequent involuntary discharge of semen without orgasm. Typically, semen is produced by ejaculation of orgasm and is not discharged from the man's body at any other time. If a man loses the mechanism of ejaculation, sperm may discharge involuntarily.

sperm count Used as a measure of male fertility, an estimate of the number of sperm in ejaculated semen. In a total ejaculate, about 300 to 500 million is considered normal; fewer than 60 million equates to sterility, or an inability to reproduce. If a sperm count is very low, there is a likelihood of lower fertility. The presence of infection or the use of drugs or alcohol can decrease fertility. Sperm count is unrelated, however, to a man's virility.

spermicide An agent that kills spermatozoa (sperm). Some sexually active people use creams and jellies that contain chemical spermicides, often in conjunction with a diaphragm.

states with confidential HIV reporting According to the Centers for Disease Control's Division of HIV/AIDS Prevention, the states with confidential reporting as of December 2001 were Alabama, Alaska, Arizona, Arkansas, Colorado, Connecticut (confidential reporting for pediatric cases only), Florida, Idaho, Indiana, Iowa, Kansas, Louisiana, Michigan, Minnesota, Mississippi, Missouri, Nebraska, Nevada, New Jersey, New Mexico, New York, North Carolina, North Dakota, Ohio, Oklahoma, Oregon (confidential infection reporting for children younger than six), South Carolina, South Dakota, Tennessee, Texas (confidential reporting for children 13 and younger), Utah, Virginia, West Virginia, Wisconsin, and Wyoming.

As of December 2001, eight areas—Hawaii, Illinois, Kentucky, Maryland, Massachusetts, Puerto Rico, Rhode Island, and Vermont—had begun a code-based system for case surveillance for HIV. Delaware, Maine, Montana, Oregon, and Washington had started a name-to-code system (names are collected, and after any needed public health follow-up, they are converted to codes).

statistics on AIDS   The information that follows is based on AIDS cases reported to the Centers for Disease Control and Prevention through December 2001. The cumulative number of AIDS cases reported to CDC was 816,149. Adult and adolescent AIDS cases totaled 807,075: 666,026 cases in males and 141,048 cases in females. Through the same period, 9,074 AIDS cases were reported in children below 13. Total deaths of persons with AIDS were 467,910, including 462,653 adults and adolescents, 5,257 children below age 15, and 388 persons whose age at death is unknown.

Of total number of AIDS cases through December 2001, ages at time of diagnosis:

Below 5: 6,975
5–12: 2,099
13–19: 4,428
20–24: 28,665
25–29: 105,060
30–34: 179,164
35–39: 182,857
40–44: 136,145
45–49: 80,242
50–54: 42,780
55–59: 23,280
60–64: 12,898
65 or older: 11,555

Adult cases as of December 2001 by exposure category:

Men who have sex with men: 368,971
Injection drug use: males, 145,750, females, 55,576
Men who have sex with men and inject drugs: 51,293
Hemophilia/coagulation disorder: 5,000 males, 292 females
Heterosexual contact: 32,735 males, 57,396 females
Recipient of blood transfusion, blood components, or tissue: 5,057 males, 3,914 females
Risk not reported or identified: 57,220 males, 23,870 females

Children by exposure category:

Hemophilia/coagulation disorder: 236
Mother with or at risk for HIV infection: 8,284

Receipt of blood transfusion, blood components, tissue: 381
Risk not reported or identified: 173

The 10 states or territories reporting the most cumulative AIDS cases among residents as of June 2001 were New York, 149,341; California, 123,819; Florida, 85,324; Texas, 56,730; New Jersey, 43,824; Pennsylvania, 26,369; Illinois, 26,319; Puerto Rico, 26,119; Georgia, 24,559; Maryland, 23,537.

STD   See SEXUALLY TRANSMITTED DISEASE.

STD exams   Medical screenings that identify sexually transmitted diseases so that individuals who have them can be treated successfully.

STD facts   See INTRODUCTION.

STD stigma   A mark of disgrace that is associated with having an STD, which makes people want to live in denial of the truth. The individual who suspects she or he has a sexually transmitted disease may not confide in family or friends and may be even less inclined to talk to a doctor about the problem. It is often very difficult for patients to tell their doctors their fears or suspicions that they have a sexually transmitted disease; their reluctance can lead to delayed diagnosis and treatment.

In research on the experiences of people at a sexual health clinic who received an STD diagnosis, researchers studied the effect of using counseling in semistructured interviews. Some of the STD-infected reported feelings of anxiety, stigma, and isolation, a factor that should be remembered by those who work with this group in various health care facilities.

stress   Stress can play a role in reducing the strength of a person's immune system, making it more vulnerable to disease, such as infection that is sexually transmitted. Stress is also a factor in the global picture of sexually transmitted diseases. At the 2002 National Sexually Transmitted Disease

Prevention Conference, sponsored by the Centers for Disease Control and Prevention and the American Social Health Association, in San Diego, California, on March 5, 2002, the presenter Laurie Garrett, author of *Betrayal of Trust: The Collapse of Global Public Health*, spoke on "STD Prevention in Societies under Stress: A Global Perspective," outlining key problems in addressing the spread of sexually transmitted diseases in a world where the stressors are many, far-reaching, and extensive. She pointed to problems in public health, such as the increasingly individualized picture of health—a challenge to everyone in public health because it could reach an extreme: "No two people would have the same prescription needs except if they were clones or identical twins." The other challenge, said Garrett, is the FDA's change in regard to consumer advertising for pharmaceutical drugs. In 1995, a law that allowed companies to use print and TV ads was enacted. Drug companies have drastically increased spending for advertising to the public and outreach to physicians, with the result that less money is allocated to development of new drugs. She referred to the "market failure" involved when "the health needs of the planet are not the same as the profitable potentials of the planet." In other words, as she put it, "On the one hand, you can make a Viagra that turns a 98 percent profit in a single year, and on the other hand, you can make a new antimalarial that saves two million lives a year. But, they're all poor people (the ones who need the drug)."

Few experts can agree on anything except that there is a need for "creative thinking," a fact mentioned by Microsoft CEO Bill Gates, at a human retrovirus meeting when he was asked what to do about creating some new sense of incentives.

Laurie Garrett underscores Americans' desperate need for a new drug for tuberculosis because the incidence of the disease is climbing, and more people had active TB in 2001 than ever before in human history: 8.5 million active cases, according to the CDC, and 2 million deaths. And drug resistance is skyrocketing. Garrett also points to a CDC–World Health Organization joint survey of 58 nations that was published in the *New England Journal of Medicine* in 2001 that looked at 1995–99 trends in multidrug-resistant TB and found that every nation had had a huge increase.

Many people are experiencing a rise in drug resistance and seeing antibiotics rendered less and less useful. Garrett attributes this to "an exploding black market" in other countries, where peddlers with no medical training are selling antibiotics (some of which were expired drugs) that were sent in for humanitarian relief and were stolen from Red Cross warehouses.

She also underscores the inappropriate use of drugs in various industries, such as the beef industry and aquaculture—"They out-use 10 to 1 what we use as antibiotics for medicinal purposes in human beings," says Garrett.

But even the antibiotic problem and our diminished ability to treat gonorrhea, syphilis, chlamydia, and so on "is dwarfed by the significance of HIV and the dilemmas this poses for all of us in dealing with sexually transmitted diseases and the future of this horrible life expectancy gap and wealth gap globally." As 40 million are living with the disease and 5 million are newly infected in a single year, HIV has "eclipsed the Black Death of the 14th century to become the biggest pandemic in the history of our species."

She also explored the devastation of HIV in Africa, where the greater numbers can be attributed to a huge population of girls and women with HIV and AIDS, a prevalence of rape of female children and teens, and a superstition that a man having sex with a female virgin can cure HIV infection.

This leads to a critical point—HIV as a national security threat that destabilizes societies, economies, and futures. Parts of Africa, Asia, and the former Soviet Union have so many young adults with HIV that some believe the United States must find a way to intervene and help. "Because, when you have no sense of future, no sense of values, and you've never been parented," says Garrett, "it's impossible to imagine a sense of social responsibility attached to sex . . . and it's impossible to imagine a sense of social responsibility attached to your children and to the raising of your children."

Dr. King Holmes, at the same conference, noted that the challenge is for the global community to find solutions to global public health problems and their underlying structural causes—because the emerging infectious diseases such as HIV, AIDS, malaria, and TB are becoming part of the structural problems themselves. Even in the United States, where there are many health interventions and prevention programs, the partner notification process appears flawed in the realm of STDs. One nationwide survey of health departments indicated that the percentage of cases interviewed for partner notification for HIV was only 52 percent, highlighting the need for more resources. It was estimated that a 600 percent increase in funding would be required to provide coverage to those who have STDs who are not interviewed for partner notification. Clearly, "societies under stress" see the effect of stress on public health and desperately need "creative thinking."

surveillance data   Material gathered and assimilated by surveillance programs whose goal is to gather all information obtainable on HIV and AIDS, from epidemiologic factors to modes of transmission to stage of disease at diagnosis. Public health agencies use the information to improve HIV prevention, treatment, and dissemination of health caveats for sexually active Americans. Surveillance data are key to promoting an improved state of the general public health.

surveillance programs   The Centers for Disease Control and Prevention, in September 1997, asked all states and territories to conduct HIV surveillance as an extension of their existing AIDS surveillance programs. This was done as a necessary response to the impact of advances in highly active antiretroviral therapy (HAART), the implementation of new HIV treatment guidelines, and the increasing need for epidemiologic data on people in all stages of HIV.

Recommended surveillance practices included the following:

- Local and state programs' collection of a standard set of surveillance data for all cases that meet reporting criteria for HIV and AIDS. A *standard set* features patient identifier; earliest date of HIV diagnosis; earliest date when an AIDS-defining condition was noted; demographics at diagnosis; facility of diagnosis; date of death; and state of residence at that time. State and local programs are to collect information on infants with perinatal exposures to HIV. Local surveillance programs can also cross-match HIV/AIDS surveillance data with other public health data and collect supplemental data on all or a sample of cases. Surveillance information, without patient identifiers, is to be encrypted and forwarded to CDC through the existing HIV/AIDS Reporting System.

- Published evaluations of non-name-based HIV surveillance in two states.

- Use of HIV/AIDS surveillance data to identify rare modes of HIV transmission and unusual clinical or virologic manifestations.

- Direction of surveillance efforts to collection of data from private and public sources of HIV testing and care services. Statistics on people tested anonymously are not to be entered into the Reporting System; they are to be reported anonymously to the HIV Counseling and Testing database.

- The regular publishing of surveillance data in a format that makes this information usable for all public health agencies—federal, state, and local.

- Regular assessments of performance of surveillance system.

- Requirement that state and local surveillance systems use prescribed reporting methods.

It was also set forth that security and confidentiality policies of surveillance programs should meet the precise standards set by the Centers for Disease Control and Prevention.

swollen glands   Lymph node swelling, which can sometimes be seen in the sexually transmitted diseases genital herpes, chancroid, HIV, lymphogranuloma venereum, syphilis, and trichomoniasis. This symptom should signal the need for a medical evaluation.

syphilis Syphilis is a complex sexually transmitted disease that has been called the "great imitator" because so many symptoms are indistinguishable from those of other diseases, according to the Centers for Disease Control and Prevention. Syphilis is a systemic disease; the rate of primary and secondary syphilis reported in the United States is now the lowest since mandatory reporting to the CDC was begun in 1941. The rate of syphilis cases in the United States declined by 89.2 percent from 1990 to 2000. However, the number of cases rose from 5,979 in 2000 to 6,103 in 2001. This was the first increase since 1990.

Cause

A very fragile bacterium called *Treponema pallidum* causes the disease syphilis, which moves through the body and can damage organs over time. The time between infection with syphilis and the appearance of a symptom averages about 21 days but can range from 10 to 90 days.

Symptoms

The early symptoms of syphilis mimic those of many other diseases; that is one reason some people do not take the initial sore or odd rash that appears seriously. Most disturbing is that early symptoms often are unnoticed because they are so mild. They also disappear soon after they are first seen. (Anyone who has been treated for another sexually transmitted disease probably should be tested for syphilis, too.)

In primary syphilis, the sign is often a chancre—an indurated, punched-out ulcer that is painless or only slightly painful and is located at the infection site. Sometimes there is a single sore; other times, many. The chancre (pronounced "shan-ker") is the classical first symptom of primary syphilis, usually a painless open sore that shows up on the penis or around or in the vagina. Other possible sites are the anus, hands, or area near the mouth. A chancre is typically one to two centimeters in diameter. These can appear as shallow ulcerations with noninflamed margins; they occur most commonly on mucous membranes that are irritated during sexual activity. The chancre lasts three to six weeks and heals on its own, without scarring, whether or not the person is treated. If a person does not receive adequate treatment, the infection progresses to the secondary stage.

The second stage of syphilis starts when one or more areas of the skin break into an itchless rash. Often the rash appears as the chancre is fading, but sometimes it may be weeks before it appears. The rash is characterized by scaly, red or reddish-brown spots on the palms of the hands and the bottoms of the feet; it can also be distributed on the torso and extremities. The rash sometimes appears on other body parts with different characteristics that resemble those of other diseases. The widespread, transient rash features brown, penny-sized sores. These sores contain active bacteria, so it is imperative to avoid sexual or nonsexual contact with the broken skin of another person during this stage.

The rash, which heals spontaneously in a few weeks or months, can be accompanied by low fever, muscle aches, fatigue, headaches, sore throat, patchy hair loss, and swollen lymph glands. Such symptoms are often mild and may come and go during the year or two after initial infection. Sometimes the rashes are not even noticeable. In secondary syphilis, a person may also have condylomata lata, oral or genital mucous patches, systemic symptoms, and symmetric adenopathy.

If the patient does not receive treatment, syphilis can proceed into a latent period—a time that is symptom-free, when contagion is not possible. Many who are not treated are fortunate in that they suffer no more consequences of syphilis.

In both primary and secondary states, when symptoms are present, a person can readily pass the disease to sex partners. The latent (hidden) stage of syphilis begins when the secondary symptoms disappear. Untreated, the infected person still has syphilis even though no signs or symptoms are apparent at that time, but it remains in the body and may start damaging the internal organs, including the nerves, brain, eyes, heart, blood vessels, liver, bones, and joints. This internal damage may show up years later in the late, or tertiary, stage of syphilis. Late-stage signs are an inability to coordinate muscle movements, paralysis, numbness, dementia, and gradual blindness. The damage may be serious enough to result in death.

Latent syphilis that was acquired in the preceding year is called *early latent syphilis*. All other latent-syphilis cases, though, are late latent syphilis or syphilis of unknown duration.

Testing

To confirm diagnosis, a doctor looks for signs of syphilis, asks whether the patient has experienced any of the symptoms, performs blood tests, and checks for microscopic identification of syphilis bacteria. The latter is accomplished by taking a scraping from the ulcer or chancre to be studied under a special dark-field microscope in order to look for the organism.

Although blood tests do produce false-negative results up to three months after infection, they can also provide evidence of infection. Shortly after infection, the body produces syphilis antibodies that can be detected by an inexpensive blood test. Furthermore, low-level antibodies remain in the blood for months (sometimes years) after successful treatment of syphilis.

Confirming a syphilis diagnosis can be hard because interpreting the results of blood tests for syphilis is difficult. Commonly used initial tests are the Venereal Disease Research Laboratory (VDRL) test and the rapid plasma reagin (RPR) test. Typically, false-positive results occur mainly in those with certain viral infections, autoimmune disorders, and other conditions. That means if the first test result shows up positive, another test must be done to confirm the result.

One test used for confirmation is the fluorescent treponemal antibody-absorption (FTA-ABS) test. Another is the *T. pallidum* hemagglutination assay (TPHA). Both tests can detect syphilis antibodies. They are not used for diagnosing a new case of syphilis in patients who have had the disease, because once a person has had a reactive result to one of these two tests, in most cases, that individual will continue to have a reactive result for life. (It is important to note that these antibodies do not protect against a new infection of syphilis.) Sequential serologic tests should be done by using the same testing method (VDRL or RPR), and it is best that they be done by the same lab.

HIV-infected patients can have abnormal serologic test results—unusually high, unusually low, or fluctuating titers—so if they have clinical syndromes that suggest early syphilis, other tests (biopsy and direct microscopy) may be needed. However, for most HIV-positive people, serological tests are accurate in diagnosing syphilis.

Serologic findings are always positive in secondary syphilis. If the syphilitic patient is in the latent or late stage, a doctor may have to do a spinal tap to check for infection of the nervous system. Because untreated syphilis of a pregnant woman can infect and possibly lead to the death of her baby, every pregnant woman should be tested for syphilis.

Congenital Syphilis

Untreated early syphilis during pregnancy results in perinatal death in up to 40 percent of cases. If the disease is acquired during the four years preceding pregnancy, it may lead to infection of the fetus in more than 70 percent of cases, according to STD Surveillance 2000, from the Department of Health and Human Services, Centers for Disease Control and Prevention. Although the outcome actually depends on the length of time a pregnant woman has had syphilis, she does have a high likelihood of having a stillbirth (syphilitic stillbirth) or of giving birth to a baby who dies shortly after birth. An infected infant may be born without symptoms and if not treated immediately may experience them in a few weeks. Babies who are not treated may suffer developmental delays, have seizures, or die. Some babies have symptoms at birth; others have them in subsequent weeks. They may experience sores, rashes, fever, hoarse crying, swollen liver and spleen, yellowish skin (jaundice), anemia, and deformities. In handling an infant with congenital syphilis, the caregiver must be careful not to touch the infectious moist sores.

In a few rare instances, an infant has syphilis that is not detected, and therefore, not treated. As the years pass, late-stage symptoms—damaged bones, teeth, eyes, ears, and/or brain—can develop.

The Centers for Disease Control and Prevention reported a decrease of 20.7 percent from 2000 to 2001, for a congenital syphilis rate of 11.1 per 100,000 live-born infants, compared to rates of 14.0 in 2000 and 27.8 in 1997. In 2000, it was also noted that racial and ethnic minorities had the highest congenital syphilis rates: 49.3, African Americans; 22.6, Hispanics; 13.2, Native Americans/ Alaska natives; 5.9, Asians/Pacific Islanders; compared with 1.5 among non-Hispanic whites.

It is clear that substantial progress has been made in the United States insofar as eliminating syphilis. In 2001, the number of congenital syphilis cases was the lowest since the revised case definition of 1988, and it is believed that proactive campaigns targeting syphilis (prevention, detection, and treatment) in women of reproductive age probably played a large role in the decline. The cornerstones of elimination are early detection and treatment with penicillin, which is widely available, cheap, effective, and safe for mothers and fetuses.

The CDC recommends syphilis testing for all women during early pregnancy. In areas of high syphilis prevalence and among high-risk women, testing should also be performed in the third trimester, including once at delivery. The CDC also advocates syphilis screening in jails, prisons, emergency departments, and other settings that provide health care to high-risk women.

Other Complications

One major downside of syphilis is that it facilitates the transmission of HIV. Genital sores of syphilis make sexual transmission and acquisition of HIV infection easier. A person with syphilis has a twofold to fivefold greater risk of contracting HIV than does a person without syphilis.

About one-third of people who have had secondary syphilis do proceed to the next stage— tertiary syphilis, with the complications that are inherent in that multiyear period. Over those years, the bacteria can damage the heart, eyes, brain, nervous system, joints, bones, and other body systems.

Late syphilis—final-stage syphilis—can cause mental illness, blindness, neurologic problems, heart abnormalities, and death. The full course of the disease usually spans many years.

Chronic infections such as syphilis and tuberculosis can lead to the development of an aortic aneurysm, which is a bulging or ballooning of part of the wall of the aorta (blood flows out of the heart through the aorta to the rest of the body). Syphilis was once the most common cause of thoracic aortic aneurysms, but this fact has almost been forgotten in the Western world, as penicillin and other antibiotics turned syphilitic aneurysms into relics of the past. However, since syphilitic aortitis usually appears as late as 10 to 30 years after primary infection, doctors must watch for a possible increased incidence of associated aneurysms because of the increase in syphilis in HIV patients. Successful treatment of ruptured thoracic aortic aneurysms is dependent on rapid diagnosis and immediate operation.

Treatment

Amazingly, a person who has had syphilis for less than a year can be cured with a single dose of penicillin. This is injected. Larger doses of penicillin are used to treat patients who have had syphilis longer than a year. Stage and manifestations of the disease determine the preparation used (procaine, benzathine, aqueous crystalline), the dosage, and the length of the treatment regimen. If an allergy to penicillin exists, another antibiotic is used.

While a person is receiving treatment for syphilis, he or she must not have sexual contact with new partners until all sores are completely healed and treatment is completed. It is important for anyone who has syphilis to notify sex partners so they can be tested and treated. Do note that although penicillin can kill the syphilis bacterium and prevent further health damage, it does not repair the damage already done. Because organisms are dividing at a slower rate, late latent syphilis and tertiary syphilis are believed to require a longer period of treatment.

CDC recommendations suggest that a patient with penicillin allergy who has syphilis and whose compliance with taking medications cannot be ensured be desensitized and then treated with benzathine penicillin. For other penicillin-allergic patients, there are several other medications that can be used for early syphilis, but their efficacy is not well studied. Parenteral penicillin G is the only way to treat neurosyphilis effectively, and it is also used to treat pregnant women who have syphilis.

Prevention

In almost every case, syphilis is spread via sexual contact with someone who has an active syphilis infection. To prevent contracting syphilis, people who are sexually active should avoid contact with sores, infected tissues, and body fluids and should use condoms during sexual intercourse.

An uninfected person who is monogamous and has sex only with a partner who is uninfected and monogamous is not at risk for contracting syphilis. If the STD status of a partner is unknown, it is important to use a latex condom with every sex act. However, people should also be aware that condoms do not provide complete protection because syphilis sores are often on areas that are not covered by a condom. Another caution: not all syphilis sores can be seen; they may be hidden in the vagina, rectum, and mouth.

It is important to know that past syphilis infection does not protect someone from contracting a new infection. Antibodies are produced as a person reacts to syphilis, and after treatment, these antibodies provide partial protection from reinfection if exposure occurs immediately. This is a very short period of protection.

The disease is described as having four stages: primary, secondary, latent, and tertiary (late). If an individual has syphilis and is untreated, he or she can infect others during the first two stages—typically, a period of one to two years.

Follow-up testing is a good idea since some people do not respond to the normal penicillin doses. Double-checking to make sure the infectious agent is destroyed is key. An individual who has neurosyphilis may require testing for two years after completion of treatment.

To prevent infants from contracting congenital syphilis from mothers who are infected, testing in early pregnancy helps to ensure that the mother is treated. A pregnant woman with syphilis can pass this bacterium to her fetus, causing severe mental and/or physical defects in the baby. (See the section Other Complications.)

Research

The National Institute of Allergy and Infectious Diseases reports that researchers have under way new tests that are designed to improve prompt diagnosis and define infection stage. A vaccine is also being researched. One high priority is development of a diagnostic test that can be done with urine or saliva rather than a blood sample. Researchers are working on a single-dose oral antibiotic because injections frighten some people. In addition, about 10 percent of Americans cannot take penicillin because they are allergic to it.

syringe   An instrument used for injecting or withdrawing fluids. *Syringe* is a pivotal word in the war against HIV/AIDS because, as of December 2001, the epidemic in the United States was being fueled by injection drug use. The CDC attributes one-fourth of AIDS cases to injection drug use. Thus, many prevention programs seek to reduce syringe-borne HIV, but these efforts have proved difficult because of the lack of availability of clean syringes.

In the context of HIV/AIDS, it is important to note that it has been determined that HIV-1 can survive in syringes used by injectors of illicit drugs longer than six weeks. In a study documented on Medscape Hematology-Oncology Journal Scan (from the AIDS Reader), it was found that the percentage of syringes with viable virus varied depending on volume of blood remaining in the syringes and the temperature of their storage spot. These experiments, of course, support the need for needle exchange programs and other HIV prevention efforts that promote greater availability of clean syringes and the removal from circulation of those syringes that are potentially infectious.

T-20 In the realm of AIDS therapies, much excitement surrounded the introduction of T-20, a fusion inhibitor first available in 2003. Some experts in the field of HIV/AIDS research believe that T-20 controls the replication of the AIDS virus better than anything used to date.

talking with a sex partner Sexually active couples need to be aware of the importance of discussing condom use as early in the relationship as possible, preferably before they are in the heat of passion. Speaking directly and honestly is the best approach.

When a man claims he will not use condoms because he does not like them, or sex does not feel as good with them, his partner can respond that using a condom will make him or her feel more relaxed and, thus, enjoy sex more. A woman should tell her partner she wants to have sex without risking an unwanted pregnancy or an STD. It is not a matter of trust, and it is not wise to take the risky approach of "pulling out in time."

For a woman, having intercourse without protection is like Russian roulette. If her partner protests that wearing a condom feels too much like "taking a shower with a raincoat," she should nevertheless be proactive in insisting on protection via condoms. A loving relationship places emphasis on protecting the other partner. Disregard of a partner's health and well-being is clearly not a loving, caring approach to sexual activity.

Both partners are wise to keep in mind that only one unprotected instance of sex can result in a sexually transmitted disease—and pregnancy. It happens all the time.

Being involved sexually with an individual who is cavalier about harming a partner's health is a bad choice. A man with a selfish approach to sex is asking his partner to deal with the grim possibility of an STD and/or pregnancy, and these stark and life-changing realities could be ones that she will be left alone to face after he has moved on to impregnate and share STDs with other partners.

One fact is certain: people have trouble talking about sex—parents and children, sex partners, even friends and relatives. It is an odd irony when one considers the barrage of sexual messages that Americans are bombarded with by the media every day of the week. Although couples talk freely about past relationships, few are willing to ask about a history of sexually transmitted disease, homosexual activity, or unprotected sex. Similarly, people are reluctant to inquire about drug use via shared needles and syringes, even though most know that this constitutes a major HIV risk.

There is no doubt that having a frank discussion with a partner will help to reduce the likelihood of contracting STDs, as well as the possibility of an unwanted pregnancy. Conversely, the individual who enters into a sexual relationship with a stranger increases his or her chances of getting a sexually transmitted disease.

Parents can encourage sexually active teens to initiate this kind of difficult communication when they are in sexual situations. Sexually transmitted diseases are endemic, and the only way to protect oneself is to have no sexual contact (to practice abstinence). If the teen is unwilling to do so, he or she must initiate a candid talk with a potential sex partner.

Some people being counseled ask when this "talk" should take place. Certainly, a passionate scenario is the wrong time because this is not fertile ground for any kind of conversation, much less the safe-sex kind, which may be embarrassing. However, the subject can be broached at a "cooler" time, when it appears likely that sexual activity is on the horizon. A sexually active person who is not careful has very high odds of getting a sexually transmitted disease or more than one, and that fact may provide the courage to have that slightly awkward talk at some point before having sex.

If a partner resists all attempts to communicate, that is a sign of trouble: either the person has an STD and wants to conceal it or he or she is not concerned with the partner's health. If a sex partner has something to hide or is not interested in maintaining good health, that is a red flag that this individual is not a good sexual partner. The person who goes blindly forward is likely to end up in a doctor's office being tested for an STD and hearing confirmation that he or she does indeed have one. Even the person who has never before been gutsy should make this kind of situation the first assertive moment of his or her life.

Some people are most comfortable in taking a lighthearted approach to bringing up safe sex talk: "I don't really know you, so I'll have to hear some of your bed history before we have sex." Or, "I value my health, so I'm not going to have sex with you until we've talked."

If this makes the other person mad, that is a signal that this potential partner looks at you as short-term gratification, not a serious possibility for a long-term relationship. The upshot of a situation in which someone is not being cherished or respected as a person can be a rapid dampening of passionate feelings.

It is important to know a sex partner because many people contract STDs because they were "tricked" into having sex before the bad news came out. For example, a person who is aware of having herpes may be less moved by a desire to be honest than by an urge to have sex. He assumes that if he informs his date, she will lose interest in him, so when she raises the subject of safe sex, he denies having sexually transmitted diseases. When she discovers that she has a herpes infection a week later, the horrible realization hits that she has had sex with a liar and an STD-infected individual—obviously, a very poor prospect for a long-term

partner. This begs the question many people ask: since so many people will not be truthful, why bother having a sex-history talk at all?

One reason is that this provides an opening for someone to insist on having safe sex exclusively—a time to make it clear that either a condom be used or there will be no sexual activity. The following are some ways that sexually active people can talk to new partners about safe sex:

- Get yourself ready for the "big talk" by practicing some lines. You can easily anticipate responses you will hear from your partner.

- Reassure yourself that you should not feel weird if you feel uncomfortable talking about sex. Few people talk freely about this during childhood—usually, sex is an underground, snickered-about topic.

- Get real. Forget the idea that sex needs to be glitzy and glamorous. Although sex is used to sell beauty products, CDs, and clothing, it does not follow that you do not need to take a practical approach to it when you need to.

- Remember that it is smart to be realistic, to face the fact that in the real world, sex is not risk-free. The version used by the media to sell products is not realistic or practical.

- Seek knowledge. If you are a teen, look for sources that have better information than most people your age actually have. Typically, seeking knowledge from a peer does not yield what you need to know. In fact, a person may be misinformed and inadvertently pass on incorrect information.

- Be aware that you can pick up incorrect information on sex in books and magazines, on television, or on the Internet. Look at the credentials of the person dispensing tips; if he or she is not a medical professional such as a physician or nurse practitioner, look elsewhere.

- Ask for information from your health care provider. Be direct and make sure you get your questions answered.

- If your partner complains to you that talking about STDs is "unsexy," your response can be, "Sexually transmitted diseases are not sexy, either."

Here are guidelines for parents:

- A parent should start talking to a child about sex during the early years (age nine or 10). Talking about it will not be so difficult in preadolescence.

- Make sure your child is well informed; information tends to make young people postpone the initiation of sexual activity. (It is a myth that such discussions lead to earlier participation in sex.) Young people who have taken sex education classes are less likely to engage in sex while they are very young, or if they do, they are more likely to use condoms. The heightened awareness does, indeed, make a difference.

- Never assume that because your teen is very smart, he or she will make smart choices about sex. Sex is an emotionally charged area that makes it hard for most adults, much less people who are young and inexperienced, to make good decisions. You can help to protect your teen by providing good information that will help in making smart decisions.

tattoos Indelible designs or figures on the skin made by a tattoo artist by inserting pigment under the skin with a needle. In the realm of sexually transmitted diseases, the reuse of equipment in a tattoo parlor is a potential means of transmitting a disease if equipment is not sterilized between clients. Tattoos can usually be removed through a series of expensive laser treatments done by a medical professional, such as a plastic surgeon or a dermatologist, but removal will not affect the presence of an STD.

T cell A blood cell—the CD4+ T cell (helper cell)—which is key to the normal function of the human immune system—is destroyed by HIV. Loss of these cells in an HIV-infected person is a powerful predictor of the course of the disease and development of AIDS.

testicular torsion The spermatic cords and blood vessels to the testicle are twisted and must be surgically repaired as soon as possible to prevent loss of the testicle. Sudden severe pain and swelling on one side of the scrotum are the two main symptoms of torsion of the testicle—a medical condition that occurs suddenly and is most common in adolescents. If a young man experiences these symptoms, he should be rushed to the emergency room.

tests Various types of lab tests are used to confirm the presence of sexually transmitted diseases in an individual. In some instances, two tests are necessary to confirm the diagnosis of a particular STD.

Thailand HIV vaccine trial The three-year collaborative study—the AIDSVAX Phase III trial—was led by the Bangkok Metropolitan Administration, along with VaxGen, the Mahidol University Faculty of Tropical Medicine in Bangkok, and the HIV/AIDS Collaboration, which is a longstanding research association of the Thai Ministry of Public Health and the Centers for Disease Control and Prevention. The basis for such a trial was that the development of an effective HIV vaccine is a worldwide public health priority. As a result of the escalating toll of HIV in Thailand, Thai government and health officials developed the Thai National Plan for HIV Vaccine Research, the goal of which is to find an effective vaccine to stem the tide of their country's HIV epidemic. VaxGen, Inc., is a biomedical research firm in San Francisco, California, that developed the vaccine to be evaluated, AIDSVAX, and funds most aspects of the study.

Phase I and II trials showed this vaccine to be safe for use and indicated that it could induce antibodies against HIV, but it remained a question whether the level and type of antibodies can effectively prevent HIV infection. This trial was designed to answer that question. The phase III trial—large-scale human testing—was to be the last step in the process before a vaccine could be reviewed for licensing, and now it has been determined that that phase will not go forward in Thailand.

Trial participants were uninfected injection drug users attending 17 drug treatment clinics in Bangkok. Half of 2,500 volunteers received the AIDSVAX vaccine, and the other half had placebo injections with no vaccine; this was a randomized, double-blind, placebo-controlled trial.

Researchers and participants were not informed as to which participants received placebo and which vaccine. Volunteers received counseling on protection against HIV infection so that no one would abandon safe behavior, as well as briefing on important information (the fact that no one knows whether the vaccine will be effective). Of course, researchers knew that some people would take risks, regardless of admonitions to the contrary.

In the United States, two of three participants in the U.S. AIDSVAX trial received the vaccine, and the third, a placebo. This greater proportion reflects the wider genetic diversity of HIV strains in the United States than in Thailand.

The U.S. study, begun in 1998 and completed in June 2001, had 5,009 volunteers at high risk of sexual HIV infection. In February 2003, the public was disappointed by the news that VaxGen's Phase III trial gave only 3.8 percent protection from HIV infection.

NIAID and the HVTN will continue studies on the ALVAC-HIV vaccine. HVTN 026 is evaluating that vaccine's safety and immunogenicity, as well as a gp120 MN vaccine, in populations outside the United States. A trial evaluating high doses of ALVAC-HIV began in 2002, and a trial of that vaccine and a lipopeptide (HVTN 042) is pending. The results from HVTN 203 and other studies, as well as discussion with involved parties at various sites, will help steer decisions about future development and testing of canarypox HIV vaccine candidates.

therapeutic options Methods of treatment and healing (therapy) available to cure or lessen the effects of a disease.

ThinPrep Pap smear The ThinPrep is believed to be an improvement on the standard Pap smear, which is used to screen for abnormal changes that point to cervical cancer. In the past, when a doctor collected a cervical sample for testing, most of the sample was discarded because only a small portion was retained for the smear on the slide that was to be examined for abnormal cells. Another disadvantage of the old Pap smear is that other elements collected (blood, mucus, inflammation) are included in the smear and can obstruct the view. In contrast, the newer technique—ThinPrep Pap test—results in a homogenous sampling, increasing diagnostic accuracy.

thrush Oral yeast infection (oral candidiasis) caused by various *Candida* species, especially *Candida albicans*. Thrush resembles creamy white curdlike patches on the tongue and inside the mouth, and it is typically painful. These white patches can be rubbed off. Some conditions may allow overgrowth of *Candida* species by upsetting the balance of microbes. Conditions that commonly cause thrush include antibiotic or inhaled steroid use (for asthma) and immunosuppressed states (in HIV patients and people having chemotherapy). Yeast infections can also occur in other locations, such as on the skin and in the vagina. Yeast infections usually are self-healing, but if a person has a weak immune system, more serious infections can occur; the same situation can occur in newborns. Infants often contract candidal infections during birth from their mothers. Doctors treat oral thrush with antifungal medications such as fluconazole, itraconazole, and nystatin.

timing of transmission In sexually transmitted diseases, it is difficult to pinpoint the exact date of transmission. Therefore, determining which sexual partner was the disease carrier often is hard. For this reason, a person who discovers that he or she has an STD should advise all sexual partners of the previous six months (or even longer) to be tested, evaluated, and treated, if necessary.

tooth deformities An abnormal appearance of the bony appendages in the mouth. Deformities of the teeth can result from congenital syphilis in its late stage if this disease is untreated. These characteristic deformities of the teeth are called Hutchinson's teeth and mulberry molars.

topical microbicide Germ killer that is applied directly to the affected area. In view of the fact that many sexually active people do not use condoms consistently or correctly, many drug companies have worked to make available a new class of products that can serve as viable options. Some of these are now being tested.

Topical microbicides are intended to provide some form of protection for sexually active people who do not use condoms because they do not like them. Many health care professionals believe that a vaginal microbicide that women can use is needed worldwide and should be a research priority.

toxoplasmosis Found throughout the world, a disease that stems from the protozoan *Toxoplasma gondii,* which is usually transmitted to human beings by means of undercooked meat, other contaminated foods, contaminated soil, or handling of cat litter. In most cases, a person with toxoplasmosis has mild to severely enlarged lymph nodes as the usual symptom. Sometimes the disease causes flulike symptoms: muscle aches, pain, and fever.

An immunosuppressed individual (such as someone with HIV/AIDS or a person who has been undergoing chemotherapy) or an infant may have a severe case of toxoplasmosis, and the result may be brain or eye damage. Sometimes during pregnancy a woman transmits toxoplasmosis to her infant; as a result, the newborn may be blind or mentally retarded. Although the CDC estimates that more than 60 million Americans have the *Toxoplasma* species parasite, few of these people have symptoms because the immune system keeps the parasite in check.

Often a person is infected by inadvertently swallowing *Toxoplasma* cysts from soil or other surfaces that are contaminated. For example, a person who has been gardening may inadvertently touch the mouth afterward; someone who cleans a cat's litter box may accidentally have contact with cat feces. Another route is putting hands to mouth after touching raw or partly cooked meat (pork, lamb, venison) or eating such meat. In rare instances, toxoplasmosis is contracted as a result of a transfusion or organ transplantation.

To diagnose toxoplasmosis, a doctor does a blood test. Those considered at risk are babies born to mothers who are first exposed to *Toxoplasma* infection during pregnancy or within a few months before getting pregnant and persons with weakened immune systems.

Prevention guidelines for those who are pregnant or have a severely weakened immune system are as follows:

- Have a blood test for *Toxoplasma* species if you already have a weakened immune system. If you test positive, your doctor will prescribe medication if that is necessary to prevent the infection from reactivating. If you test negative, then it is wise to take precautions to prevent infection.

- A woman who plans to get pregnant may want to be tested for *Toxoplasma* species. If she tests positive, she most likely does not need to worry about passing the infection to her infant because the positive test result means she has already been exposed. Unless a woman is exposed to *Toxoplasma* during pregnancy or shortly before, there is little risk of transmission to her infant. If she tests negative, she can take precautions to prevent infection.

- A pregnant woman should discuss her risks for this disease with her doctor, who may want to do a blood test.

- Wear gloves when you are involved in outdoor activities that put you in contact with soil. After going inside, wash your hands with soap and warm water.

- Do not handle raw meat unless you wear clean latex gloves. Carefully wash kitchen utensils and cutting boards that raw meat has touched.

- Cook meat until it is no longer pink in the middle or until juices are clear.

- Prevent your cat from contracting *Toxoplasma* parasites by keeping it indoors; do not feed your cat raw or undercooked meat.

- Avoid handling stray cats.

- Do not change a litter box if a healthy or nonpregnant person can do this for you. Otherwise, wear gloves and clean the litter box every day because the cat feces parasite is only infectious to you a few days after it is passed. Wash your hands carefully after cleaning the box.

(Note: cats who have *Toxoplasma* parasites can spread them via feces only for a few weeks after being infected. Unfortunately, you will not know whether your cat is passing this parasite, and your cat can be reinfected.)

Treatment for toxoplasmosis may or may not be necessary. Typically, if a person is healthy and is not pregnant, there is no need for treatment because toxoplasmosis is a self-correcting condition. Medication is used for pregnant women and for those with weakened immune systems.

transfusion-associated HIV   In the early days of the AIDS epidemic, in a number of cases people contracted HIV by receiving a tainted blood transfusion. This problem led to improved screening of blood and blood products, and today the likelihood of contracting HIV/AIDS from blood transfusion is extremely low, although not 100 percent impossible.

Trichomonas vaginalis   The flagellated protozoan that causes trichomoniasis.

trichomoniasis   Commonly called "trich," a sexually transmitted disease that produces an estimated 5 million new cases in the United States every year, according to a 2000 report from the Centers for Disease Control and Prevention. Mainly an infection of the urogenital tract, it usually occurs in certain sites—the urethra in men and vagina in women. It is pronounced "trick-oh-moe-nye-uh-sis." This disease is also called trichomonas ("trick-oh-moe-nass").

Cause

Trichomoniasis is caused by the single-celled protozoan parasite *Trichomonas vaginalis*. It is spread through penis-to-vagina intercourse or vulva-to-vulva contact with an infected partner. A female can contract this disease from an infected man or woman, but men usually contract it from infected women only. Women are more likely to have symptoms than are men, but both the woman and her sexual partners must be treated.

Symptoms

It is not unusual for a person with trichomoniasis to have no symptoms. When women do have symptoms, these may include burning, itching, frothy and smelly vaginal discharge (gray or yel-

low-green), vaginal or vulvar redness, painful or frequent urination, lower abdominal pain, and discomfort during intercourse. The problems appear within five to 28 days of exposure. Typically, if a woman is going to have symptoms, she has them within six months of being infected. Sometimes the symptoms are worse after menstruation.

Men, on the other hand, rarely have symptoms. If they do, these may include painful urination, a penile discharge that is white and thin, and tingling inside the penis.

Testing

To test for trichomoniasis, a health care provider does a physical examination and a lab test. A pelvic exam of a woman may reveal the characteristic small red ulcerations of the vaginal wall or cervix.

For diagnosis of trichomoniasis, a doctor collects a secretion sample from the patient's penis or vagina. This is either sent to a lab or examined under a microscope in the doctor's office to check for the presence of *Trichomonas* species. In men, the parasite is often hard to detect.

Treatment

Both sex partners need to be treated even when there are no symptoms (men can transmit the disease to sex partners). A person with trichomoniasis is treated with antibiotics—usually a single dose of metronidazole (Flagyl) given by mouth. The individual taking this drug should not drink alcoholic beverages (which may cause nausea and vomiting). In a few weeks, symptoms in infected men may disappear without treatment, but this is deceptive because a man with trichomoniasis can still infect female partners until he has been treated and cured. Therefore, it is important for both partners to be treated at the same time to eliminate the parasite, and a couple should not have sex until treatment has ended and both are symptom-free.

If a person is treated but remains infected, the doctor usually prescribes the same drug at a higher dose and for a longer period—or more than one drug may be needed. To prevent reinfection during treatment, one should avoid sexual intercourse entirely.

Complications

Trichomoniasis has been associated with an increased risk of transmission of HIV and low-birth-weight babies. The reason is that the genital inflammation of trichomoniasis may invite HIV infection if a woman is exposed to it. If a woman is HIV-positive and has trichomoniasis, too, she is more likely to transmit HIV to a sex partner.

A pregnant woman with trichomoniasis may experience premature rupture of the membranes, resulting in preterm delivery. In rare cases, a woman can give her baby trichomoniasis during delivery. If diagnosed, a child should be treated. A pregnant woman who does have trichomoniasis should consult her doctor about this problem.

When a baby or child does have trichomoniasis, it is possible that the mother spread infection during childbirth; it may point to sexual abuse if the disease is in a young child; and in a teen, it may indicate sexual abuse or sexual activity. If sexual abuse or activity is suspected, there is a need for evaluation for other sexually transmitted diseases as well. Treatment is necessary for any infant, child, or teen who has trichomoniasis.

Prevention

Trichomoniasis is spread to partners through sexual contact. Thus, use of a latex condom during every sex act provides some protection. Also, it is possible that trichomoniasis may be transmitted by infected sheets and towels, so it is a good idea not to share these items with someone who is infected. It is important for male partners to be treated even though they almost always have no symptoms.

Sexually active individuals need to know that condoms do not provide complete protection against all sexually transmitted disease; that is because sores, lesions, and infective organisms may occur in places that a condom does not cover, and thus the partner can be exposed to the infection.

Another caveat for prevention is to limit the number of sex partners and avoid alternating partners. The best course of action is sexual abstinence or sexual activity limited to one uninfected partner.

A person who believes infection may have occurred should avoid sexual contact and see a doctor for treatment. Genital symptoms such as an unusual discharge, genital itching, or burning during urination should be red flags that something is wrong.

A person who discovers that he or she has trichomoniasis (or any other sexually transmitted disease) has a responsibility to notify recent sex partners.

Also, someone who has had trichomoniasis should be aware that she or he can still be infected again. No immunity exists.

Trinidad HIV-1   A distinctive clade B HIV type 1 seen in heterosexually transmitted HIV in Trinidad and Tobago spotlighted in a study. Worldwide, the transmission of HIV-1 is mainly associated with heterosexual activity; non–clade B viruses are culpable in most cases. Researchers have found that the HIV epidemic in the Caribbean and specifically in Trinidad and Tobago has features of such heterosexual epidemics, including a prominent role for accompanying sexually transmitted diseases.

The study, documented in the *Proceedings of the National Academy of Science USA* (vol. 97, issue 19, September 12, 2000), examined the molecular epidemiologic characteristics of HIV-1 in Trinidad and Tobago when an abrupt transition from homosexual to heterosexual transmission (in the absence of IV drug use) was observed; that change was concomitant with a rapid rise in HIV-1 prevalence in the population's heterosexuals. Researchers noted that the Trinidad V3 consensus sequence "differs by a single amino acid from the prototype B V3 consensus" and was stable over the study's decade. The results show that canonical clade B HIV-1 can generate a typical heterosexual epidemic.

tubal ligation   An operation, also referred to as having the "tubes tied," that is performed on a woman's fallopian tubes to make her unable to conceive. After a tubal ligation, she should not be able to get pregnant. This means of contraception is considered permanent, but in very rare cases there are failures and a woman does get pregnant.

tubal pregnancy   Also known as an ectopic pregnancy, a pregnancy implanted accidentally in the fallopian tubes rather than in the uterus. Some sexually transmitted diseases enhance the likelihood of a woman having a tubal pregnancy.

tuberculosis Tuberculosis (TB) is caused by the bacterium *Mycobacterium tuberculosis,* which usually attacks the lungs but can attack any body part. Although TB was once a leading cause of death in the United States, scientists in the 1940s discovered the first of several drugs that could treat tuberculosis successfully. TB began to disappear in the United States. However, in the year 2000, more than 16,000 cases were reported.

The mode of spread is through the air, one person to another. When a person with TB of the lungs or throat coughs or sneezes, someone who is near that individual may breathe in the bacteria from the air and become infected. The bacteria usually settle in the lungs and grow there. From that spot, the blood can transport the bacteria to the kidney, spine, or brain.

A person with TB in the lungs or throat can be infectious. Most vulnerable to being infected by this person are those with whom he or she lives and works.

People with latent TB do not have symptoms or feel sick, and they cannot spread TB. They usually have a positive skin-test reaction, and they may have TB disease at some point. Ideally they can take medicine to prevent development of the disease. People with TB disease can be cured by treatment.

Symptoms of TB in the lungs are a bad cough (lasting two weeks or more), pain in the chest, and coughing up of blood or sputum (phlegm from deep in the lungs). Other symptoms of TB include fatigue, weight loss, lack of appetite, fever, chills, and night sweats.

A TB skin test can detect latent TB. This is a desirable course of action for those who have spent time with a person who has TB, who have HIV or another condition that puts them at high risk, who suspect they have TB, who inject drugs, who are from a country where TB is common (Latin America, the Caribbean, Africa, Asia, Eastern Europe, and Russia), or who live in a place where TB is common (homeless shelters, prisons, jails, and some senior-care facilities).

The skin test involves injection of a small amount of testing fluid—tuberculin—under the skin on the arm. In two to three days, a health care worker examines the spot for the skin's reaction. Often there is a small bump, which health care workers measure to see whether the reaction is negative or positive. When someone has a positive result, a doctor usually orders a chest X ray and possibly a test of phlegm. If it is determined that TB is present, the diseased individual requires medicine to cure TB. If a TB exposure was recent, it may be necessary to have a second skin test 12 weeks after exposure.

Bacille Calmette-Guérin (BCG) vaccine is a TB vaccine that is often given to infants and children in countries where TB is common, but in the United States, this vaccine is not widely used. However, the vaccine does not always protect people from tuberculosis.

A person who has been vaccinated with BCG may have a positive TB skin test result. This may indicate latent TB in an individual who has recently spent time with someone with TB, who is from a region where TB is common, or who spends time in a place where TB is common (homeless shelters, drug-treatment centers, health care clinics, jails).

People who have a weak immune system and are especially vulnerable to TB include babies, young children, people with HIV/AIDS, and those who have other problems—substance abuse, diabetes mellitus, silicosis, head or neck cancer, leukemia, Hodgkin's disease, severe kidney disease, low body weight—and those who are having medical treatments and procedures such as organ transplantation and corticosteroid therapy.

Those at high risk for TB disease are individuals with HIV, those who became infected with TB within the past two years, babies and young children, IV drug users, people who have a disease that weakens the immune system, elderly adults, and people who were incorrectly treated for TB in the past.

The medicine often used to treat latent TB infection is isoniazid, or INH. If this medicine is taken as prescribed, TB disease never develops. Typically the medication must be taken for six to nine months. A person who is taking INH should contact a doctor if any side effect occurs: lack of appetite, nausea, vomiting, yellowish eyes or skin, fever for three or more days, abdominal pain, or tingling in fingers and toes. Note: alcoholic beverages should not be consumed while one is taking INH.

Usually several different drugs are required to cure TB disease because of the prevalence of drug-resistant tuberculosis. Drugs used to fight TB include isoniazid (INH), rifampin, pyrazinamide, ethambutol, and streptomycin.

A person with TB in the lung or throat is probably infectious. Thus, it is important to stay home from work or school to prevent spreading TB and return to work or school only when a doctor says it is safe.

ulcer An open, craterlike lesion. This can be present in any one of a number of sexually transmitted diseases such as herpes and chancroid.

unawareness In respect to sexually transmitted diseases, the act of participating in sexual activity while failing to acknowledge risks that are inherent in being a sexually active individual today. That means not following safe-sex measures or abstinence to prevent contracting STDs.

universal precautions Precautions that are taken in order to prevent transmission of HIV and other blood-borne pathogens. Blood and body-fluid precautions are supposed to be used for all patients, especially those in emergency-care settings in which the risk of blood exposure is high and infection status is usually unknown. These precautions are also the standard for care in shelters, child care facilities, and so on, where volunteers and workers may come in contact with blood and/or body fluids of those who are known or suspected to have HIV.

The following are the universal precautions guidelines:

- Routinely use barrier precautions to prevent skin and mucous membrane exposure when contact with blood or other body fluids of a patient is anticipated. Gloves should be worn for touching blood and body fluids, mucous membranes, non-intact skin, handling of items or surfaces soiled with blood or body fluids (such as diapers or bandages), and procedures such as venipuncture. New gloves should be used for each patient. If a treatment or procedure is likely to generate droplets of blood or body fluids, workers should wear masks and protective eyewear or face shields to prevent exposure of mucous membranes of the mouth, the nose, and the eyes. If procedures may generate splashes of blood or body fluids, aprons or gowns should also be worn for protection.

- Wash hands and other skin immediately and thoroughly if contaminated with blood or other body fluids. After gloves are removed, wash hands immediately and thoroughly.

- Try to prevent injuries when cleaning scalpels and other instruments and devices, when cleaning used instruments, during needle disposal, and when handling sharp instruments. To prevent needlestick injuries, you should take care that needles are not recapped, purposely bent or broken by hand, removed from disposable syringes, or otherwise manipulated by hand. After use, disposable syringes and needles, scalpel blades, and so on should be put into puncture-resistant containers for disposal. Large-bore reusable needles must be put into a puncture-resistant container for transport to the reprocessing area.

- Make available ventilation devices, mouthpieces, resuscitation bags, and other devices in places where the need for resuscitation may arise to try to minimize the need for emergency mouth-to-mouth resuscitation.

- Workers who have weeping dermatitis or exudative lesions should not handle patient-care equipment or be involved in direct patient care until these health conditions are resolved.

- Using universal blood and body fluid precautions for all patients eliminates the need for use of the isolation category of "blood and body-fluid precautions" previously recommended by CDC for those patients known or suspected to be infected with blood-borne pathogens. Isolation precautions should be used as needed in cases in which associated conditions, such as infectious diarrhea and TB, are diagnosed or suspected. Certain precautions must be taken for any *invasive procedure*, which is defined as surgical entry into tissues, cavities, or organs or repair of major traumatic injuries in an operating or delivery room, emergency room, or outpatient setting, including physicians' and dentists' offices; cardiac catheterization and angiographic procedures; vaginal or cesarean delivery or other invasive obstetric procedure during which bleeding may occur; or cutting, manipulation, or removal of any oral or perioral tissues, including tooth structure, during which bleeding occurs or the potential for bleeding exists. The universal blood and body fluid precautions listed, combined with the precautions listed in the following, should be the minimal precautions for all such invasive procedures.

- Health care workers who participate in invasive procedures must use appropriate barrier precautions to prevent skin and mucous-membrane contact with blood and other body fluids of patients. Gloves and surgical masks must be worn during invasive procedures. Gown, or aprons of materials that provide an effective barrier should be worn, as well as protective eyewear or face shields, for procedures that may generate droplets or splashing of body fluids or blood or bone chips. Health care workers performing or assisting in vaginal or cesarean deliveries should wear gloves and gowns when handling the placenta or the infant until blood and amniotic fluid have been removed from the infant's skin and should wear gloves during postdelivery care of the umbilical cord.

- If a glove is torn or a needlestick or other injury occurs, the glove should be removed and a new glove used as quickly as patient safety permits; the needle or instrument involved in the incident should be removed from the sterile field. There are similar sets of precautions for dentistry offices, for autopsies and morticians' services, for

dialysis centers, and for laboratories, as well as extensive rules for sterilization and disinfection for housekeeping and laundry services in health care facilities.

Employers of health care workers should make sure that employees have universal precautions orientation and training and are familiar with modes of HIV transmission and prevention of HIV and other blood-borne infections, and that they understand the need for routine use of universal precautions for all patients. Employers should provide necessary equipment and supplies to minimize risk of infection by HIV and other blood-borne pathogens and should monitor employees for adherence to protective measures.

urethritis Inflammation of the urethra, which is caused by an infection that is characterized by discharge of clear to purulent material—and by burning during urination. It is not unusual to have an infection that is without symptoms. The bacterial pathogens of clinical importance in men who have urethritis are *Neisseria gonorrhoeae* and *Chlamydia trachomatis*. Doctors test to diagnose the diseases because in addition to the need for treatment both of these infections are reportable to state health departments. In addition, a diagnosis may improve patient compliance with therapy and notification of partners.

Diagnostic tools are Gram stain, culture, and urine testing. New nucleic acid amplification tests provide detection of either pathogen on first-void urine.

Nongonococcal urethritis (NGU) is more common than is gonoccal urethritis. The most common causes of NGU are *Chlamydia trachomatis* and *Ureaplasma urealyticum*. All who have urethritis should be tested for gonococcal and chlamydia infection.

Patients are treated for nongonoccal urethritis with azithromycin or doxycycline, or as an alternate regimen, erythromycin base, or ofloxacin. Gonococcal urethritis is treated with ceftriaxone, cefixime, or ofloxacin plus azithromycin or doxycycline.

It is important for someone with urethritis to return to the doctor if symptoms persist. One should not have intercourse until seven days after the start of drug therapy. Sex partners in the preceding 60 days should be evaluated and treated if necessary.

urine testing   Various lab tests that are performed on urine to detect disease, infection, or drug use. Urinalysis is a urine test that can detect infection and other problems.

vaccine for HIV No proven preventive vaccine for HIV exists today, and some experts predict that one will not be available in the United States until about 2009. The first vaccine could be found through trials in countries where transmission rates are high and expensive medications are nothing but remote avenues of help, because people in these places would embrace a preventive that was even 50 percent successful.

The vaccine puzzle's answer is elusive because there is insufficient knowledge as to how the immune system controls the virus. Nevertheless, researchers remain optimistic and undaunted, and the goal of the Dale and Betty Bumpers Vaccine Center in the National Institutes of Health complex is an AIDS vaccine by the year 2007, as reported in *Patient Care* (October 1999).

In a study funded by the National Institute of Allergy and Infectious Diseases that was reported in *Nature* magazine (May 2001), researchers described an experimental vaccine that combines genes from HIV and simian immunodeficiency virus (SIV), a virus found in monkeys that is similar to HIV, followed by a booster shot with a pox virus carrying the same genes; it appears to protect monkeys from infection with a combination immunodeficiency virus. The monkeys that were administered the vaccine still became infected with the virus combo of HIV and SIV, but the vaccine did help contain the virus for up to 62 weeks. Dr. Harriet L. Robinson of the Yerkes Regional Primate Research center in Atlanta, Georgia, contended that the experimental treatment holds "very high promise for a preventive vaccine. The protocols all combined DNA priming (of the immune system) with either protein or recombinant pox virus boosting and differed in their ability to raise neutralizing antibody and cell-mediated immune responses. We got our best and most long-lasting protection in the group that received intradermal DNA prime followed by recombinant pox virus boost." She expected to try to develop the vaccinations that led to the most favorable protection, and her group hoped to take the protocol into human trials in about a year. There are other trials with the simian version of HIV—at Harvard and one by Merck, both of which are considered important on the road to finding an AIDS vaccine.

In a report from the Office of AIDS Research, National Institutes of Health, for fiscal year 2003, a "plan for HIV-related research," it was announced that progress in vaccine research in animal models has provided "strong motivation to further explore and develop vaccine concepts, and to move additional candidate vaccines into clinical testing." Also, as a result of increased funding from NIH for development of HIV vaccines, many new approaches are being pursued, from basic research in vaccine design and studies of immune responses in small animals through actual product development.

The report notes that even though vaccines tested in animals have not prevented virus infection, researchers think that an equally important vaccine outcome is the ability to control HIV viral load early in the course of infection. They cite two reasons: cohort studies that have dealt with large numbers of infected people show that controlling viral load links with good prognosis and delayed progression to AIDS. Also, some studies have shown that uninfected partners of HIV-positive people are infected less often when there is a reduced HIV level in the blood. Further, transmission to infants of HIV-infected mothers is less likely when the viral load in the mother is low. This means that a vaccine that could control HIV viral load would have a huge impact on the AIDS epidemic.

Some of the newest vaccine efforts target dendritic cells. The alphavirus family—Sindbis virus, Venezuelan equine encephalitis virus, and Semliki Forest virus—may have an inborn propensity to move to antigen-presenting cells, macrophages, or dendritic cells, and this is important because a vaccine that uses the outer coat of the alphavirus to carry copies of HIV protein genes has been demonstrated to induce "immune responses and . . . reduced virus load in macaques (monkeys) challenged with pathogenic virus." Doubt has been cast on attenuated vaccines because of evidence of CD4 loss in the few people who had received attenuated forms of HIV, as well as observations of late disease progression in nonhuman primates that received attenuated virus with nef gene alterations, which indicated that many progressed to disease years after infection.

The upshot is that many new vaccine approaches are being investigated that are bolstered by new scientific findings on the immune response to HIV and new insights related to the structure and function relationship of the HIV virion itself. With this in mind, the following priority list for AIDS-related research was established and presented in the report from the Office of AIDS Research, focusing on goals for the year 2003:

- A top priority for testing candidate vaccines is resolving the crisis in monkey supply for studies. Most HIV/AIDS vaccine investigators have not had a sufficient number of rhesus macaques to test vaccines properly and do comparative analysis of vaccines. NIH is expected to develop creative ways to work with suppliers to beef up the breeding capacity of these animals.
- Another obstacle to be passed is the need for appropriate facilities for vaccinated animals after they are tested with HIV.
- A research priority is support of efforts to design and test vaccines that can induce antibody responses to the HIV envelope that can neutralize a large array of HIV isolates. Also, resources must be set up to speed any promising vaccine through studies to testing in human volunteers.

- NIH should support a coordinated program of quality control and assurance for testing in macaque and human studies for assays being developed and evaluated.
- NIH should develop a way to ensure licensure of HIV vaccines for adolescents, including linking adolescent cohorts to networks that anticipate quick trials.

The priority list also continues to advocate priorities that were identified in the Vaccines Plan for Fiscal Year 2002.

vaginal discharge   A discharge from the vagina. In a number of sexually transmitted diseases, the first sign a woman is an unusual vaginal discharge of some kind. (See descriptions of specific STDs and Appendix VI.) A woman who detects a discharge should see her doctor for evaluation and treatment of this condition.

vaginal intercourse   Sexual activity in which the erect male penis is inserted into the woman's vagina.

VDRL test   The Venereal Disease Research Laboratory (VDRL) test is often used to detect evidence of syphilis. Sometimes, false-positive findings occur in those who have viral infections, autoimmune disorders, and other health conditions, so for this reason, a second test such as the fluorescent treponemal antibody-absorption test is usually needed to confirm diagnosis. The other commonly used initial test is the rapid plasma reagin (RPR) test.

venereal disease   Decades ago, the common name for what are now referred to as sexually transmitted diseases (STDs). Multiple infectious diseases are transmitted mainly by sexual activity, including genital herpes, genital warts, gonorrhea, HIV, syphilis, and chlamydia. STDs can cause problems that range from rashes to infertility to death.

vertical transmission   The transmission of an infectious disease such as HIV from an infected pregnant woman to her infant.

vesicle A vesicle is a small skin blister that contains a clear fluid. In the diseases shingles and herpes, people often have vesicles.

viral culture An available testing method that is considered the gold standard of herpes testing. It starts when a doctor obtains a sample from a lesion with a sterile swab; the sample then goes to a lab, where the virus is grown for several days in a culture of healthy cells. If the swabbed sample does indeed contain herpes, this virus infects the cells of the culture, and the changes in cells can be detected via microscope.

viral load In regard to HIV the viral RNA copy number in the blood of an infected person. A key factor in treating HIV is the determination of the viral load of human immunodeficiency virus type 1 (HIV-1). When an individual is tested, the results of viral load determinations are used by doctors to make decisions regarding the initiation of antiretroviral therapy and to determine whether current antiretroviral therapy is working well or whether changes are required by the amount of virus in the blood. A reverse-transcriptase polymerase chain reaction procedure determines viral load.

viral shedding An infected person can shed the herpesvirus through the skin even when he is not having symptoms. Therefore, the sexual partner(s) are at risk of contracting herpes at these times even though there are no lesions present.

viral STDs Sexually transmitted diseases caused by viruses include hepatitis B, human papillomavirus (HPV), herpes simplex, molluscum contagiosum, and human immunodeficiency virus (HIV).

virus A microscopic agent that is capable of causing infection but can only grow and multiply in living cells. Viruses may have either RNA or DNA as their genetic material. Herpes simplex virus and human papillomavirus are examples of viruses.

visualization Also called imagery, a technique sometimes used in therapy or individually with the goal of creating a state of relaxation. In the case of a person battling HIV, visualization can be used to maximize the mind–body connection, in order to mount a defensive against disease despite an ailing immune system. The desired goal or change can be "imagined," thus giving some people a feeling of empowerment, which can make visualization a potentially helpful healing technique.

vitamins Substances that a human being needs for healthy growth, development, and metabolic processes. The body can synthesize vitamins D and K, which are also obtained from food, as are other vitamins. A deficiency of a specific vitamin can cause specific health problems. Vitamins may be water-soluble or fat-soluble.

voluntary HIV testing A term usually used to refer in particular to voluntary HIV testing of pregnant women who fear that they have been exposed and want to protect their fetus if, indeed, they are HIV-positive.

The goals of the CDC's perinatal HIV prevention program are to ensure that pregnant women and their health care providers discuss the importance of HIV testing during pregnancy; to make voluntary HIV testing available to pregnant women (especially high-risk ones) when and where they access medical care; to ensure that pregnant women who have HIV, or are at high risk for infection, get prenatal care; and to ensure that HIV-positive women can access prevention interventions to reduce vertical transmission and to ensure that these women can be treated.

vulvovaginal candidiasis See CANDIDIASIS.

warts in the mouth   A projection on the mucous membranes of the mouth that is caused by a virus. The strains of human papillomavirus that cause genital warts usually tend to stay in the genital region but are occasionally transmitted to the mouth by means of oral sex. In people with HIV, these are more difficult to get rid of because of the immune system's difficulty in fighting infection. A new remedy on the horizon that is being researched in some HIV dental clinics is a throat lozenge that contains interferon, which appears to cause reduction in warts in the mouth in some patients.

See also GENITAL WARTS.

wasting syndrome   A condition associated with AIDS in which many of those with AIDS lose protein from lean tissue mass. The syndrome often causes illness or death in those with late-stage AIDS infection. Wasting syndrome differs from malnutrition caused by a digestive disorder in that it stems from a metabolic change of AIDS that causes the body to break down protein to meet its energy needs (rather than using its fat stores first).

Low testosterone levels or excessive production of tumor necrosis factor may also contribute to wasting, but both conditions are treatable. Various treatments are used for wasting syndrome, including appetite stimulants (Megace and Marinol), anabolic steroids, and testosterone.

The Food and Drug Administration Investigational New Drug program permits treatment with human growth hormone of certain people who are suffering from AIDS-related wasting. The person must meet specific criteria to participate; one of several criteria is that the individual must have lost 10 percent of body weight in the absence of any clear-cut cause, such as an opportunistic infection (cryptosporidium or *mycobacterium avium* complex).

Western blot test   A test commonly used to determine whether a person has HIV-1 antibodies. Typically, this test can confirm (or refute) a positive ELISA test finding. The Western blot is more specific and can definitively indicate whether a person is actually HIV-positive. (Conditions such as lupus and syphilis sometimes cause a false-positive ELISA result.)

If someone has a positive Western blot result, that can be considered conclusive proof of HIV infection. A negative result within six months of the exposure to a person with HIV should not be considered the final word because of the interval that may pass between HIV infection and the appearance of anti-HIV antibodies. Thus, a person who has been exposed to HIV and is still showing negative results on ELISA and Western blot should be retested.

wet smear   An easy and reliable test of vaginal discharge used to screen for certain vaginal conditions, which can help in the diagnosis of bacterial vaginosis, trichomoniasis, and candidiasis. When a wet smear is done, the medical practitioner's ability, based on training and experience, is important. An advantage of the wet smear is that results can be obtained immediately, and the patient will know whether she has one of these conditions.

Also called a "wet prep," this test requires obtaining a sample of discharge from the vagina; this is placed in normal saline solution on a slide. Using a microscope, the lab technician or physician looks for white blood cells, trichomonads, candidal pseudohyphae, and clue cells. If the patient has bacterial vaginosis, for example, the slide will show scarce white blood cells, decreased lactobacilli, increased bacteria, and clue cells.

white blood cells The infection-fighting cells in the body's immune system.

World Health Organization (WHO) Established April 7, 1948, the World Health Organization is the United Nations' specialized health agency, which works to attain the highest possible level of health for all people. In the constitution of WHO, *health* is defined as "a state of complete physical, mental, and social well-being and not merely the absence of disease or infirmity." The governing body is the World Health Assembly, made up of representatives from WHO's 191 member states.

Among the many goals of WHO is the control and/or eradication of major diseases. Services include providing condoms, treatment, counseling, testing, sex education, and efforts to prevent vertical transmission. WHO also works to improve access to health services that are affordable and effective and stages comprehensive efforts to prevent infant, child, and maternal mortality. The WHO website estimates that the annual incidence of curable STDs, which excludes AIDS, is 333 million cases.

yeast infection   See CANDIDIASIS.

yeast infection in men   An infection caused by a yeast, most commonly *Candida albicans.* Although less talked about, yeast infections do occur in men. A woman's vulvovaginal candidiasis (yeast infection) can be transmitted to a man's genital area via sexual intercourse. Also, men can contract a fungal infection in the groin area called *tinea cruris* that is characterized by a red and itchy rash.

yogurt douche   A feminine hygiene practice that involves "cleansing" the vagina with a mixture of yogurt and water. Some women follow the old wives' tale that recommends the practice of vaginal douching with a yogurt mixture to relieve yeast infections. This does not help get rid of yeast infections; furthermore, douching of any kind is not recommended because it upsets the natural ecosystem of the vagina. Also, some people try the option of eating yogurt or taking acidophilus tablets to enhance the vagina's *Lactobacillus* species content, but this is not believed to work either.

Youth Risk Behavior Survey   Studies underscore that the most effective prevention programs are comprehensive ones that include a focus on delaying sexual activity and provide information on how sexually active young people can protect themselves. Trends that were revealed in the eight-year Youth Risk Behavior Survey showed a decline in sexual risk behaviors and increased use of condoms in young people who are sexually active in the United States. The percentage of sexually experienced high school students decreased from 54.1 percent in 1991 to 49.9 percent in 1999, and condom use increased from 46.2 percent to 58.0 percent. The findings point to a reversal in the 1970s upswing in sexual risk taken by teens and also show how successful prevention efforts have been in delaying the first instance of intercourse in teens and in increasing condom use in young people who are sexually active.

A report of teen sexual activity in 1997 indicated that about half of teens were having sex, and about half were not using protection when they had sex. These were the findings of the 1997 Youth Risk Behavior Surveillance, a study that looked at 16,262 U.S. high school students (grades nine through 12). The study showed that of adolescents, 49 percent of boys and 48 percent of girls had had sexual intercourse, but only 62.5 percent of boys and 50.8 percent of girls had used a condom at last intercourse. These figures had changed by the time of the 1999 survey.

The 1999 Youth Risk Behavior Surveillance showed that 50 percent had had sexual intercourse in their lifetime; 16 percent had had sexual intercourse with four or more partners; 36 percent had had sexual intercourse during the previous three months; 58 percent of students who were currently sexually active had used condoms for their last intercourse; and 16 percent of the currently sexually active used birth control before last intercourse. Black students (70 percent) were much more likely to use condoms than were Hispanics or whites (55.2 percent and 55 percent, respectively). Of the students surveyed nationwide, 90.6 percent reported that they had been taught about HIV/AIDS in school.

It is clear that a substantial morbidity rate and social problems result from the approximately 1 million pregnancies per year that occur in females 15 to 19 and the estimated 3 million cases of sexually transmitted diseases each year in those ages 10 to 19. Of the estimated 12 million cases of STDs other than HIV that are diagnosed every year in the United States, about two-thirds occur in people below the age of 25.

APPENDIXES

APPENDIX I
RESOURCES FOR INFORMATION ON SEXUALLY TRANSMITTED DISEASES

The Internet has hundreds of websites that deal with sexually transmitted diseases. The following are some that contain news, information, updates, and links on STDs such as HIV/AIDS, genital warts, syphilis, gonorrhea, and genital herpes. A listing of hotlines for information on sexually transmitted diseases follows.

STD INTERNET RESOURCES

Acquired Immunodeficiency Syndrome (AIDS) and Human Immunodeficiency Virus (HIV)
http://www.niddk.nih.gov/fund/program/
    A-Elist.htm#AIDS

This site by the National Institute of Diabetes & Digestive and Kidney Diseases describes research programs on various AIDS complications.

AIDS Animal Models
http://www.ncrr.nih.gov/compmed/cmaids.htm

The AIDS animal models website offers information on research using animal models to find better ways to treat HIV and AIDS. Researchers hope that breakthroughs will lead to the development of an effective HIV vaccine. According to this site by the National Center for Research Resources, chimpanzees and specific-pathogen-free macaque monkeys are used in AIDS investigations.

AIDS Clinical Trials Information Service (ACTIS)
(800) TRIALS-A
(800) 874-2572
http://actis.org

A service of the United States Department of Health and Human Services, this site provides current information on HIV/AIDS treatments and drugs, as well as federally and privately sponsored clinical trials for those with AIDS and HIV.

AIDS Education Global Information System
http://www.aegis.com

AIDS Education Global Information System is one of the best and largest sources of HIV/AIDS information on the Web. It features the "HIV Daily Briefing," with updates on new information of interest.

AIDS Healthcare Foundation
http://www.aidshealth.org

Features information from AIDS and HIV specialists on home health care centers and disease management, for those with HIV and AIDS.

AIDS Information
http://aidsinfonyc.org

This is a linked collection of informative pages for those who are living with HIV and AIDS. The material is from community-based groups in New York City. It features a newsletter, an HIV Treatment Registry Database, a data network, and more.

AIDS International Training and Research Program
http://www.nih.gov/fic/programs/aitrp/aitrp.html

This site features contacts and international locations for current HIV/AIDS programs and listings for programs that are recruiting.

AIDS Neurological Manifestations
http://www.ninds.nih.gov/health_and_medical/
    disorders/aids.htm

This is a fact sheet on the effects of AIDS on the brain and spinal cord.

AIDS Treatment News
http://aids.org/index.html

The home of AIDS Treatment News and Direct Access Alternative Information Resources (DAAIR), this site lists more than 3 million Web pages related to HIV/AIDS treatment.

AIDS Related Malignancies

http://cancernet.gov

Gives specifics on AIDS-related cancers, clinical trials, alternative medicine, and tips on coping. Free publications are offered.

AIDS Report, IAPAC

http://www.iapac.org

Daily reports on new drugs and treatments for HIV/AIDS from the International Association of Physicians in AIDS Care.

AIDS Research Programs

http://rover.nhlbi.nih.gov/resources/aids

The National Heart, Lung, and Blood Institute programs focus on heart, blood, and chest complications from AIDS, as well as the nation's blood supply and HIV-related lung disease.

AIDS Therapeutics Toxicity Studies Program

http://ntp-server.niehs.nih.gov/Main_Pages/AIDS/
    AIDSpage.html

This links to scientific reports on AIDS therapeutic evaluations conducted with rodent research models.

The American College of Obstetricians and Gynecologists

(202) 863-2518
http://www.acog.org

This site, sponsored by the American College of Obstetricians and Gynecologists features women's issues, news releases, and a search engine for the public.

American Foundation for AIDS Research (amFAR)

(212) 806-1600
(800) 38-amFAR
(800) 382-6327
http://www.amfar.org

This site covers activities and information disseminated by the American Foundation for AIDS Research, commonly referred to as amFAR.

The Body

http://www.thebody.com

Features are "Ask the Experts," HIV/AIDS information organized in more than 550 topic areas, and CDC news updates.

CDC Morbidity and Mortality Weekly Report

http://www.cdc.gov

Click on MMWR for the *CDC Morbidity and Mortality Weekly Report,* where you can find data on specific diseases as reported by state and territorial health agencies/departments and reports on the diseases.

CDC-National Center for HIV, STD and TB Prevention-Divisions of HIV/AIDS Prevention Home Page

http://www.cdc.gov/nih_aids/dhap.htm

This page presents the Centers for Disease Control and Prevention's HIV mission—prevention and reduction of the incidence of this disease.

CDC National Prevention Information Network

(800) 458-5231
http://www.cdcnpin.org/hiv/start.htm

This website (CDC National Prevention Information Network-HIV/AIDS Resources) is the former National AIDS Clearinghouse.

Center on AIDS and Other Medical Consequences of Drug Abuse

http://www.nida.nih.gov/OOA/OOAHome.html

The site provides information on drug abuse and HIV/AIDS, and related epidemics, with statistics and links.

Center for Mental Health Research on AIDS

http://www.nimh.nih.gov/oa

This site describes the center's research on the physiologic and neurobehavioral effects of HIV/AIDS transmission and infection on the individual who is infected, the family, and the community.

ClinicalTrials.gov

http://www.clinicaltrials.gov

The site lists information from the U.S. National Institutes of Health on clinical research studies.

Critical Path AIDS Project

http://www.critpath.org/critpath

A site that spotlights news, research, articles, and treatment information.

Dale and Betty Bumpers Vaccine Research Center

http://www.niaid.nih.gov/vrc

Features vaccine research information from the National Institutes of Health, updates on HIV vaccine research, and information and enrollment guidelines for an HIV vaccine clinical trial.

Department of Disease Prevention and Promotion of Health and Human Services

http://www.healthfinder.gov

This site provides HIV/AIDS-related information from news articles, medical journals, educational sites, support groups, state agencies, and organizations.

Division of Acquired Immunodeficiency Syndrome, National Institute of Allergy and Infectious Diseases
http://www.niaid.nih.gov/research/daids/default.htm

This site has information on NIAID-funded research, HIV vaccines, and HIV/AIDS prevention and treatment

Division of AIDS (DAIDS)
http://www.niaid.nih.gov/daids

Offers varied material, including division overview; information on clinical trials and research; resources and programs; publication and meeting summaries; information on vaccines, prevention, and treatment for HIV/AIDS; and funding opportunities.

Division of Extramural Research, Infectious Diseases and Immunity Branch—AIDS Research Program
http://www.nidr.nih.gov/research/extramural/aids.asp

This spotlights a program that examines the oral complications of HIV/AIDS. Readers can find facts on oral infections and AIDS.

Doctor's Guide Global Edition
http://www.docguide.com

This website provides links to medical news sites and information, discussion groups, newsgroups, and related sites. It has an HIV/AIDS section.

Elton John AIDS Foundation
http://www.ejaf.org

Find out about events, merchandise, and how to donate to this famous AIDS charity.

Gay and Lesbian Medical Association
(415) 255-4547
(415) 255-4784
http://www.glma.org

A site that focuses on addressing the needs of gays and lesbians and supplying information pertaining to STDs and other health issues.

Gay Men's Health Crisis
(212) 367-1000
http://www.gmhc.org

A well-known group that focuses on HIV/AIDS and its impact on homosexual men; addresses various aspects of living with HIV/AIDS; new treatments; and health information. Special sections include "Drugs, Sex and HIV" and "Take Action," AIDS awareness products, and special events listings.

Hemophilia and AIDS/HIV Network for the Dissemination of Information (HANDI)
(800) 424-2643; English, x3051; Spanish, x3054.

Informational site for those with hemophilia and HIV/AIDS.

Herpes Information
http://www.viridae.com/publicsns.htm

Look for updates on herpes treatments and information on living with herpes simplex virus.

HIV, AIDS, and Older People
http://www.aoa.dhhs.gov/aoa/pages/agepages/aids.html

This site reaches out to seniors with HIV/AIDS.

HIV/AIDS Information
http://sis.nlm.gov/aidswww.htm

This Specialized Information Systems (SIS) site has trial, drug, and treatment information; articles; and Web links. SIS coordinates treatment information access with other agencies.

HIV/AIDS Office of Special Health Issues, FDA
http://www.fda.gov/oashi/aids/hiv.html

Features information from the Food and Drug Administration on HIV and AIDS.

HIV/AIDS Treatment Information Service
(888) 480-3739
http://www.hivatis.org

Offers information on HIV/AIDS treatments. Calls and service are free and confidential. The Health Care Financing Administration provides funding for this service.

HIV and AIDS Malignancy Branch
http://www-dcs.nci.nih.gov/branches/aidstrials

This is a branch of the U.S. National Institutes of Health. Describes research including pediatric investigations and current pediatric and adult trials.

HIV and AIDS Treatment Prevention Information on HIV Infoweb
http://www.infoweb.org

A good starting point for those who want to do searches for HIV/AIDS treatment and prevention information.

HIV Counseling Program
http://www.cc.nih.gov/swd/hiv_index.html

This site is a confidential counseling service for NIH Clinical Center patients and NIH staff. For the general public, there is information on seminars and training on HIV/AIDS.

HIV InSite, University of California, San Francisco
http://hivinsite.ucsf.edu

A site with information on HIV treatment, prevention, and social issues. It is based at the University of California at San Francisco and San Francisco General Hospital.

HIV Prevention Web Site, National Institute of Allergy and Infectious Diseases (NIAID)

http://www.niaid.nih.gov/daids/prevention

Reviews NIAID support for HIV/AIDS prevention (non-vaccine) research, including links to a worldwide collaborative clinical trials network.

HIV Vaccine Clinical Trial, Dale and Betty Bumpers Vaccine Research Center, NIAID

http://www.vrc.nih.gov/VRC/clinstudies.htm

Features information on studies.

HIV Vaccines Explained—Making HIV Vaccines a Reality

http://www.niaid.nih.gov/publications/pdf/
    HIVvaccinebrochure.pdf

This consumer-friendly brochure looks at HIV vaccine research, history of vaccines, information for HIV vaccine volunteers, and ways people can help to advance research on vaccines.

HIV Vaccines Web Site

http://www.niaid.nih.gov/daids/vaccine/

This site is sponsored by the National Institute of Allergy and Infectious Diseases to update the public on AIDS vaccine efforts.

International Association of Physicians in AIDS Care

http://www.iapac.org

The Web page of doctors who specialize in taking care of AIDS patients.

Johns Hopkins AIDS Service

http://www.hopkins-aids.edu

This is a collection of resources from one of the country's top clinical centers.

Journal of the American Medical Association HIV/AIDS Information Center

http://www.ama-assn.org/special/hiv/hivhome.htm

Produced by the premier medical publication *The Journal of the American Medical Association (JAMA)*, this website offers daily news updates, abstracts from HIV/AIDS articles scanned from journals, and links to resources.

Journal of the American Medical Association Sexually Transmitted Disease Information Center Library

http://www.ama-assn.org/special/std/std.htm

This is designed as a resource site for physicians and other health professionals.

Journal of the International AIDS Society

http://www.aidsonline.com

Shows sample documents from the journal's technical articles that deal with HIV research and other issues.

Keep Your Body Healthy

http://www.drugabuse.gov/drugpages/psahome.html

The National Institute on Drug Abuse highlights its campaign that addresses drug use and HIV/AIDS risks.

Library of the National Medical Society

http://www.medical-library.org/library.htm

Features a variety of articles on health topics, including sexually transmitted diseases of all kinds.

Mayo Health Oasis

http://www.mayoclinic.com/index/cfm

A website with information on diseases and conditions, including STDs, with answers and self-care guides.

MEDLINEplus AIDS information

http://www.nlm.nih.gov/medlineplus/aids.html

This site gives Web browsers news from the National Institutes of Health, scientific groups, and the media; it also has clinical trial listings and information on alternative therapies, disease management, and nutritional and other AIDS advice. Some material in Spanish is included.

Medscape HIV/AIDS

http://hiv.medscape.com/home/topics/aids/aids.html

One of the specialty sites of this multispecialty medical information Web resource. Contains articles, treatment updates, and conference summaries. Free access, with required registration.

National AIDS Treatment Advocacy Project

http://www.natap.org/natap

The site provides HIV, AIDS, and hepatitis treatment information and news on drugs and research. It also maintains a calendar of events.

National Association of People With AIDS

http://www.napwa.org

Find out about programs and events for those with HIV and AIDS.

National Cancer Institute: Cancer Information Service

(800) 4 CANCER
http://www.nci.nih.gov

Resource for cancer information.

National Institute of Allergy and Infectious Diseases (NIAID)
http://www.niaid.nih.gov

Offers information on sexually transmitted diseases.

National Institute on Drug Abuse (NIDA)
http://www.nida.nih.gov

Addresses drug use and HIV/AIDS risks.

National Institutes of Health
http://www.nih.gov

Provides a wealth of health information, as well as assorted resources and an NIH search engine.

National Institute of Mental Health
http://www.nimh.nih.gov

Addresses mental health problems, some of which are linked to sexually transmitted diseases, such as HIV/AIDS.

NIAID and Clinical Center HIV Program
http://www.niaid.nih.gov/hivclinic

Provides information on enrolling in trials (HIV/AIDS) as well as a list of current trials under way. Has contact info in Spanish.

Office of AIDS Research (OAR), NIH
http://www.nih.gov/od/oar

The OAR oversees the National Institutes of Health's AIDS research programs.

Office of AIDS Research Fiscal Year 2003 Plan for HIV-Related Research
http://www.nih.gov/od/oar/public/pubs/fy2003/
    i_overview.pdf

This summarizes the National Institutes of Health's AIDS research agenda, including budget figures. Three new areas of emphasis have been added: microbicides, HIV prevention research, and women, girls, and HIV/AIDS.

Overview of the Immune Responses and Oncology Portfolio
http://www.nih.gov/ninr/research/dea/science/
    immune.htm

This is a list of HIV/AIDS-related nursing research areas, from improving immune function to handling symptoms.

Pediatric, Adolescent, and Maternal AIDS Branch
http://www.nichd.nih.gov/crmc/pama/pama.htm

The website of the National Institute of Child Health & Human Development. A research agenda focuses on HIV/AIDS in mother and child, adolescents at risk and HIV-infected, and high-risk pediatric groups, such as hemophiliac children.

Pediatric AIDS Foundation
http://www.pedaids.org

This website has information pertaining to children with HIV/AIDS.

Project Inform
http://www.projinf.org
(800) 822-7422

A national nonprofit organization that is community-based and provides free, confidential information. Hotline hours: Monday-Friday, 9 A.M.–5 P.M.; Saturday, 10 A.M.–4 P.M. (Pacific Time).

Protein Expression Laboratory
http://www.grants.nih.gov/guide

This site spotlights a program wherein NIH scientists study HIV proteins.

Regional Primate Research Centers
http://www/ncrr.nih.gov/compmed/cmrprc.htm

A national network of centers assists scientists in using nonhuman primate models for research on HIV/AIDS and other diseases. This site has a directory of primate research resources and training and research programs available to outside scientists.

SexHealth.com
www.sexhealth.com/sexhealth/user/display.cfm

Information on sexually transmitted diseases, contraception, sexuality, dating, and relationships.

Sexually Transmitted Diseases, Centers for Disease Control and Prevention
http://www.cdc.gov/nchstp/dstd/dstdp.html

Offers information updates, treatment guidelines, and disease facts.

Sexually Transmitted Diseases Condition Center
http://www.medinformation.com/mf/
    community.nsf.STDs

Spotlights symptoms, news, prevention, and other topics for those interested in learning more about sexually transmitted diseases.

Sexually Transmitted Disease in the United States
http://www.siecus.org/pubs/fact/fact0008.html

Fact sheets from the Sexuality Information and Education Council of the United States.

Sexually Transmitted Disease Research
http://www.niaid.nih.gov/dmid

Click on STDs. Information is provided by the National Institute of Allergy and Infectious Diseases, National Institutes of Health.

Statistics on Global Health
http://www.globalhealth.gov

This site addresses global health issues and the link between domestic and international issues. Health portal for the U.S. Department of Health and Human Services.

STDs-InteliHealth
http://www.intelihealth.com/IH/iht1H/8799/8799/
  8799.html

Features Harvard Medical School's consumer health information on sexually transmitted diseases.

Studies of Ocular Complications of AIDS (SOCA)
http://www.nei.nih.gov/neitrials/socaintro/htm

A site that provides patient information on treatments, clinical trials, publications, and contacts for information on AIDS-related eye diseases (primarily cytomegalovirus infection).

UNAIDS
http://www.unaids.org

A joint United Nations Program on HIV/AIDS that pools resources from six international groups working to alleviate the pandemic.

WebMED.org
http://www.webmed.org

This site has sections for consumers, physicians, nurses, and health instructors. Features an HIV/AIDS information center.

STD HOTLINES

AIDS Clinical Trials Information Service (ACTIS)
(800) TRIALS-A (874-2572)
(800) 243-7012 (TTY)

AIDS Treatment Information Service/CDC (ATIS)
(800) HIV-0440 (800-448-0440)

American Foundation for AIDS Research (amFAR)
733 Third Avenue, 12th Floor
New York, NY 10017
(212) 682-7440
(800) 764-9346

American Public Health Association
1015 15th Street
Washington, DC 20005
(202) 789-5600

American Red Cross AIDS Education Office
1730 D Street, NW
Washington, DC 20006
(202) 737-8300

American Social Health Association
P.O. Box 13827
Research Triangle Park, NC 27009
(800) 227-8922

The Americans with Disabilities Act Information and Assistance Hotline
(800) 949-4232 (V/TTY)

AZT Information Hotline
(800) 843-9388

Business & Labor Information Service (CDC NAC)
(800) 458-5231
(800) 243-7012 (Deaf/TDD)

Links business groups and labor groups with resources for developing HIV/AIDS-in-the-workplace programs.

Centers for Disease Control and Prevention (CDC)
1600 Clifton Road NE
26 Executive Park
Atlanta, GA 30333
(404) 639-3311

The Centers for Disease Control Hotline
(800) 343-AIDS
(800) 342-2437

The Centers for Disease Control and Prevention National AIDS Information Clearinghouse "Materials Catalog" and "Business Responds to AIDS" Resource Services
P.O. Box 3003
Rockville, MD 20849-6003
(800) 458-5231 (in Maryland)
(800) 243-7012 (TDD/Deaf Access)
(301) 763-5111 (9 A.M.–7 P.M. M–F)
(301) 217-0023 (International)

Department of Health and Human Services
Office of the Secretary
200 Independence Avenue, NW, Room 615-F
Washington, DC 20201
(202) 245-6296

Experimental Treatment Infoline
(800) 633-7444 (New York State only)
(212) 239-5523 (other states)

Food and Drug Administration (FDA)
5600 Fishers Lane
Rockville, MD 20857
(301) 443-2410

FDA Center for Drug Research
Office of Director
5600 Fishers Lane, Room 13B-45
Rockville, MD 20857
(301) 443-2894

Gay Men's Health Crisis
129 West 20th Street
New York, NY 10011
(212) 807-6664
AIDS Hotline: (212) 807-6655 (M–F, 10 A.M.–9 P.M.;
Sat., 12–3 P.M.)

**Hemophilia and AIDS/HIV Network
for the Dissemination of Information (HANDI)**
110 Greene Street
Suite 303
New York, NY 10012
(212) 431-8541
(800) 42-HANDI

Herpes Resource Center
(800) 230-6039

Lesbian AIDS Project (LAPS)
(212) 337-3532

National AIDS Hotline
(800) 342-2437 (24 hours daily)
(800) 243-7889 (TTY/TDD)
(800) 342-AIDS (English)
(800) 344-SIDA (Spanish)
(301) 217-0023 (International)

National AIDS Network
729 Eighth Street, SE
Suite 300
Washington, DC 20003

National AIDS Treatment Advocacy Project
72 Orange Street, #3C
Brooklyn, NY 11201
(718) 624-8541

National Association of People with AIDS
1413 K Street, NW, 7th Floor
Washington, DC 20005
(202) 898-0414
(800) 673-8538

National Cancer Institute
Bldg. 31, Room 11A-48
6003 Executive Boulevard
Bethesda, MD 20892
(301) 496-4000

**National Clearinghouse for Alcohol and Drug
Information's Center for Substance Abuse
Prevention**
(800) 729-6686

National Gay and Lesbian Task Force
1734 14th Street, NW
Washington, DC 20009-4309
(202) 332-6483
(800) 221-7044

National Hemophilia Foundation
(212) 219-8180

National Herpes Hotline
(919) 361-8488 (9 A.M.–7 P.M. EST weekdays)

National HIV Telephone Consultation Service
(800) 933-3413

National Indian AIDS Hotline
(800) 283-2437

National Institute of Drug Abuse
(800) 662-HELP

**National Institutes of Allergy
and Infectious Diseases**
Office of Communications
Bldg. 31, Room 7A-32
Bethesda, MD 20892
(301) 496-5717

National Institutes of Health Clinical Center
(800) AIDS-NIH
(800) 243-7644

**National Institutes of Health (NIH) Office
of the Director**
Bldg. 1, Room 344
6003 Executive Boulevard
Bethesda, MD 20892
(301) 496-4000 (main information number)
For information on AIDS clinical trials at the NIH
Clinical Center:
(800) AIDS-NIH (243-7644) (M–F, 12–3 P.M. EST)

National Library of Medicine

Three online AIDS databases: AIDSLINE, AIDSDRUGS,
and AIDSTRIALS. For an information packet, call (800)
638-8480.

National Minority AIDS Council
1931 13th Street, NW
Washington, DC 20009
(202) 483-6622
(202) 544-1076

**National Native American AIDS Prevention
Center**
3515 Grand Avenue
Suite 100
Oakland, CA 94610
(510) 444-2051

**National Pediatric and Family HIV
Resource Center**
30 Bergen Street ADMC #4
Newark, NJ 07103
(973) 972-0410
(800) 362-0071

**National Sexually Transmitted Disease
Hotline/CDC**
(800) 227-8922 (8 A.M.–11 P.M. EST, weekdays)

Native American AIDS Information Hotline
(800) 283-2437

Rural AIDS Network
1915 Rosina
Santa Fe, NM 87501
(505) 986-8337

Teen AIDS Hotline
(800) 283-2473

AIDS information and grief counseling, 8:30 A.M.–1 P.M.
and 2–5 P.M. M–F

**U.S. Centers for Disease Control's National STD
Hotline**
(800) 227-8922 (services: free materials and referrals
to clinics)

U.S. Public Health Service
200 Independence Avenue, SW
Washington, DC 20006
(202) 293-7330

Women's AIDS Network
(415) 821-7984

Women Alive
(800) 554-4876

Hotline staffed by HIV-positive women volunteers
Mon., Wed., and Fri., 11 A.M.–6 P.M. (PT), 2–9 P.M. (ET)

Women and HIV/AIDS—Sister Connect
(800) 747-1108

APPENDIX II
HIV/AIDS TIMELINE

1980

- Kaposi's sarcoma occurs in epidemic proportions in homosexual men.

- From 1980 to 1981, an unusual health situation is noted in Los Angeles, California, where five young homosexual men are treated for *Pneumocystis carinii* pneumoni—a rare occurrence in people who are not severely immunosuppressed; two die. All five have previous or current cytomegalovirus infection and candidal mucosal infection. These individuals do not know each other and share no common contacts; they report having no sex partners with similar illnesses. Two of them report frequent sexual encounters with various partners. All five use inhalant drugs; one is an intravenous drug user.

1981

- In New York and California, clinical investigators note an unusual clustering in young gay men of rare diseases such as Kaposi's sarcoma and opportunistic infections such as *Pneumocystis carinii* pneumonia, as well as cases of persistent lymphadenopathy for which there is no explanation.

- In Africa, from 1981 to 1983, there are epidemics of life-threatening enteropathic diseases ("slim disease"), cryptococcal meningitis, progressive Kaposi's sarcoma, and esophageal candidiasis (Rwanda, Tanzania, Uganda, Zaire, Zambia). The first AIDS cases in Africans are reported.

- When unusual infections in IV drug users are noted by physicians as unprecedented in num-

ber, investigators begin trying to figure out why so many intravenous drug users and homosexual men are exhibiting severe immune suppression. Doctors had previously observed only subtle defects in immunity in such cases. The situation raises concern since these young, formerly healthy men have no underlying history of immunosuppressive therapy or disease, and these diseases have always been rare in the United States.

- June 5: The Centers for Disease Control and Prevention in Atlanta, Georgia, publishes "Pneumocystis Pneumonia—Los Angeles," in *Morbidity and Mortality Weekly Report,* which speaks of a new disease affecting gay men, and doctors report that the lung infection *Pneumocystis carinii* pneumonia has struck "five young men, all active homosexuals, in Los Angeles." This article—the first on AIDS to appear in the medical literature—essentially marks the beginning of what would become the AIDS pandemic.

- The first case of AIDS is officially recorded. On June 16, the first AIDS patient seen at the National Institutes of Health is admitted under Dr. Thomas Waldmann's National Cancer Institute Omnibus Metabolism Branch protocol.

- A drug technician at the Centers for Disease Control and Prevention notes an unusually high number of requests for pentamidine—a drug used in treating *Pneumocystis carinii* pneumonia, which leads to the above-mentioned medical report of *Pneumocystis carinii* pneumonia in five L.A. gay men. Researchers begin to search for the cause of the infections and the cases of Kaposi's sarcoma seen increasingly among gay men in New York.

Most think it is a result of the use of poppers, or nitrate inhalants; some contend that an infectious agent is the cause. *Pneumocystis carinii* pneumonia later begins to appear in drug addicts.

- Before 1981, disseminated *Mycobacterium avium* complex disease is rare—only 32 people have been described in medical literature up to that year—but it is seen often in the first AIDS patients.

- *The New York Times* (July 3) runs a short article reporting the outbreak of a rare cancer in 41 gay men in New York and California.

- August: The CDC reports a total of 108 cases of the "new disease" in the United States.

- Cases of Kaposi's sarcoma and pneumocystis increase nationwide, according to the Centers for Disease Control. Most of these cases are being diagnosed in gay men.

- September 15: The National Institutes of Health sponsors a conference in Bethesda, Maryland, on Kaposi's sarcoma and opportunistic infections, and 50 clinicians attend.

- In the fall of 1981, simian acquired immune deficiency syndrome (simian AIDS) is identified in macaques in two of the National Institutes of Health's Regional Primate Centers.

- October: The CDC declares the new disease an epidemic.

1982

- Some scientists tag the new set of symptoms *gay-related immune deficiency* (GRID) (the term *HIV* is not yet used). Evidence begins to suggest the symptoms are caused by an infectious agent, possibly a blood-borne virus.

- January 12: The Gay Men's Health Crisis (GMHC) is formed in New York in order to deal with the spread of the new "gay cancer."

- AIDS Project Los Angeles is organized; its first service, a hotline, is housed in the Gay and Lesbian Community Services Center. The first benefit raises $7,000, but in the decade to come,

APLA will raise more than $77 million for services for people with AIDS.

- Dr. Anthony Fauci sees the second AIDS patient admitted to the National Institutes of Health (National Institute of Allergy and Infectious Diseases).

- March 3: A conference sponsored by the U.S. Public Health Service at the Centers for Disease Control and Prevention in Atlanta is held to discuss AIDS. Attendees debate whether the mysterious new disease is caused by a transmissible or immune-suppressing agent(s).

- NIAID intramural scientists do a study of adenovirus in patients with AIDS.

- The National Cancer Institute establishes an Epidemiology Working Group on Kaposi's sarcoma.

- NCA intramural researchers do a field study to determine the immunological status of healthy homosexual men.

- An article in the *Wall Street Journal* looks at the fact that physicians are also seeing gay-related immune deficiency in women and male heterosexual drug users. Hemophiliacs and Haitian refugees in Miami also appear to be suffering from the same syndrome.

- The first blood transfusion recipient with AIDS in the United States is identified, as are the first infants with AIDS.

- The National Institute of Neurological and Communicative Disorders and Stroke collaborate to study simian AIDS.

- June 30: A meeting at the New York Department of Health spotlights evidence supporting the contention that AIDS seems to be caused by an infectious agent. It is announced that AIDS cases have been seen in IV drug users, homosexuals, hemophiliacs, and Haitians.

- July 27: The disease is named *acquired immunodeficiency syndrome* (AIDS).

- September: The CDC reports 593 U.S. AIDS cases (243 deaths).

- The CDC defines AIDS as a disease that is at least moderately predictive of a defect in cell-mediated immunity when it occurs in someone who has no known cause for diminished resistance to the disease.

- November: The CDC sends out formal recommendations to protect those involved in lab and health care activities from contracting AIDS. These guidelines are based on guidelines for hepatitis B.

- By December 31, 3,863 Americans with hemophilia or other coagulation disorders are diagnosed with AIDS.

- Fourteen nations report AIDS cases.

- The National Library of Medicine begins compiling a bibliography on manifestations of AIDS.

- Federal funds of $5.6 million are allocated for AIDS research.

- PBS broadcasts a national TV special, "AIDS: The Mysterious Disease."

- The National Heart, Lung, and Blood Institute sets up an intraagency agreement with the Centers for Disease Control and Prevention to evaluate immunological changes that follow transfusion with blood or blood products in patients with hemophilia, sickle-cell disease, and thalassemia.

- The CDC reports a case of AIDS that is the result of a blood transfusion in a previously healthy infant.

- The National Institutes of Health's intramural study of the history of immunodeficiency and opportunistic infections has 25 enrollees with AIDS.

1983

- The Centers for Disease Control and Prevention warns blood banks of a suspected problem with the blood supply.

- The CDC establishes a national AIDS hotline.

- The first AIDS discrimination trial is held in the United States.

- It becomes apparent that heterosexuals are also at risk for AIDS when two women contract AIDS from infected sex partners. The heterosexual

transmission risk is reported in the *New England Journal of Medicine.*

- The Buddy Program becomes the first direct client service.

- The AIDS Medical Foundation is established in New York by Robert Mehl. Later the group becomes amfAR.

- The first U.S. Conference on AIDS is held in Denver, Colorado, and the People with AIDS Coalition results from that conference.

- ABC's *20/20* does its first segment on AIDS.

- March: A report underscores epidemiologic evidence that AIDS chiefly affects gay men in San Francisco and New York City, and that in New Jersey, those with AIDS are mostly drug users and Haitians, and 68 percent are Latinos and African Americans.

- The CDC publishes guidelines adopted by the Public Health Service asking people at high risk for AIDS not to donate blood.

- The CDC, the FDA, and the National Institutes of Health issue prevention recommendations on how to prevent sexual, drug-related, and occupational transmission of the AIDS infection.

- Human T cell leukemia virus (HTLV) is identified in patients with AIDS.

- May: A report of experimental evidence linking a retrovirus and AIDS is published. At the Institut Pasteur in France, Dr. Luc Montagnier's research group isolates a new virus that becomes known as lymphadenopathy-associated virus (LAV). They do not claim that LAV is the cause of AIDS, however.

- June: The CDC reports 1,972 cases of AIDS (759 deaths) in the United States. By September, the figures rise to 2,259 cases and 917 deaths.

- September: The NIAID and NCI launch the very important Multicenter AIDS Cohort Study (MACS) and the San Francisco Men's Health Study, with the goal of establishing large, comprehensive longitudinal studies of at-risk-for-AIDS populations. (Shortly thereafter, NIAID takes over all responsibility for the program.)

- In the United States, the mysterious plague shows up in different ways in different areas. In New Jersey, for example, IV drug users are about half of those with the disease, and gay men are the minority of cases. In other parts of the United States, the disease has become an epidemic in gay communities.

- In Europe, AIDS epidemics show links to Africa and to gay men who have visited the United States. The United Kingdom Department of Health makes an official report of AIDS in the United Kingdom; three UK people have died. Also, in Melbourne, the first Australian death from AIDS is recorded.

- The possibility of household transmission of AIDS is raised by a report of AIDS in children that is interpreted incorrectly. Fear spreads, and in San Francisco, it is reported that some bus drivers begin wearing facemasks. Casual transmission as a means of transmission is dispelled only through years of education prompted by this misinformation.

- As more children with AIDS are reported in 1983, it becomes clear that they have acquired the infection from mothers infected with the virus, either in the womb or during childbirth.

- AIDS cases are reported in 33 countries, and 3,000 Americans now have AIDS (1,283 have died).

- It becomes clear that the AIDS-causing virus can be transmitted through blood transfusions. Thus, officials from the Centers for Disease Control and Prevention meet with directors of blood banking groups in Atlanta to work on proposals to screen out those donors at high risk for AIDS. One idea advanced is screening (interviews or questionnaires) to allow prospective donors to identify themselves as participants in high-risk activities.

1984

- January: The CDC reports 3,000 U.S. cases of AIDS (1,283 deaths).

- The different modes of HIV transmission are identified.

- Thousands of lesbians and gays march at the Democratic convention in an effort to spotlight the need for increased federal spending for AIDS.

- Scientists report the isolation of a virus that gives monkeys an AIDS-like illness.

- Serologic tests for antibodies to HIV are developed; the tests allow researchers in later years to conduct hundreds of seroprevalence surveys worldwide. The tests enable researchers to show that when AIDS-like illnesses occur in different populations, disease follows the appearance of HIV antibodies.

- Scientists observe that never-married San Francisco men are 2,000 times more likely to contract Kaposi's sarcoma than in the years 1973 to 1979.

- It is hypothesized that the clustering of AIDS cases and the occurrence of these in diverse risk groups make sense only if AIDS is caused by an infectious microorganism that is transmitted as the hepatitis B virus is: by sexual activity, inoculation with blood or blood products, and mother-to-infant transmission.

- April 23, 1984: The U.S. Health and Human Services secretary, Margaret Heckler, announces that Dr. Robert Gallo of the National Institutes of Health has discovered the cause of AIDS, the retrovirus named HTLV-III. At the same time, it is announced that a diagnostic blood test has been developed for identification of HTLV-III. Dr. Gallo has accomplished this isolation at the National Cancer Institute. Blood testing begins to detect virus antibodies.

- The journal *Science* publishes four papers from Dr. Gallo's laboratory that show the cause of AIDS to be the retrovirus HTLV-III.

- More data lead researchers to look closely at evidence for a retroviral cause of AIDS. National Institutes of Health researchers isolate a cytopathic T lymphotropic virus from 48 people—18 of 21 with pre-AIDS (older term synonymous with AIDS-related complex), three of four clinically normal mothers of children with AIDS, 26 of 72 children and adults with AIDS, and one (who later had AIDS) of 22 healthy homosexuals. The virus, named HTLV-III, is not found in 115 healthy heterosexual subjects. Also, antibodies reactive with HTLV-III antigens are found in serum samples of 88 percent of 48 patients who have AIDS, 79 percent of 14 homosexuals with pre-AIDS, and less than 1 percent of hundreds of healthy heterosexuals. Soon after, researchers find that 100 percent of AIDS patients test positive for HTLV-III antibodies in a study in which none of 14 controls has antibodies.

- Around this same time, HTLV-III is isolated from AIDS patients' semen, producing findings consistent with data showing AIDS transmission via sexual contact.

- One of the earliest suggestions of an infectious cause is published in a report in the *American Journal of Medicine* (1984;76:487–492), which explains that cases of AIDS among gays are not happening randomly but are clustered among sexual contacts. There are 40 people identified who show linked transmission over three generations of infection. Four theories of cause being investigated at this time are (1) the possibility that multiple and repeated infections with cytomegalovirus lead to immune suppression; (2) that people are experiencing immunologic exhaustion from multiple previous infections; (3) that alloimmunization to lymphocytes is due to intrarectal sperm injection; and (4) that toxic effects are produced by components of genital lubricants or inhalant drugs. It turns out that theories (2) through (4) are incompatible with the observed transmission mode, and no one can produce credible evidence to back up theory (1).

- San Francisco researchers report their isolation of a retrovirus they call the AIDS-associated retrovirus (ARV); it is isolated from AIDS patients in different risk groups and from asymptomatic people in AIDS risk groups. As is the case with HTLV-III and LAV, AIDS-associated retrovirus grows substantially in peripheral blood mononuclear cells and kills CD4+ T cells. This same group in San Francisco isolates AIDS-associated retrovirus from genital secretions of women with antibodies to the virus, data consis-

tent with the observation that men can contract AIDS after contact with a virus-infected female.

- June: In a joint press conference Dr. Robert Gallo and Dr. Luc Montagnier announce their belief that Gallo's HTLV III and Montagnier's LAV are identical. The same month, the CDC reports 4,918 U.S. cases of AIDS (2,221 deaths).

- Gaetan Dugas, called Patient Zero (the one who supposedly "brought" AIDS to the United States), dies.

- All gay bathhouses in San Francisco are closed.

- The U.S. Health and Human Services secretary, Margaret Heckler, predicts that researchers will have a vaccine in a few years and that a cure for AIDS will be discovered before 1990.

- AIDS Project Los Angeles is instrumental in the founding of AIDS Action Council, a group set up to lobby the government for increased funding and services for HIV/AIDS.

- There are 6,993 Americans with AIDS by the end of 1984, and 3,342 deaths.

1985

- The FDA approves the first AIDS antibody test, which is then used to screen the U.S. blood supply.

- A national poll reflects Americans' fears regarding HIV. The poll shows that 72 percent of Americans favor mandatory HIV testing, 51 percent favor quarantine of those infected, and 15 percent favor tattoos for those who are HIV-positive.

- The California legislature makes a move to guarantee confidentiality of HIV testing in that state, and the concept is then adopted nationwide.

- Reports are circulated that condoms can prevent the sexual transmission of AIDS, and "safe sex" is widely promoted for sexually active people.

- Participants gather for the first International Conference on AIDS in Atlanta.

- The FDA approves Dr. Robert Gallos's AIDS diagnostic kit, which is based on the Western blot technique. Soon after, the first commercial kit for antibodies is licensed.

- The American Foundation for AIDS Research (amfAR) is founded in Los Angeles.

- The Pasteur Institute files a lawsuit against the National Cancer Institute because they believe they are entitled to a share of the royalties from the NCI's patented AIDS blood test.

- The actor Rock Hudson dies of AIDS, causing numerous people to call hotlines and pursue HIV screening.

- AIDS Project Los Angeles holds the world's first AIDS Walk; the event raises $673,000.

- Ryan White, a 13-year-old hemophiliac with AIDS, is barred from school in Indiana.

- In Uganda, AIDS is known locally as "slim disease," descriptive of the wasting effect characteristic of the final stage of the disease. By 1985, large numbers of people in Central Africa have AIDS.

- A World Health Organization definition of AIDS in Africa is adopted so that African countries can assess and report cases of AIDS.

- Cases of AIDS are reported in 51 countries.

- May: The CDC reports that there have been 10,000 AIDS cases in the United States and that 4,942 have died. The CDC revises its AIDS definition to include more disease conditions and to exclude people from being identified with AIDS if they test negative for serum antibody to HTLV-III/LAV.

- State and local health departments are funded nationwide to implement HIV prevention programs.

- The first guidelines for blood screening are issued.

- The FDA licenses ELISA.

1986

- A possible transmission of the virus from dentist to patient is reported.

- January: The CDC reports 16,458 U.S. AIDS cases, with 8,361 deaths.

- Health experts agree that the viruses LAV, HTLV-III, and ARV are the same, so the International Committee of Viral Taxonomy rules that the use of the other names be replaced by use of the one name *human immunodeficiency virus* (HIV).

- Preliminary reports of using the drug zidovudine (AZT) to treat AIDS are made at the International AIDS Conference II in Paris.

- A global AIDS strategy is launched by the World Health Organization. At a WHO meeting, participants join in issuing a recommendation that all countries help to prevent the spread of AIDS by providing sterile needles and syringes to drug abusers.

- The U.S. surgeon general, C. Everett Koop, publishes a major report on AIDS, the "Report on Acquired Immune Deficiency," and calls for AIDS education and condom use.

- The Ugandan minister of health declares an AIDS epidemic in his country, and other African countries follow. These countries request assistance from the World Health Organization.

- The Zambian ministry of health launches an AIDS campaign to educate its people.

- Congress adds $47 million to the federal budget in order to create the research units to be known as the AIDS Clinical Trial Groups.

- The CDC reports that AIDS cases are increasing in all parts of the United States and in all racial and ethnic groups—but that the cumulative incidence among blacks and Hispanics is more than three times the incidence for whites.

- December: The CDC reports 28,098 cases of AIDS in the United States, with 15,757 deaths.

1987

- A public information campaign, America Responds to AIDS, is launched.

- February: The World Health Organization launches its Global Programme on AIDS.

- Comprehensive U.S. school-based education on HIV/AIDS is funded.

- The FDA approves AZT as the first antiretroviral drug to be used in treating AIDS. The cost for an individual to use this drug therapy is about $12,000 a year.

- President Ronald Reagan makes a public address on AIDS.

- Vice President George Bush calls for mandatory HIV testing.

- The CDC revises its AIDS definition to place more emphasis on HIV infection status.

- The CDC National AIDS Clearinghouse is established.

- May: The CDC reports that in the years from 1981 to 1987, nine health care workers contracted HIV (these individuals worked with AIDS patients and had no other risk factors).

- August: The CDC reports 40,051 AIDS cases in the United States, with 23,165 deaths. Also that month, NIAID researchers begin the first U.S. clinical trial at the National Institutes of Health to test an experimental HIV vaccine in humans.

- The first Counseling and Testing Guidelines are issued.

- The British government launches a major ad campaign, featuring an educational leaflet delivered to every home.

- Princess Diana opens the first specialized AIDS hospital ward in England. Her shaking hands with AIDS patients affects existing attitudes about people with AIDS, who are sometimes treated as pariahs.

- President Kaunda of Zambia announces that his son has died of AIDS.

- The United States passes legislation prohibiting entry into the United States of HIV-infected immigrants, aliens, and short-term visitors.

- A U.S. family is burned out of their home by arsonists who seek to keep their sons with AIDS out of the local schools.

- By November: The number of AIDS cases worldwide (officially reported to the World Health Organization) is 62,811, representing people in 127 countries. Most experts believe that the figure reported is a gross understatement of the true number of AIDS cases.

- In 1985, when the antibody test is first made available commercially, many believe that a positive result means infection with HIV even in children infected at birth. But two years later, it becomes clear that the test is only measuring antibody passed from the mother—not the child's own antibody. By 18 months old, many children clear their mother's antibody; that means that many children first deemed HIV-positive actually are not.

- The group ACT UP is organized to work for AIDS services, drug approvals, and research funding. Members prepare for activist action.

- Senator Jesse Helms introduces legislation to prevent funding of AIDS education programs that "encourage or promote homosexual activity," and the bill is passed. The action becomes known as the "no promo homo" rule.

- The American Medical Association rules that doctors must provide treatment for those with AIDS.

- The famous pianist Liberace dies of AIDS.

- The FDA approves the first Western blot blood test to diagnose HIV.

- After ACT UP stages mass civil disobedience on New York's Wall Street, the FDA announces a two-year shortening in the drug-approval process.

- Delta Airlines tries to ban passengers with AIDS, but the threat of a national boycott makes the airline back down.

- The CDC expands its definition of AIDS to encompass more diseases, including dementia and wasting syndrome.

- The AIDS Memorial Quilt is begun in San Francisco.

1988

- The American Medical Association urges doctors to violate confidentiality and warn the sexual partners of those who are being treated for AIDS.

- February 12: Trimetrexate is the first AIDS drug given preapproval distribution status, under new FDA regulations. The drug is used to treat *Pneumocystis carinii* pneumonia in AIDS patients unable to tolerate other treatments.

- The United States bans discrimination against federal workers with HIV.

- The National Institutes of Health establishes the Office of AIDS Research; Dr. Anthony Fauci is named acting director.

- The United States mails to households nationwide 107 million copies of "Understanding AIDS," an informative booklet by Surgeon General C. Everett Koop.

- The CDC substantially expands state and local prevention funding.

- The FDA puts into effect new regulations that they believe will shorten the time required to develop new treatments for AIDS.

- The United Kingdom funds expansion of needle exchange programs, and in the United States, New York begins such a program. For the first time, the number of cases of new HIV infection transmitted by shared needles surpasses the number of those that are newly sexually transmitted.

- In London, a world summit of health ministers devises a common AIDS strategy to fight the epidemic. Delegates of 148 countries work on AIDS prevention programs.

- April: The NIAID funds six national vaccine development groups to work on developing an HIV vaccine.

- June: The CDC reports that it is receiving news of a new AIDS case every 14 minutes.

- June: Universal precautions are established for all U.S. health care workers.

- August: The CDC reports 72,024 AIDS cases in the United States and announces that about 1 to 1.5 million Americans have HIV. The following month, the World Health Organization reports 111,000 cases of AIDS worldwide. WHO states that this figure is probably underreported by about half.

- National Institute of Dental and Craniofacial Research investigators report their finding that saliva serves to inhibit the transmission of HIV.

- November: One CDC study shows that three of 1,000 college students are HIV-infected.

- The World Health Organization institutes World AIDS Day, an annual event, on December 1.

1989

- New drugs are offered for the treatment of opportunistic infections. The price of AZT (Burroughs Wellcome) is lowered by 20 percent. The FDA authorizes dideoxyinosine, a new antiretroviral drug intended for use by patients who cannot tolerate AZT.

- A federal study shows that AZT slows the progression of HIV infection in people who have no or few symptoms.

- DIVA TV is formed; the Damned Interfering Video Activists are video makers who document the events sponsored by ACT UP.

- The FDA authorizes preapproval distribution of AZT for treatment of pediatric HIV cases.

1990

- Ryan White dies in the United States at age 19. A hemophiliac who contracted HIV via infected blood products, he had become well known through his fight to be allowed to attend a public school. A few months after his death, Congress passes the Ryan White CARE Act, which is meant to provide systems of care for people with AIDS who lack adequate health insurance or other resources. The bill authorizes $881 million in emergency relief to 16 cities that have suffered devastation from the AIDS epidemic; however, Congress appropriates less than $350 million.

- The needle exchange program in New York is closed down.

- In San Francisco, people meet for the Sixth International Conference on AIDS, which occurs amid worldwide protests about U.S. immigration policies regarding those who are HIV-positive.

- A large number of children in Romanian orphanages are reported to have HIV as a result of multiple blood transfusions.

- It is estimated that about 8 to 10 million worldwide are living with HIV. Of those, 5 million are men and 3 million are women. These women have had about 3 million infants, more than 700,000 of whom have HIV. Vertical transmission before or during birth is already a known risk, and now breast-feeding is added to the list of means of transmission of HIV.

- Congress passes two acts important to those with HIV: the Americans with Disabilities Act, which prohibits discrimination against those with HIV, and the AIDS Housing Opportunities Act, which sets aside $156 million to expand affordable housing for those with HIV-related illnesses.

- AZT is tested in combination with dideoxyinosine (ddI), dideoxycytidine (ddC), alpha-interferon, and granulocyte macrophage colony-stimulating factor (GM-CSF), and researchers find that each grouping has increased benefits.

- December: More than 307,000 AIDS cases have been reported to WHO; the actual number, however, is believed to be about 1 million.

1991

- The actor Jeremy Irons is the first celebrity to wear an AIDS-awareness red ribbon when he appears at the Tony Awards, putting the Red Ribbon campaign on the map as an international symbol of AIDS awareness.

- Public concern about transmission in medical and dental settings is raised by the notorious case of the dentist David Acer, who has transmitted HIV to some of his patients. As his infected patient Kimberly Bergalis nears death, she testifies before Congress and writes to the American Medical Association in her campaign to ensure mandatory testing of health care workers.

- Earvin "Magic" Johnson makes a public announcement that he is HIV-positive and is retiring from pro basketball. He will become an AIDS-awareness spokesman.

- Freddie Mercury, lead singer for the rock group Queen, dies of AIDS.

- The location for the 1992 international AIDS conference is changed from Boston, Massachusetts, to Amsterdam, as a result of the U.S. pol-

icy that requires short-term visitors to declare their HIV status.

- May 30: The FDA authorizes preapproval distribution of dideoxycytidine (ddC) under an Investigational New Drug protocol for the treatment of patients with AIDS or advanced AIDS-related complex who cannot be maintained on zidovudine (AZT).

- September 27: The FDA approves foscarnet (Foscavir) for treating cytomegalovirus retinal infections in those with AIDS.

- October 9: The FDA approves didanosine (ddI) (Videx) for treating advanced HIV patients (adults and pediatric patients older than six months).

- The first combination test for detecting HIV-1 and HIV-2 antibodies is licensed.

- November 8: The FDA authorizes preapproval distribution of atovaquone under the Investigational New Drug protocol to patients with *Pneumocystis carinii* pneumonia (for those unable to tolerate the standard treatment—trimethoprim sulfamethoxazole).

- By the end of 1991, the second 100,000 AIDS cases have been reported in the United States, as well as 133,000 deaths due to AIDS.

1992

- The International Olympic Committee rules that HIV-infected athletes cannot compete in the Olympics.

- The Business Responds to AIDS program is launched.

- March 6: The FDA authorizes preapproval distribution of rifabutin under the Investigational New Drug protocol for preventing or delaying onset of *Mycobacterium avium* complex.

- The first clinical trial of multiple-drug therapy is launched.

- The major conventions of both the Democratic and Republican Parties feature moving speeches delivered by people with AIDS.

- May 27: The FDA licenses the 10-minute diagnostic test (SUDS HIV-1), which health professionals can use to detect the presence of HIV-1.

- June 19: The FDA approves zalcitabine (ddC) for use in combination with zidovudine (AZT) as a treatment for adults with advanced HIV who have signs of deterioration (clinical or immunologic). Zalcitabine (Hivid) is the first drug approved under the FDA's proposed accelerated drug approval policy.

- September 11: The FDA approves itraconazole (Sporanox) for treating blastomycosis and histoplasmosis in immunocompromised and nonimmunocompromised patients.

- October 5: Stavudine (d4T) is the first drug made available for expanded investigational use under the parallel track policy.

- October 8: The FDA approves new labeling for nonprescription drugs for vaginal candidiasis to warn women that frequent or persistent cases of vaginal fungal infections are sometimes an early sign of HIV infection.

- November 25: The FDA approves atovaquone (Mepron) for treating *Pneumocystis carinii* pneumonia patients with mild to moderate disease if these people cannot tolerate the usual therapy—trimethoprim-sulfamethoxazole.

- December 22: The FDA approves dronabinol (Marinol) for treating AIDS-associated anorexia and weight loss.

- December 23: The FDA approves rifabutin (Mycobutin) for prophylaxis against *Mycobacterium avium* complex.

- The tennis star Arthur Ashe announces that he contracted HIV through a blood transfusion in 1983.

- Congress appropriates funds for Housing Opportunities for People with AIDS.

1993

- Cases of resistance to AZT are reported.

- January: The Russian ballet star Rudolf Nureyev dies from complications of AIDS.

- February 8: Arthur Ashe dies of pneumonia, a complication of AIDS.

- The CDC expands its AIDS definition to include invasive cervical cancer, T cell counts of less than 200, pulmonary TB, and recurrent bacterial infections. This new definition is expected to make figures on new AIDS cases swell by up to 100 percent.

- AIDS advocates draft a bill to reorganize the National Institutes of Health and create new Office of AIDS Research to streamline and supervise the many federal AIDS research projects. Congress passes the bill.

- European researchers show that AZT monotherapy is not effective for treatment early in the disease.

- May 7: The FDA approves the Reality Female Condom—a barrier product that women can use to protect themselves so partner cooperation or complicity is not a factor in protection.

- June: Sexual transmission tops IV drug use as the means by which women are most likely to contract HIV.

- September 10: The FDA approves megestrol acetate (Megace) for treating anorexia, cachexia, and unexplained weight loss in those with AIDS.

- The film *Philadelphia* raises Americans' consciousness of AIDS. For his role as an attorney dying of AIDS in this film, Tom Hanks wins an Oscar in 1994.

- Studies on discordant couples show that condoms appear to be 98 percent effective against HIV.

- A community planning process is instituted in order to target local prevention efforts more successfully.

- A European trial (Concorde) finds that AZT is not a useful therapy for HIV-positive people who have not yet experienced symptoms.

- December 14: The FDA publishes an interim rule establishing a requirement for certain infectious disease testing, donor screening, and record keeping in order to help prevent the transmission of HIV and hepatitis B and C through human tissue used in transplantation.

- December 17: The FDA approves trimetrexate glucuronate (Neutrexin) for moderate to severe *Pneumocystis carinii* pneumonia.

- December 23: The FDA approves clarithromycin (Biaxin) for treating disseminated mycobacterial infections due to *Mycobacterium avium* and *Mycobacterium intracellular* (*Mycobacterium avium* complex).

- December 27: The FDA licenses immune globulin intravenous, human (Gamimune) for use in HIV-infected children; the goal is to decrease frequency of bacterial infections, increase the time free of serious bacterial infections, and decrease frequency of hospitalizations.

- The Centers for Disease Control and Prevention expands its AIDS definition after criticism that its existing definition actually undercounts women, as well as others with serious HIV-related illnesses. The new definition's broader scope corrects the underreporting of AIDS cases in the United States.

1994

- After the identification of the first preventive regimen, perinatal HIV prevention guidelines are issued.

- January 7: The FDA approves trimethoprim-sulfamethoxazole (Bactrim and Septra) for prevention of *Pneumocystis carinii* pneumonia in those who are immunosuppressed and considered at high risk for this kind of pneumonia.

- February 4: U.S. Secretary of Health and Human Services Donna Shalala announces the appointment of 18 members of the National Task Force on AIDS Drug Development, which includes experts from academia, industry, medicine, government, and the HIV/AIDS-affected communities.

- March 29: The FDA asks all condom makers to start using an air-burst test on all latex condoms. The test is designed to measure condom strength and gauge resistance to breakage during its use.

- June 24: Stavudine (d4T) (Zerit) is approved for use in treating adults with HIV who cannot tolerate or no longer respond to other antiviral drugs.

- August 5: The FDA approves new labeling for zalcitabine (ddC) (Hivid) to include its use as monotherapy for HIV-infected adults.

- August 8: The FDA approves new labeling for zidovudine (AXT) (Retrovir) to include its use in preventing vertical transmission of HIV.

- November 7: The FDA approves a polyurethane condom that can be used by those individuals who are allergic to latex and thus unable to use latex condoms.

- December 20: The FDA authorizes preapproval distribution of Serostim, a mammalian derived recombinant human growth hormone, under an Investigational New Drug (IND) protocol to those patients experiencing AIDS-related wasting.

- December 22: The FDA approves oral ganciclovir (Cytovene) for treating cytomegalovirus retinitis in individuals who have a compromised immune system.

- December 23: The FDA approves the first non-blood-based collection kit using oral fluid for detecting antibody to HIV-1.

- A study reveals that AZT reduces the risk of vertical transmission (from mother to infant) by two-thirds.

- AIDS is the leading cause of death in Americans in the age bracket 25 to 44; 400,000 people in the United States have contracted AIDS since 1981, and more than 250,000 have died.

1995

- By 1995, 500,000 cases of AIDS have been reported in the United States.

- The Delta trial—a major clinical trial of combination antiretroviral therapy—shows that combining AZT with ddI or ddC provides major improvement over using AZT alone. When the success of this approach is confirmed by other studies, the gold standard for treating HIV becomes dual-combination therapy.

- February 23: The FDA revises the guidelines for Home Specimen Collection Kit Systems Intended for Human Immunodeficiency Virus (HIV-1 and/or HIV-2) Antibody Testing.

- March 24: The FDA clears for marketing the first blood test to measure latex antibodies. This identifies those who should not use latex condoms because they are allergic to them and must use other barrier products to prevent HIV transmission.

- June: The FDA publishes "An FDA Guide to Choosing Medical Treatments."

- June 6: The FDA revises blood donor criteria to exclude prisoners from donating blood, blood components, and plasma for 12 months after last date of incarceration.

- August: The FDA recommends that blood establishments implement donor screening for HIV-1 antigen using licensed test kits. Although there are no tests currently approved for HIV-1 antigen(s) donor screening, the FDA issues the recommendation in advance of the availability of such tests in order to provide plenty of time for blood and plasma banks to get ready for this testing.

- September 1: The FDA authorizes preapproval distribution of intravenous cidofovir (Vistide) under an Investigational New Drug (IND) protocol for HIV-infected persons with relapsing cytomegalovirus retinitis that has continued to progress despite treatment.

- September 8: The FDA publishes a proposed rule in the *Federal Register* that will change its regulations on investigational new drug applications (INDs) and new drug applications (NDAs). The rule is proposed in response to one of the recommendations made by the National Task Force on AIDS Drug Development. The rule clearly defines in the NDA format and content requirements the need to present effectiveness and safety data for important demographic subgroups—gender, age, race.

- October 12: The FDA approves clarithromycin (Biaxin) for prevention of *Mycobacterium avium* complex.

- October 27: The FDA grants marketing approval for oral ganciclovir (Cytovene) capsules as prophylactic treatment for preventing HIV-related cytomegalovirus disease.

- November 17: The FDA approves doxorubicin hydrochloride liposome injection (Doxil) for treating Kaposi's sarcoma.

- November 20: The FDA gives accelerated approval for lamivudine (3TC) (Epivir) to be used with zidovudine (AZT) (Retrovir) in treating AIDS/HIV.

- December 6: The FDA approves saquinavir (Invirase), the first protease inhibitor, for use with other nucleotide analog medications. This application is approved only 97 days after the FDA receives the marketing application.

- December 12: The FDA releases the report "Timely Access to New Drugs in the 1990s, An International Comparison." This documents that the FDA's high standards do not delay consumer access to important new drugs compared with situations in other countries, and that the United States makes available valuable drugs as soon as (and often sooner than) do counterparts worldwide.

- December 21: The FDA grants traditional approval for stavudine (d4T) (Zerit) for treating adults with HIV who have had prolonged prior AZT therapy.

- The WHO global program on AIDS is closed and replaced by UNAIDS.

- The Olympic gold medalist Greg Louganis reveals that he is HIV-positive.

1996

- A short-course regimen is identified for reducing perinatal HIV transmission in the developing world.

- January: The Joint United Nations Program on AIDS (UNAIDS) is launched.

- Magic Johnson returns to pro basketball, rejoining the Los Angeles Lakers.

- The heavyweight boxer Tommy Morrison, shown to be HIV-positive in testing before a fight, is barred from boxing.

- Researchers present their belief that Kaposi's sarcoma is caused by HHV-8, a herpesvirus.

- By the time of the 11th International Conference on AIDS in Vancouver in July 1996, many researchers and physicians share a belief that triple-combination therapy is superior to dual-combination therapy.

- March 1: The FDA gives full approval for ritonavir (Norvir), to be used alone or in combination with nucleoside analog medications for people with advanced HIV disease.

- March 4: The FDA grants full approval for an intravitreal implant (Vitrasert) with ganciclovir (Cytovene) for treating CMV retinitis.

- March 13: The FDA gives accelerated approval for indinavir (Crixivan) for use alone or in combination with nucleoside analog medications in those with HIV or AIDS. After receipt of the marketing application, the FDA approves the drug in only 42 days.

- March 14: The FDA approves the Coulter HIV-1 Antigen Assay, which is a test kit that can be used to screen blood donors for HIV-1.

- April 8: The FDA grants full approval for a daunorubicin citrate liposome injection (Dauno-Xome) for first-line cytotoxic treatment of advanced HIV-associated Kaposi's sarcoma.

- May 14: The FDA approves the first over-the-counter (OTC) HIV test for at-home use. Components of the Confide HIV Testing System are an over-the-counter home blood collection kit; HIV-antibody testing at a certified lab; and a test-result center that provides test results, counseling, and referral, all of which are done anonymously.

- June 12: The FDA approves azithromycin (Zithromax) to prevent or delay the onset of infection with *Mycobacterium avium* complex (MAC).

- June 21: The FDA grants accelerated approval for nevirapine (Viramune) for use with nucleoside analog to treat those with HIV who have clinical and/or immunological deterioration.

- June 26: The FDA approves cidofovir (Vistide) as an intravenous treatment for AIDS-related cytomegalovirus retinitis.

- July 17: The FDA sends a letter to health care workers to inform them of about 15 case reports of spontaneous bleeding in HIV-positive people with hemophilia being treated with HIV protease inhibitors at the time of the event.

- August 6: The FDA approves the first HIV test based on use of urine samples. It detects the presence of antibodies to HIV-1 with an enzyme-linked immunosorbent assay (ELISA) method.

- At year's end, UNAIDS reports that safer sex practices have led to a decline in the number of new HIV infections in many countries, including the United States, Australia, New Zealand, northern European countries, and parts of sub-Saharan Africa. Worldwide, however, the rate of infections continues to grow rapidly.

- In San Francisco, the first AIDS hospice founded is closed because fewer people are dying of AIDS thanks to new treatments.

1997

- February: The first decline in AIDS deaths is reported.

- March 14: The FDA grants accelerated approval for nelfinavir (Viracept), the first protease inhibitor available for use by children as well as adults. The FDA also grants pediatric labeling for the protease inhibitor ritonavir (Norvir).

- April 4: The FDA gives accelerated approval to delavirdine (Rescriptor), which is a nonnucleoside reverse transcriptase inhibitor that can be used in combination with other antiretroviral drugs for treating HIV-1.

- June 11: The FDA issues a public health advisory regarding reports of diabetes and hyperglycemia in patients receiving protease inhibitors for treatment of HIV-1.

- August 4: The FDA approves paclitaxel (Taxol) for second-line treatment of Kaposi's sarcoma that is AIDS-related.

- September 26: The FDA approves Combivir, a combination of zidovudine (AZT) and lamivudine 3TC, antiretroviral drugs already approved for treating HIV.

- The FDA sends out a warning to consumers and pharmacists about two unapproved and fraudulently marketed home-use test kits advertised on the Internet for home testing of HIV and hepatitis A.

- A final ruling is made by the FDA requiring labeling of latex condoms with an expiration date; the ruling is based on testing that was done after the product received various latex-aging tests.

- November 7: The FDA approves a new formulation of saquinavir (Invirase) (Fortovase) for treatment of HIV-1.

- It becomes clear that the number of people affected by the side effects of protease inhibitor drugs is greater than once believed. Because some of these side effects are serious, the FDA issues a warning concerning diabetes and hyperglycemia in patients receiving protease inhibitors.

- At the end of 1997, UNAIDS reports an HIV epidemic far worse worldwide than had previously been thought. Surveillance shows that about 30 million are living with HIV/AIDS, and about 16,000 new infections occur daily.

- Worldwide, 1 in 100 adults in the 15 to 49-year-old age group is believed to be HIV-positive, but only 1 in 10 of them is aware of the infection. It is estimated that by the year 2000, the number of those with HIV/AIDS could be as high as 40 million. It is believed that about 2.3 million have died of AIDS: nearly half of those are women and 460,000 children younger than 15. A report by UNAIDS states that the full impact of the epidemic, in terms of AIDS mortality rate, is just beginning to be felt.

1998

- Analysis of a blood sample from the person with the oldest documented HIV case (1959) shows that the first such infection probably occurred decades before.

- The Congressional Black Caucus provides additional funding for minority AIDS-prevention programs.

- The United Nations issues recommendations that urge HIV-infected mothers not to breast-feed their infants.

- May 28: The FDA approves Cambridge Biotech HIV-1, a Western blot test with a new indication for urine specimen testing.

- August 26: The FDA approves fomivirsen sodium intravitreal injectable (Vitravene) injection to treat cytomegalovirus retinitis in those with AIDS who have proved intolerant of or unresponsive to other treatments.

- September 17: The FDA approves efavirenz (Sustiva) to treat HIV and AIDS.

- December 17: The FDA approves abacavir (Ziagen) for HIV-1 in adults and children.

- In Canada, an outbreak of HIV infection occurs among IV drug users in Vancouver.

- After a Thailand trial shows zidovudine's (AZT's) effectiveness in preventing mother-to-child transmission, Glaxo Wellcome cuts the price of AZT by 75 percent.

- AIDSVAX starts the first human trial of an AIDS vaccine using 5,000 volunteers in the United States.

- In South Africa, the AIDS activist Gugu Diamini is beaten to death by neighbors after revealing her HIV-positive status on television. This occurs on the heels of Deputy President Thabo Mbeki's request for people to "break the silence about AIDS" to quell the epidemic's spread.

- UNAIDS estimates that during 1998, 5.8 million people have contracted HIV, and half of these are younger than 25. About 70 percent of all new infections and 80 percent of all deaths are in sub-Saharan Africa.

- After being called upon to lift the ban on federal funding for needle exchange programs, U.S. Health and Human Services Secretary Donna Shalala announces findings that such programs probably would decrease the spread of HIV/AIDS, that such programs do not necessarily lead to increased drug use, but that federal funding will not be advanced for financing needle exchanges.

- The Centers for Disease Control and Prevention announces a drop in AIDS deaths of 47 percent from 1996 to 1997, but the fact remains that new infections amount to about 40,000 a year.

1999

- January 5: The FDA approves atovaquone (Mepron) for prevention of *Pneumocystis carinii* pneumonia.
- February 2: The FDA approves alitretinoin (Panretin) for topical treatment of cutaneous lesions in patients with AIDS-related Kaposi's sarcoma.
- February 17: A businessman is sentenced to more than five years for selling bogus HIV testing kits.
- A large-scale study of HIV infection among young gay men in New York City shows that large numbers of these men have become HIV-infected in the past two years.
- The Leadership and Investment in Fighting an Epidemic Initiative is introduced to address the global AIDS pandemic.
- The number of AIDS cases acquired by perinatal transmission declines to 144 annual cases, an all-time low.
- In the United Kingdom, the number of HIV-positive prisoners reaches an all-time high.
- In the United States, a doctor who injected his former lover with AIDS-infected blood is sentenced to 50 years in prison.
- University of Alabama researchers claim that they have discovered that the source of HIV is a chimpanzee in West Central Africa.
- AIDS produces the fourth-highest total of deaths worldwide, according to the annual World Health Report.
- The Ugandan Ministry of Health begins a voluntary door-to-door HIV screening program in an effort to squelch the AIDS epidemic that has claimed 700,000 lives in the country. Since 1986, the government has launched several successful initiatives. In 1992 about 30 percent of people in Kampala have HIV; by 1999, the figure is 12 percent.

- South Africa wages a battle with U.S. and multinational pharmaceutical companies to force a drug price cut.
- Initial findings from a joint Uganda-U.S. study spotlight the viability of a new drug regimen, a single oral dose of the antiretroviral drug nevirapine, remarkable for its greater affordability and effectiveness in reducing vertical transmission of HIV.
- HIV vaccine development suffers a setback when health care authorities announce that people infected with a weakened form of HIV more than 17 years ago have begun to show signs of AIDS.
- Russia's official AIDS prevention center reports a 12-fold increase in the rate of new HIV cases in Moscow.
- March 2: The FDA approves a supplement to Amplicor HIV-1 Monitor Test. The FDA also approves another supplement for patient monitoring, which can be used to help manage those individuals on highly active antiretroviral therapy (HAART).
- March 29: A couple is sentenced for distributing an ozone generator marketed as a way to oxidize body toxins, curing everything from gangrene to cancer to AIDS. The previous year, in a Florida court, Kenneth Thiefault and his wife, Mardol Barber, had been convicted on conspiracy, distribution of an ozone generator, mail and wire fraud, and tax violations.
- April 15: The FDA gives accelerated approval to amprenavir (Agenerase) 50-mg and 150-mg capsules and oral solution; this protease inhibitor can be used with other antiretroviral agents for treating HIV-1.
- June 29: The FDA approves ritonavir (Norvir) 100-mg soft gelatin capsules.
- August 17: The FDA issues its final ruling on over-the-counter drug products containing colloidal silver; it is stated that certain products

containing colloidal silver or silver salts are not recognized as safe and effective and are mislabeled as appropriate for treating HIV/AIDS and other diseases.

- By the end of 1999, UNAIDS estimates that 33 million people worldwide have HIV/AIDS.

2000

- Launched on Valentine's Day, 2000, the AIDS Channel on the Internet features live broadcasts from the house of a Canadian AIDS activist, Richard Hollingsworth, who tries to auction his corpse on eBay and whose HIV-infected blood is used in some paintings. The point, says Hollingsworth, is for webcasts of his home life with his wife and five stepchildren to raise AIDS awareness. The site, http://www.aidschannel. com, also features HIV/AIDS information.

- June 19: The FDA and Cal-Tech Diagnostics sign a consent decree to stop manufacture and sale of HIV in vitro diagnostic test kits until manufacturing problems are corrected.

- July: The XIII International AIDS Conference in Durban, South Africa, stuns the 12,000 participants, as they visit "ground zero" of the epidemic in 2000. At the conference, 5,000 doctors and scientists sign the Durban Declaration, which confirms their belief in the overwhelming evidence that HIV is the cause of AIDS.

- September 15: A lopinavir and ritonavir combination (Kaletra) is approved for combination use with other antiretroviral agents for treating HIV in adults and children six months and older.

- October: The Global AIDS Program is created to coordinate the Centers for Disease Control and Prevention's international HIV/AIDS programs.

- October 31: The new formulation of dideoxy-inosine (ddI) enteric coated capsule (Videx EC) is approved for use in combination with other antiretrovirals for adults with HIV-1 whose management requires once-a-day administration of didanosine or an alternative didanosine formulation.

- November 14: Trizivir, a fixed-dose combination of abacavir (ABC) (Ziagen), zidovudine (AZT) (Retrovir), and lamivudine (3TC) (Epivir), receives new-formulation approval for treating HIV in adults and adolescents. Because it is a fixed-dose tablet, it cannot be used in treating those whose weight is less than 40 kilograms.

- December 22: The FDA alerts health care providers and patients about a potential safety concern involving an unapproved experimental product for HIV/AIDS, goat antiserum: it has allegedly been stolen from a "storage facility."

2001

- Figures are released by the U.S. government on the HIV/AIDS epidemic as of December 31, 2001:

  People living with HIV/AIDS: about 900,000

  People who may not know they are HIV-positive: about 300,000

  Number of new HIV infections per year: about 40,000

  Percentage of new HIV infections in males: 70 percent

  Percentage of new HIV infections in females: 30 percent

  Cumulative AIDS cases (through December 2001): 816,149

  Cumulative number of those who have died of AIDS as of December 31, 2001: 467,910

- The CDC announces the new HIV Prevention Strategic Plan to cut annual HIV infections in the United States by half within five years.

- January 5: The FDA and Bristol Myers Squibb issue a caution for HIV combination therapy with stavudine (Zerit) and didanosine (Videx) in pregnant women.

- July 20: The FDA announces that a scientific review panel has confirmed that condoms are effective against HIV/AIDS, but epidemiologic studies are insufficient to confirm that they provide protection against other sexually transmitted diseases.

- September 21: The FDA approves the first nucleic acid test systems to screen plasma for HIV and hepatitis C. The FDA licenses the first nucleic acid test (NAT) systems intended for screening plasma donors. These are expected to ensure further the safety of plasma-derived products by permitting earlier detection of HIV and hepatitis C infections in donors.

- September 26: The FDA approves TrueGene HIV-1 Genotyping Kit and Open Gene DNA Sequencing System (Visible Genetics, Inc.) for use in pinpointing drug resistance in HIV patients.

- October 26: Accelerated approval is granted to tenofovir disoproxil fumarate (Viread) for treating HIV-1 along with other antiretroviral medicines. This is the first nucleotide analog approved for HIV-1 treatment.

- The South African government appeals a high court ruling that state hospitals must dispense nivirapine to HIV-positive women who give birth in state hospitals. The health minister, however, agrees to assess its policy, regardless of the outcome of the appeal. The government's fear is that the ruling will lead to legal action demanding antiretroviral drugs for all 4.7 million HIV-positive South Africans. The government ultimately loses its case: the Pretoria High Court orders it to provide nevirapine to all pregnant HIV-positive mothers and their infants. The state is also required to provide formula milk to prevent infection through breast-feeding. The prominent AIDS activist group Treatment Action Campaign takes the health department to court.

- New research shows that more than three-quarters of U.S. AIDS patients may be becoming resistant to one or more of their drugs within three years of initiating treatment. Knowledge that drug-resistant HIV is spreading faster than expected serves to reinforce concern about the waning usefulness of treatments that extend lives. One scientist reports that on the basis of blood tests conducted on 1,647 patients in 1999, three years after beginning medical care, 78 percent carried a virus resistant to at least one drug in the cocktail of medicine they took, and half were resistant to more than one class of drug.

- An HIV conference in Thailand addresses the needs and rights of those with HIV/AIDS.

- Roche announces plans for enlarging access to its experimental fusion inhibitor (T-20), a new HIV treatment. A worldwide open-label safety study, code-named T-20 305, is scheduled to begin between January and April 2002.

- Defying pressure by pharmaceutical companies, Nigeria becomes the first African country to import cheap knockoffs of patented AIDS drugs. Nigeria announces plans to begin distributing drugs produced by the Indian company Cipla at a fraction of the prices that major drug firms charge.

- Iran announces a jump in HIV figures, and health officials say that the main cause of transmission is use of unclean needles to inject drugs, especially in jails.

- The U.S. National Institutes for Health recommend that people taking antiretrovirals for HIV not use the dietary supplement garlic, which prevents many antiretrovirals from working correctly. Researchers have found that garlic supplements sharply reduce blood levels of the protease inhibitor saquinavir.

- The British charity ActionAid helps to launch a survivors' group called Widows of the Genocide (Avega), with more than 25,000 Tutsi women members in Rwanda, in response to the traumatic aftermath of the Hutu genocide of Tutsis in Rwanda in 1994, when thousands of women were gang-raped by Hutu soldiers and members of militias that led the slaughter of 800,000 Tutsis and Hutus. Women coping with the trauma of 1994 discover that the murderers have given them HIV; of 1,400 members of Avega tested in 2001, two-thirds are HIV-positive.

- Continuing to deny the extent of the AIDS crisis in Africa, South Africa's president Thabo Mbeki rebukes his predecessor, Nelson Mandela, for insisting that drugs be made available to the millions of South Africans with HIV.

- The Chinese health minister Zhang Wenkang predicts that China may have 10 million HIV carriers by the year 2010—"if the current 30-percent annual growth rate is not curbed."

- March: Reports indicate that many of the 75 infertility clinics in Britain demonstrate bias against treating people with HIV.

- Of the 5 million infected with HIV in 2001, 3.5 million live in sub-Saharan Africa, where women's powerlessness makes any insistence on condom use futile.

- Scientists and health care workers announce that a global condom shortage and the continuing reluctance of men to use condoms are two conditions causing a worldwide explosion in HIV/AIDS.

- December: UNAIDS, the UN's HIV/AIDS branch, reports that there are 50 million living with HIV/AIDS. Also in 2001, there are 3 million AIDS-related deaths and 5 million new HIV infections. Of the 5 million new infections, 3.5 million occur in sub-Saharan Africa. The 14,000 new infections occurring each day are mostly (95 percent) in developing countries; of those, 2,000 are in children younger than 15. The regions with the fastest growth in new infections are Eastern Europe and Central Asia, with 250,000 new infections. In the Russian Federation, new reported diagnoses have almost doubled from 1998 to 2001. Of adults in Botswana, 36 percent have HIV; in Zimbabwe, 25 percent. AIDS has orphaned more than 12 million children in sub-Saharan Africa.

- Researchers find that cholesterol-lowering drugs may slow the advance of HIV. Research published in the journal *Proceedings of the National Academy of Sciences* shows findings that removing cholesterol from cells in a test tube may severely inhibit the action of HIV.

- A legal ruling makes it a crime to knowingly infect someone with HIV. After a trial at Glasgow High Court in Scotland, a jury decides that Stephen Kelly has acted culpably and recklessly by having unprotected sex with Anne Craig, even though he knows he is HIV-positive. Kelly receives a five-year sentence.

- At the World Trade Organization (WTO) Doha meeting, November 2001, developing countries win a coup in relaxing drug patents, a move that proponents expect will reduce the costs of reme-dies for treating diseases that kill millions of indigent people yearly. Countries can seek a waiver on public health grounds from strict WTO rules that guarantee drug patents for 20 years.

- A rural South African rumor that having sex with a virgin cures AIDS leads to a trial of six men who are accused of raping a nine-month-old baby; the trial draws attention to the 80 percent increase in child sexual abuse in one year. In 2000, more than 67,000 cases of rape and sexual assault against children are reported, compared to 37,500 in 1998.

- A new anti-HIV drug derived from coal is tested in military clinics in Tanzania; about 350 HIV-positive soldiers take it. Developed by a subsidiary of CEF, the South African state oil company, the drug is supposed to strengthen the immune system.

- A seaweed derivative is studied in the United States to see whether it contains the key to killing the human immunodeficiency virus. The microbicide Carraguard, derived from the seaweed *Chrondus crispus,* is already used in cosmetics and foods. Researchers want to discover whether it can be used in a microbicidal gel that women can use, and are testing it in chemical cocktails to determine whether it can kill HIV and other sexually transmitted diseases. Four studies are in human trials.

- Researchers identify a new strain of HIV that resists treatment by AZT. It appears that this strain has an inherent capacity to resist treatment. In the past, this level of resistance was seldom seen in patients who had not been taking any drugs to fight HIV. Tests show that this strain can become AZT-resistant in two weeks, whereas normal HIV strains require months to do so.

- Leaders of Asian nations join forces to seek avenues for cutting the costs of AIDS treatments, in an effort to buy drugs in bulk and negotiate collectively with pharmaceutical companies. More than 1.5 million people in Southeast Asia have HIV.

- A former Japanese health ministry official is found guilty of negligence for failing to prevent the sale of untreated blood products. A Tokyo court sentences Akihito Matsumura to one year in prison. Since the early eighties, more than 1,800 hemophiliacs in Japan have contracted HIV from untreated blood, and more than 500 have died.

- May: About 80 percent of Rwandan women have HIV. Many were infected by rape by troops during the 1994 genocide of 1 million Tutsis and Hutus.

- The South African president, Thabo Mbeki, says that the West blames the South African AIDS epidemic on "lustful, lower-order, germ-carrying" blacks—a statement that shocks and disappoints AIDS experts. Mbeki has openly expressed doubts about the link between HIV and AIDS, and he also doubts the scale of the epidemic, even though South Africa has the highest number of AIDS/HIV sufferers in the world, estimated at about 4.7 million.

- Human rights advocates are outraged when Colombian guerrillas force an entire municipality in their government-granted safe haven to take AIDS tests. Three are forced from their homes after a positive test result. The much-feared field marshal Jorge Briceno of the Revolutionary Armed Forces of Colombia forces the testing.

- Medical experts in Thailand predict that Myanmar's AIDS epidemic will soon eclipse the worst in Africa. The AIDS specialist Dr. Chris Beyrer, a U.S. researcher at Johns Hopkins University, estimates that about 4 to 7 percent of the population of Myanmar has HIV.

- For the first time, Ireland reports that most new HIV infections are in heterosexuals, two-thirds of whom are women. Daily, the small country has one new case.

- It is reported that an uncommon form of hepatitis—hepatitis G—appears to make those with HIV fare better. HIV patients without hepatitis G are shown to be 3.6 times more likely to die over a two-year period than are those who have both viruses. Researchers are studying this finding to discover whether it may provide a new way to block HIV.

- The head of the United Nations' AIDS program announces a belief that racial prejudice is helping to spread HIV worldwide. Dr. Peter Piot tells delegates at the world racism conference in South Africa that if the AIDS epidemic had centered in Europe and mainly affected whites, the response would have been faster and more generous. He emphasizes that laws against prejudice and AIDS should encourage patients to feel safe in revealing their status. Dr. Piot opines that unequal access to lifesaving HIV treatments is one of the worst global examples of discrimination.

- Scientists at an international conference in Philadelphia say that an HIV vaccine is now feasible. Many potential vaccines are being tested, but much research remains to test safety and effectiveness. David Baltimore, a conference organizer, says he is more optimistic than in the past that a vaccine now being tested will provide a level of immunity that will make a difference.

- In the United States, VaxGen announces that it is in the final stages of large-scale human trials that involve the inoculation of thousands of gay men in North America and IV drug users in Thailand. It is believed that even if it is only 40 percent effective, the vaccine will be in great demand. Unfortunately, in preliminary trials, some volunteers become infected with HIV.

- The European Commission announces its intention to accelerate new drug approval and to ease the ban on advertising prescription drugs, thus allowing pharmaceutical companies to market drugs directly to those who suffer from diabetes, AIDS, and asthma. The new fast-track program, based on that of the United States, may reduce the time required for companies to win approval for drugs from 18 months to nine to 12 months.

- The United States moves to block European Commission proposals to get cheap drugs into developing countries. Advisers to President George W. Bush object to the campaign to relax key trade agreements on intellectual property rights.

- In Brazil, the health minister, José Serra, asks the public health lab to produce a generic version of nelfinavir, a drug patented by the Swiss firm

Roche, with the goal of reducing the cost by 40 percent. This could make Brazil the first country to break a patent on a drug used to treat AIDS. Brazil is estimated to have the highest number of people with AIDS in Latin America—about 200,000. Of them, 25 percent use nelfinavir.

- U.S. and South African doctors begin a human trial of an AIDS vaccine using a horse disease (Venezuelan equine encephalitis) to combat the most prevalent strain of HIV in South Africa.

- The Swedish Institute for Infectious Disease Control announces that the number of new HIV cases in Sweden has increased by 48 percent in the first half of 2001 compared to the same period the previous year. It is believed that many of the 155 new cases can be attributed to IV drug use.

- U.S. Surgeon General David Satcher angers conservative Christians and causes the administration to do a distancing act when he publishes a report that recommends more comprehensive sex education and distribution of condoms in schools. The report also rejects as unsubstantiated the claim that homosexuality is a reversible lifestyle choice and states that stigmatizing gay men and lesbians could result in mental health problems. President George W. Bush says he wants federal funds to be spent on programs that promote the idea of avoiding sex before marriage.

- GlaxoSmithKline extends its offer of cheap AIDS drugs to 63 countries.

- The FDA warns companies that make AIDS drugs to modulate the optimistic tone of their ads for antiretroviral drugs. Some people contend that many such ads are misleading, failing to point out the limitations of drugs and featuring photos of healthy-looking people who do not accurately depict typical AIDS sufferers. Initial complaints are lodged by AIDS activists in San Francisco, who are protesting magazine and billboard ads that feature healthy-looking models performing athletic feats such as mountain climbing, when, in fact, those who take highly active antiretroviral drugs actually experience side effects that are often debilitating, and these individuals do not remotely resemble the models in the advertising. Companies are given 90 days to comply with the directive to modify ads.

- The United States, the first country to pledge money to the United Nations fund set up to provide economic support for countries that have the worst AIDS epidemics, donates $200 million to the multibillion-dollar global AIDS effort.

- The legal case of 39 large drug companies against the South African government collapses, setting off rejoicing in the developing world. The result is that drugs these companies supply to South Africa will be supplied at drastically reduced prices; for example, a year's supply of triple-therapy drugs will be sold for $600–$700 a year, compared to $10,000 in the United States. South Africa will also be able to import cheap drugs from Brazil and India, where some patents for drugs that are copied have expired (this includes some that treat opportunistic infections).

- President George W. Bush appoints Scott Evertz, a gay man, director of the Office of National AIDS Policy.

- The Centers for Disease Control and Prevention reports that the incidence of HIV in those older than 50 is increasing at twice the rate of increase in younger people.

- Chengdu, a city in the central province of Sichuan in China, prohibits HIV-positive people from marrying and orders compulsory HIV testing of those in high-risk groups who are arrested. It also bans HIV-positive people from teaching and segregates them in prisons.

- The FDA approves tenofovir disoproxil fumarate tablets (Viread) in combination with other antiretroviral drugs for treatment of HIV-1.

2002

- At University Hospital Lausanne, in Switzerland, scientists identify a gene that may partly explain why some people with HIV respond better to treatment than do others. The hope is that this discovery will help doctors develop individually tailored treatments. Researchers find that in patients with the gene MDR1 3435C/T, a far greater increase in key immune system cells occurs after treatment, and this could be evidence that the body chemical produced by the gene, called P-glycoprotein, may be important to the success of antiretroviral drugs. *Lancet* reports that it will be some time before this study results in new medications.

- U.S. doctors come up with a new technique to boost the immune system in fighting HIV. The treatment calls for removing the immune cells that HIV targets from the body of a person with HIV and modifying these to make them more HIV-resistant, then returning the cells to the body. No full clinical trial has tested this on HIV patients as yet. Scientists know that the chemical component of HIV called gag must attach to the membrane, and they know that it

attaches to areas rich in cholesterol. HIV, after finding its way through the membrane, is able to replicate and exit to infect other cells. Researchers are now trying to find a way to block HIV and gag, perhaps with cholesterol-lowering drugs.

2003

See developments reported in early 2003 in the introduction.

Sources: AVERT Website, the AIDS-Arts Forum Website, National Institute of Allergy and Infectious Diseases "AIDS History" on Website, AIDS Project L.A. Website, CDC: "Milestones in the U.S. HIV Epidemic" online, CDC: "NIH Researchers Recall Early Years of AIDS," White House Website, U.S. Food and Drug Administration Website "Milestones."

APPENDIX III
HOME CARE FOR HIV/AIDS PATIENTS

The following are guidelines from the U.S. Centers for Disease Control and Prevention for providing effective care to people who have AIDS.

Sign up for a home care course so that you can learn all you can about managing various situations. These courses are offered by the Red Cross, state health departments, the Visiting Nurses' Association, and HIV/AIDS service groups.

Read about HIV and AIDS so that you understand the ins and outs of opportunistic infections. In caring for someone who has AIDS, remember that HIV is in blood, semen, vaginal fluid, and breast milk. On the other hand, you do cannot contract HIV from air, food, water, insects, animals, dishes, knives, forks, spoons, toilet seats, feces, nasal fluid, saliva, sweat, tears, urine, or vomit, unless blood is present in or on any of the items. You can, however, get germs from contact with some of these things, so it is important to be extremely careful.

Avoid touching infected blood, and do not allow it to splash in your eyes, nose, mouth, or an open cut or sore. When caregivers for people with AIDS have become infected in rare cases, it is believed that this resulted from sharing a razor, getting blood from the sick person in an open cut or sore, or having contact with the blood in some other way. Thus, you must protect yourself from infection by following universal precautions.

It is key for caregivers to understand the changes that often accompany HIV and AIDS. The patient gradually becomes sicker and sicker, and in some people, HIV damages the brain, making it hard to think clearly. A change from feeling well to being very sick can be a quick one. Thus, at the outset of caregiving, try to get some answers you may need to know at some point. Consider the following:

- Find out what the AIDS patient wants you to do. Some people are comfortable with having a caregiver provide all sorts of assistance in daily living, but others find too much help intrusive.

- Encourage the person you are taking care of to continue to take part in activities he or she enjoys.

- Promote the ideas of healthy diet and exercise, and discourage the use of cigarettes, illegal drugs, and alcoholic drinks.

- Take care to respect the patient's privacy and encourage his or her independence.

- Ask the patient before do things to help whether assistance will be welcome.

- Inquire about what you can do to make your friend, relative, or partner more comfortable; let him or her know you are willing to assist him or her on trips to the bathroom if he or she wants, to provide help with dressing, and so on.

- Have a talk with the individual's doctor, nurse, social worker, case manager, or other health care worker to find out what you should and should not do. Before you visit any of those involved in her or his care, get written permission from the patient, because most health care professionals require this before talking to you.

- Jot down notes on proper dosages of medications and any side effects you should expect to see. Also, find out any danger signals you should watch for: Is a cough or fever sufficient reason to call the doctor? Or diarrhea? You need to know the kinds of problems and warnings that indicate that the patient needs his or her medication changed or needs hospitalization.

- Have a handy list of phone numbers of people you might need to call if the patient appears to need medical attention.

- Try to keep the home looking clean and cheerful, as you would for anyone who is ill.

- Make arrangements so that the patient is close to a bathroom.

- Have helpful items within the patient's reach: tissues, towels, blankets, trash can, and so on.

- Help the bed-ridden patient to change positions often, at least every four hours. This can help to stave off problems such as bedsores, stiffness, and pneumonia. Ask a nurse to show you how to use a sheet to help roll the patient from side to side in bed. If necessary, have a "medical trapeze" installed over the bed to allow the person to change positions independently (this does require some strength, however).

- Keep sheets dry, and put something very soft under the person with AIDS: a water mattress, egg-crate foam, or sheepskin. If you see red or broken skin, report this to the medical professional in charge of this person's care.

- If the patient is confined to a bed, help him or her do range-of-motion exercises to improve circulation.

- Give massages and back rubs.

- If the person cannot get up, have a bedpan within easy reach.

- Seek information from an attorney or an AIDS organization about being named the person's *care coordinator.* According to the Centers for Disease Control and Prevention, you may need this or power of attorney to handle insurance-claim filing, applications for government aid, and other business.

- If you need help in getting through the emotionally draining job of taking care of someone with AIDS, you can join a support group or see a counselor. On the same note, be sure to look after your own health needs: nutrition, exercise, rest, and regular outings with friends and family.

- Get information from AIDS service groups on respite care: arrangements for people who can care for the patient when you need to go somewhere.

- Provide emotional support. Make sure you understand the patient's need to feel involved in his or her care and not feel himself or herself a helpless sufferer. Chat about normal topics: books, movies, world events.

- Have quiet times: watching TV, reading, laughing, and so forth.

- Be a good listener if the person wants to talk about the disease and feelings of fear, loneliness, and anger.

- Invite the patient's friends to visit.

- Give comfort. Do not hesitate to hug, kiss, pat, and hold hands.

- If your friend or relative can get out, take him or her on walks or rides, or just out on the porch.

- Wash your hands often and thoroughly (at least 15 seconds with warm, soapy water) so that you do not transfer germs to the patient. Make sure that you are methodical about doing this before preparing food and after using the bathroom. If you touch your nose, mouth, or genitals, or if you touch anyone's blood, semen, urine, vaginal fluid, or feces, wash your hands. Use hand cream if your hands become red or raw from the repeated washings.

- Keep your cuts and sores covered with bandages. Anytime that you have cold sores, fever blisters, or another skin infection, do not touch the patient or anything that he or she uses. If you must take care of him or her at this time, wear disposable gloves. (Remember, too, that gloves can be used only one time.)

- Keep people away from the patient if they have boils, impetigo, and/or shingles. Ask visitors who are sick to return after they are well. Remember, an AIDS patient cannot fight colds, flu, and other common ailments. If you become sick and you are the only person available to care for the AIDS patient, you must wear a surgical mask that covers your mouth and nose.

- Keep chickenpox germs away because this disease is very dangerous for someone with AIDS; it can be fatal. Once chickenpox sores have completely crusted over, the person then can enter the room of the AIDS patient. Even someone who has been exposed to chickenpox should stay away for three weeks.

• Anyone who has shingles (herpes zoster) should not enter the patient's room until all the sores have healed over. The shingles germ can also cause chickenpox.

• If the AIDS patient is accidentally exposed to measles, shingles, or chickenpox, call the doctor to get a prescription for a preventive medication.

• Make sure that anyone who is helping with care or living in the house of the AIDS patient has had regular childhood shots.

• Anyone living with an AIDS patient who has to get a polio vaccination should ask for an injection with *inactivated virus,* according to the Centers for Disease Control and Prevention. This is because a regular oral polio vaccine has weakened polio virus that can spread from the one who had the shot to the AIDS patient and give him or her polio.

• Make sure that each person in the house with the AIDS patient gets a flu shot and a tuberculosis test yearly.

• Do not share anything that might have any blood from the person with HIV: razors, toothbrushes, pierced jewelry, tweezers, and so on.

• Take care with pets. Have the person with AIDS wash his or her hands after playing with the pet, and make sure litter boxes are emptied daily. If the pet becomes sick, keep it away from the ill individual and take it to the vet.

• When washing sheets and clothes that have blood, semen, feces, urine, vomit, or vaginal fluid on them, use disposable gloves and use a normal wash cycle, hot or cold water. If you cannot wash these things right away, store them in plastic bags.

• Keep the house clean and mop floors often. Keep the toilet clean with a commercial cleaner or a bleach-and-water solution (one-quarter cup bleach to one gallon of water). Replace plastic urinals and bedpans once a month. Make up a new batch of bleach-and-water solution each time because it is effective for only 24 hours.

• Follow food cautions: no raw eggs or milk; no raw fish or shellfish; meat cooked with no pink in the middle; utensils washed before reusing with other foods; washing of cutting board between uses for different foods and after use; prevention of contact of blood from meats with other foods; careful washing of fruits and vegetables; avoidance of organic lettuce and organic vegetables that cannot be peeled or cooked; washing of dishes with hot water and soap; avoidance of food preparation if you have diarrhea; serving of hot foods hot and cold foods cold; prompt storing of leftovers.

• If the patient with AIDS has a persistent cough, inform the doctor so the patient can be given a TB test. If the result is positive, everyone in the household should be checked for TB infection because medication may be required.

• If the patient gets jaundice or has chronic hepatitis B, everyone in the house and anyone who has had sex with the patient should check with a doctor to find out whether they need medication. Children in the house should get the hepatitis AB vaccine even if they are not in close proximity with the person with AIDS.

• Do not kiss or touch fever blisters or cold sores on the mouth or nose of the patient. If you need to touch them, you must wear gloves and wash your hands after removing them. Dispose of the gloves each time.

• Always wash your hands after you have touched the saliva or urine of an AIDS patient because many people with and without AIDS have cytomegalovirus. If a pregnant woman gets CMV, she can infect her unborn child, causing birth defects.

• In buying gloves, get the disposable, hospital-type latex or vinyl variety; do not reuse even if the package says they can be reused. The other option is to use household rubber gloves, good for housekeeping but not appropriate for use with a person with AIDS because of their bulk. Rubber gloves can be cleaned and reused; use hot, soapy water and a bleach–water mixture (one-quarter cup bleach to one gallon water).

• In removing gloves, peel them down by turning inside out to keep the wet side on the inside, away from your skin and the skin of other people. After removing them, immediately wash your hands well.

- Clean up spilled blood as soon as possible.

- If you accidentally get any blood-tinged body fluid in your eyes, nose, or mouth, quickly flood water into the spot that has been splashed. Call a doctor and ask what else you need to do.

- If you administer medicine with needles and syringes, take great care not to stick yourself. A needle and syringe are good for one use only. Do not replace caps on needles; do not pick up a needle with your fingers (use tweezers); do not take needles off syringes; do not break or bend needles. You should hold the sharp end of a needle away from you and touch needles and syringes by the barrel only. Put used needles and syringes into a puncture-proof container that is provided by health care professionals and AIDS organizations. If you do not have one, a coffee can will work. Ask the AIDS patient's doctor or nurse how to dispose of the container that holds used needles and syringes.

- If you are stuck by a needle, place the needle into the appropriate container and immediately wash where you stuck yourself. Use warm, soapy water and then call the doctor or a hospital emergency room and ask what you need to do. If the doctor wants you to take AZT, you must do so within a few hours.

- Get rid of all liquid waste that has blood in it by flushing it down the toilet. All items that cannot be flushed—sanitary pads, paper towels, dressings and bandages, diapers, and so on—should be put into a bag and sealed closed. Ask health care professionals where you should dispose of these. Wear gloves during this process.

- Follow strict safe-sex precautions if you are having sex with a person who has HIV infection.

- If you see signs of dementia (short attention span; trouble with speaking, moving, and think-ing; poor memory; mood swings; malaise), check with the patient's health care provider to find out what you should do. Also, remove dangerous objects from his or her reach, and remember to speak in simple sentences to promote ease of understanding.

- In children with HIV or AIDS, watch for breathing problems, diarrhea, unusual sleepiness, and changes in appetite. Check with the doctor before having any immunizations. Oral polio vaccine is contraindicated for these children.

- Provide toys that are plastic and washable. Keep stuffed toys washed and clean. Make sure the child stays away from the cat's litter box and any sandbox a pet might have been inside. If a child with HIV or AIDS is exposed to chickenpox, contact the doctor immediately for advice. Keep cuts and scrapes bandaged and use gloves if the child bleeds. Provide lots of hugs and kisses and rocking. Let the child be around other kids.

- Be prepared for the late stages of AIDS, which require certain precautions. You will see signs that the AIDS patient is in the final phase of the disease. He or she will sleep more and be harder to waken. You will note some mental confusion and restlessness. The patient will lose bladder and bowel control and may require a catheter and require frequent cleanups. His or her skin may feel cool and may darken on the side of the body touching the bed. Do not use electric blankets but do keep the patient covered with blankets. He or she may experience trouble seeing and hearing. He or she may stop eating and drinking, so you will need to wipe his or her mouth with a wet cloth frequently and apply lip moisturizer. He or she may urinate infrequently. Breathing can become noisy; that can be helped by putting extra pillows under his or her head or raising the head of the bed. Feed ice chips if the person can swallow. Call the doctor if the patient's breathing becomes irregular or if it appears that he or she stops breathing for a minute.

APPENDIX IV
STATE REQUIREMENTS ON STD/HIV/AIDS EDUCATION (DECEMBER 2001)

In 40 states, public schools require education about sexually transmitted diseases, including HIV and AIDS. The following are specific state-by-state requirements:

Alabama: STD/HIV/AIDS education required; must stress abstinence and contraception.

Alaska: STD/HIV/AIDS education required; no specific content requirements to follow.

Arizona: No STD/HIV/AIDS education required; if taught, instructors must stress abstinence.

Arkansas: No STD/HIV/AIDS education required; if taught voluntarily, teachers must stress abstinence.

California: STD/HIV/AIDS education required; must stress abstinence and contraception.

Colorado: No STD/HIV/AIDS education required; if taught voluntarily, teachers have no state-specific content to follow.

Connecticut: STD/HIV/AIDS education required; no state-specific content requirements exist.

Delaware: STD/HIV/AIDS education required; teachers must teach abstinence and contraception.

District of Columbia: STD/HIV/AIDS education required; teachers must cover contraception.

Florida: STD/HIV/AIDS education required; teachers have no state-specific content requirements.

Georgia: STD/HIV/AIDS education required; teachers must teach abstinence and localities may teach contraception.

Hawaii: STD/HIV/AIDS education required; teachers must stress abstinence and contraception.

Idaho: STD/HIV/AIDS education required; teachers have no state-specific content requirements.

Illinois: STD/HIV/AIDS education required; instructors must stress abstinence and contraception.

Indiana: STD/HIV/AIDS education required; must stress abstinence.

Iowa: STD/HIV/AIDS education required; no state-specific content requirements.

Kansas: STD/HIV/AIDS education required; no state-specific content requirements.

Kentucky: STD/HIV/AIDS education required; must teach abstinence.

Louisiana: No STD/HIV/AIDS education required; if taught voluntarily, teachers must stress abstinence.

Maine: STD/HIV/AIDS education required; teachers must stress abstinence and contraception.

Maryland: STD/HIV/AIDS education required; teachers must stress abstinence and contraception.

Massachusetts: No STD/HIV/AIDS education required; if taught voluntarily, teachers have no state-specific content.

Michigan: STD/HIV/AIDS education required; teachers must instruct in abstinence.

Minnesota: STD/HIV/AIDS education required; teachers have no state-specific content requirements.

Mississippi: No STD/HIV/AIDS education required; if taught, instructors must stress abstinence. If localities teach contraception, they must include information about failure rates or effectiveness. Localities may override required topics including abstinence, but they may not contradict required exclusions.

Missouri: STD/HIV/AIDS education required; must stress abstinence and contraception.

Montana: No STD/HIV/AIDS education required; if taught voluntarily, teachers have no state-specific content requirements.

Nebraska: No STD/HIV/AIDS education required; if taught voluntarily, teachers have no state-specific content requirements.

Nevada: STD/HIV/AIDS education required; no state-specific content requirements.

New Hampshire: STD/HIV/AIDS education required; no state-specific content requirements.

New Jersey: STD/HIV/AIDS education required; must stress abstinence. If localities teach contraception, they must include information on failure rates or effectiveness.

New Mexico: STD/HIV/AIDS education required; must stress abstinence and contraception.

New York: STD/HIV/AIDS education required; teachers must stress abstinence and contraception.

North Carolina: STD/HIV/AIDS education required; teachers must stress abstinence. If localities teach contraception, they must include information about failure rates or effectiveness.

North Dakota: STD/HIV/AIDS education required; teachers have no state-specific requirements.

Ohio: STD/HIV/AIDS education required; teachers must stress abstinence.

Oklahoma: STD/HIV/AIDS education required; teachers must teach abstinence and contraception.

Oregon: STD/HIV/AIDS education required; must stress abstinence and contraception.

Pennsylvania: STD/HIV/AIDS education required; must stress abstinence and contraception.

Rhode Island: STD/HIV/AIDS education required; must stress abstinence and contraception.

South Carolina: STD/HIV/AIDS education required; must stress abstinence and contraception.

South Dakota: No STD/HIV/AIDS education required; taught voluntarily, no state-specific content requirements. Abstinence is taught in character education.

Tennessee: STD/HIV/AIDS education required; teachers must stress abstinence.

Texas: No STD/HIV/AIDS education required; if taught voluntarily, must stress abstinence. If localities teach contraception, they must include information about failure rates or effectiveness.

Utah: STD/HIV/AIDS education required; must stress abstinence. Prohibits advocacy of use of contraceptive methods or devices. Teachers may not respond to students' questions in ways that conflict with these requirements.

Vermont: STD/HIV/AIDS education required; must teach abstinence and contraception.

Virginia: No STD/HIV/AIDS education required; if taught voluntarily, must teach abstinence and contraception.

Washington: STD/HIV/AIDS education required; teachers must stress abstinence and contraception.

West Virginia: STD/HIV/AIDS education required; teachers must stress abstinence and contraception.

Wisconsin: STD/HIV/AIDS education required; no state-specific content requirements.

Wyoming: STD/HIV/AIDS education required; no state-specific content requirements.

Source: Kaiser Family Foundation State Health Facts Online. Data source: Sex Education in the U.S.; Policy and Politics, Issue Update, September 2000.

APPENDIX V
MINORS' RIGHT TO CONSENT TO HIV/STD SERVICES (JANUARY 2003)

In all 50 states and the District of Columbia, minors have the right to consent to HIV/STD evaluation and treatment services. The following states have no specific rulings in regard to this right: Alaska, Arizona, Indiana, Massachusetts, Nebraska, South Dakota, Utah, West Virginia, and Wisconsin. Most states, however, have specific rulings regarding this right:

Alabama: Minor must be at least 12. State officially classifies HIV/AIDS as an STD or infectious disease, for which minors may consent to testing and treatment. Doctor may notify parents.

Arkansas: Doctor may notify parents.

California: Minor must be at least 12. Law explicitly authorizes minor to consent to HIV testing. Law does not apply to HIV treatment.

Colorado: Law explicitly authorizes minor to consent to HIV testing and/or treatment.

Connecticut: Law explicitly authorizes minor to consent to HIV testing and/or treatment.

Delaware: Minor must be at least 12. Doctor may notify parents. Law explicitly authorizes minor to consent to HIV testing and/or treatment.

Florida: State officially classifies HIV/AIDS as an STD or infectious disease, for which minors may consent to testing and treatment.

Georgia: State officially classifies HIV/AIDS as an STD or infectious disease, for which minors may consent to testing and treatment. Doctor may notify parents.

Hawaii: Minor must be at least 14. Doctor may notify parents.

Idaho: Minor must be at least 14. State officially classifies HIV/AIDS as an STD or infectious disease, for which minors may consent to testing and treatment.

Illinois: Minor must be at least 12. State officially classifies HIV/AIDS as an STD or infectious disease, for which minors may consent to testing and treatment. Doctor may notify parents.

Iowa: Law explicitly authorizes minor to consent to HIV testing and/or treatment. Parent must be notified if HIV test result is positive.

Kansas: Doctor may notify parents.

Kentucky: State officially classifies HIV/AIDS as an STD or infectious disease, for which minors may consent to testing and treatment. Doctor may notify parents.

Louisiana: Doctor may notify parents.

Maine: Doctor may notify parents.

Maryland: Doctor may notify parents.

Michigan: Doctor may notify parents. Law explicitly authorizes minor to consent to HIV testing and/or treatment.

Minnesota: Doctor may notify parents.

Mississippi: State officially classifies HIV/AIDS as an STD or infectious disease, for which minors may consent to testing and treatment.

Missouri: Doctor may notify parents.

Montana: Doctor may notify parents. Law explicitly authorizes minor to consent to HIV testing and/or treatment.

Nevada: State officially classifies HIV/AIDS as an STD or infectious disease, for which minors may consent to testing and treatment.

New Hampshire: Minor must be at least 14.

New Jersey: Doctor may notify parents.

New Mexico: Law explicitly authorizes minor to consent to HIV testing. Law does not apply to HIV treatment.

New York: Law explicitly authorizes minor to consent to HIV testing and/or treatment.

North Carolina: State officially classifies HIV/AIDS as an STD or infectious disease, for which minors may consent to testing and treatment.

North Dakota: Minor must be at least 14. Parent must be shown the informed consent form for an HIV test before the minor signs it.

Ohio: Law explicitly authorizes minor to consent to HIV testing. Law does not apply to HIV treatment.

Oklahoma: State officially classifies HIV/AIDS as an STD or infectious disease, for which minors may consent to testing and treatment. Doctor may notify parents.

Oregon: State officially classifies HIV/AIDS as an STD or infectious disease, for which minors may consent to testing and treatment.

Pennsylvania: State officially classifies HIV/AIDS as an STD or infectious disease, for which minors may consent to testing and treatment.

Rhode Island: Law explicitly authorizes minor to consent to HIV testing and/or treatment.

South Carolina: Any minor 16 and older may consent to any health service. Health services may be provided to minors of any age without parental consent when the provider believes the services are necessary.

Tennessee: State officially classifies HIV/AIDS as an STD or infectious disease, for which minors may consent to testing and treatment.

Texas: State officially classifies HIV/AIDS as an STD or infectious disease, for which minors may consent to testing and treatment. Doctor may notify parents.

Vermont: Minor must be at least 12. State officially classifies HIV/AIDS as an STD or infectious disease, for which minors may consent to testing and treatment.

Virginia: State officially classifies HIV/AIDS as an STD or infectious disease, for which minors may consent to testing and treatment.

Washington: Minor must be at least 14. State officially classifies HIV/AIDS as an STD or infectious disease, for which minors may consent to testing and treatment. Includes surgery.

Wyoming: State officially classifies HIV/AIDS as an STD or infectious disease, for which minors may consent to testing and treatment.

The Kaiser Family Foundation State Health Facts Online (http://statehealthfacts.Kff.org). Data Source: Alan Guttmacher Institute, January 2003 (available at http://www.agusa.org/pubs/spib_MASS.pdf).

APPENDIX VI
SEXUALLY TRANSMITTED DISEASES AT A GLANCE

Sexually transmitted diseases are an enormous public health problem. For that reason, the U.S. surgeon general has issued a "call to action to promote sexual health and responsible sexual behavior." Underscoring areas of concern, the surgeon general spotlights the following:

- Of the 10 most commonly reported infectious diseases in the United States, five are sexually transmitted.

- About 50 million people in the United States have genital herpes, and every year, there are 1 million new cases.

- About 15 percent of cases of infertility in U.S. women can be attributed to problems arising from chlamydia and gonorrhea.

- Four types of human papillomavirus (HPV)—the sexually transmissible virus that causes genital warts—cause about 80 percent of cervical cancer cases.

- In the United States, about 800,000 to 900,000 people are living with HIV. Approximately 40,000 new HIV infections occur yearly. About one-third of Americans do not know their HIV status because they have not been tested.

- The AIDS epidemic is shifting toward women. According to the CDC, women made up 32 percent of those reported with HIV from July 1999 to June 2000, whereas women accounted for only 28 percent of HIV cases reported since 1981.

- About 104,000 children fall prey to sexual abuse each year in the United States.

- Antihomosexual attitudes sometimes lead to antigay violence. Two dozen studies spotlight the fact that about 80 percent of gay men and lesbians were harassed verbally or physically because of their sexual orientation, 45 percent had received a threat of violence, and 17 percent had been attacked physically.

- About half of all U.S. pregnancies are not planned; considerable costs—increased welfare dependency, reduced employment and educational opportunities, and child abuse and neglect—are the result.

- In 1996, there were about 1,366,000 induced abortions in the United States.

STDs at a Glance

BACTERIAL VAGINOSIS

Bacterial vaginosis (BV) is considered a sexually associated infection because it is not officially classified as a sexually transmitted disease. A suspected link with sexual activity exists because BV is prevalent in sexually active women and rarely seen in virgins. A very common vaginal infection in women of childbearing age, BV is also called nonspecific vaginitis and gardnerella-associated vaginitis.

SIGNS/SYMPTOMS

Half of the women with BV have no symptoms. Others report a thin, bad-smelling white or gray vaginal discharge, burning with urination, and vaginal itching. After intercourse, they may note a fishlike odor. Three of the following are required for a BV diagnosis: clue cells (seen under a microscope), vaginal pH higher than 4.5, homogenous vaginal discharge, vaginal discharge that has a fishy odor if a drop is placed in 10 percent potassium hydroxide.

TRANSMISSION

Unclear. Most likely to contract BV is a woman who has multiple sex partners or who has a new sex partner. BV is not prevalent in monogamous couples. BV is not transmitted by objects or toilet seats.

TEST

Wet prep (microscopic examination of vaginal discharge).

TREATMENT

Antimicrobial medication. Although BV may clear up on its own, you should seek treatment because of the possibility of complications. Women who are not pregnant can use topical or oral metronidazole (Flagyl). Take all of the antimicrobial medicine prescribed. Flagyl should not be used during the first trimester of pregnancy.

PREVENTION

Use latex condoms and barriers (dental dams), limit your number of sex partners, and avoid douching, which upsets the vagina's natural ecosystem. Usually a male sex partner does not need treatment, but female partners can spread the disease between them.

COMPLICATIONS

If you are pregnant and have BV, you are more likely to have a preterm delivery (and, thus, a premature baby) or postpartum endometritis. Also, there is a possibility of pelvic inflammatory disease, which can lead to infertility or an ectopic pregnancy. BV heightens a woman's susceptibility to HIV and other STDs.

CANDIDIASIS (YEAST INFECTION)

SIGNS/SYMPTOMS

Inflammation, itching, and curdlike, cheesy white vaginal discharge. Sometimes people have beefy red plaques in the groin area that spread to the scrotum or labia; red lesions on thighs; or curdy white patches in the vaginal area. A man may experience painful urination and red, itchy skin with pustules. Frequently candidiasis can be diagnosed by physical exam alone.

TRANSMISSION

Sometimes sexually transmitted but most often results from overgrowth of *Candida* organisms, which are normally in the vagina.

TEST

Physical exam and microscopic examination of vaginal discharge.

TREATMENT

To alleviate symptoms, you can use over-the-counter antifungal topical agents if you are sure you have candidiasis because you have had it in the past and recognize the symptoms. Or your doctor can prescribe oral fluconazole (Diflucan) pill. Note: these treatment creams can destroy the latex of condoms and, thus, make them ineffective for prevention of STDs and pregnancy.

PREVENTION

Risk factors for repeated candidiasis include pregnancy, diabetes, antibiotic or steroid use, immunosuppression, HIV infection, wearing of tight clothing, and use of silk or nylon underpants.

CHANCROID

SIGNS/SYMPTOMS

Within a week of exposure, a man may have painful open sores (with ragged borders) on the genitals; lesions resemble the kind caused by syphilis or genital herpes. Other signs include fever, headaches, malaise, and swollen lymph nodes in the groin. A woman may have vaginal discharge, painful urination, painful intercourse, or rectal bleeding. Areas that chancroid can affect are the vulva, vagina, cervix, urethra, penis, and anus.

TRANSMISSION

Sexually transmitted.

TEST

Gram stain, culture, biopsy, blood test.

TREATMENT

Antibiotics.

PREVENTION

Consistent use of latex condoms and barriers (dental dams).

COMPLICATIONS

Increased risk of transmission of HIV. These lesions are thought to be a huge risk factor for heterosexual spread of HIV.

CHLAMYDIA

Four million new cases of chlamydia are diagnosed each year. For that reason, this has become the most commonly reported infectious disease in the United States, with 783,242 cases reported in 2001.

SIGNS/SYMPTOMS

People frequently have no symptoms or symptoms do not appear for weeks or months after chlamydia has been contracted from a sex partner. Then some men and women have an abnormal yellowish genital discharge and burning during urination. A woman may have pain during intercourse, a red and swollen cervix, and bleeding between menstrual periods. A man may have a discharge from his penis tip.

TRANSMISSION

Sexual intercourse and oral sex or contact with bodily fluids that are infected followed by touching an eye, thus allowing entry of chlamydia and causing an eye infection. A mother can give her baby chlamydia during delivery. This disease is not contracted from contact with toilet seats, towels, and other objects.

TEST

Physical exam and a swab of the vagina or penis to obtain secretions for lab analysis. Urine testing is also used sometimes.

TREATMENT

Antibiotics. Chlamydia should be treated aggressively because of the drastic complications that can result. If your symptoms do not end after a week of treatment, return to your doctor for follow-up. If you have chlamydia, make sure all of your sex partners are tested and treated, if necessary. Do not have sex until a follow-up test confirms that you are cured and until your partners have been checked and treated.

PREVENTION

As of 2002, the CDC recommended annual screening for young adult women and teens and older women at risk for chlamydia; the CDC also recommended rescreening three months after completion of treatment. Inconsistent use of condoms is commonly behind transmission of chlamydia, so be sure to use condoms and barriers (dental dams) consistently. If you have multiple sex partners, have frequent testing for chlamydia.

COMPLICATIONS

Untreated chlamydia puts a woman at high risk for pelvic inflammatory disease. Future ectopic pregnancy and infertility are possible problems. Women who have chlamydia are much more likely to become infected with HIV if they are exposed to the virus. In a man, untreated chlamydia may lead to inflammation of the urethra and epididymis. Chlamydia can cause an inflamed rectum, inflamed eye lining, and trachoma—the most common preventable cause of blindness.

CYTOMEGALOVIRUS INFECTION

An incurable herpesvirus infection, cytomegalovirus poses major problems mainly for babies and people with an impaired immune system or those who are undergoing chemotherapy.

SIGNS/SYMPTOMS

Usually none, but fever, fatigue, and swollen lymph glands are possible.

TRANSMISSION

Spread via sexual contact and kissing. It is often found in semen and cervical secretions. It is also transmitted from mother to infant via breastfeeding, from person to person (for example, at day care centers), and by blood transfusion or tissue transplantation.

TEST

ELISA blood test.

TREATMENT

Certain antiviral drugs (ganciclovir, foscarnet, and cidofovir) are helpful. Treatment of people with AIDS with highly active antiretroviral therapy suppresses cytomegalovirus.

PREVENTION

Aggressive handwashing and proper diaper handling reduce risk. Although condoms have been shown to be effective at preventing sexual transmission of CMV, no type of safe sex can guarantee that you will not get CMV infection because it can be transmitted in saliva. Consistently use condoms and barriers (dental dams).

COMPLICATIONS

In the United States, CMV is the top cause of congenital infection. This can mean serious complications at birth or later in life (such as mental retardation, deafness, or epilepsy).

DONOVANOSIS (GRANULOMA INGUINALE)

SIGNS/SYMPTOMS

This extremely rare STD is characterized by bumps that usually show up within 80 days of exposure and slough into ulcers. The ulcers can be seen in the mouth or genital or anal areas. They are dark red and large and often enlarge; the affected skin may bleed easily.

TRANSMISSION

Sexually transmitted.

TEST

Biopsy of infected skin.

TREATMENT

Antibiotics for three weeks or more (follow your doctor's directions). Take all of the prescription as directed. All of your sex partners should take antibiotics for donovanosis even if they are symptom-free. Anyone you have had sexual contact with in a 60-day time frame before your donovanosis symptoms appeared should be treated.

PREVENTION

Use latex condoms and barriers (dental dams).

COMPLICATIONS

Donovanosis increases the risk of contracting HIV if exposed to the virus. You also may have permanent scarring of the urethra or other areas.

GENITAL HERPES

In the United States, about 50 million have this incurable disease, and about 1 million people are newly infected with herpes simplex virus every year. This means about one in five of the total adolescent and adult population in the United States has genital herpes, according to the Centers for Disease Control and Prevention. The most startling fact is that about 89 percent of those who have genital herpes do not know it because they have no symptoms or do not recognize the symptoms. So they can (and do) spread genital herpes unknowingly. Genital herpes is typically HSV-2; the virus that causes cold sores or fever blisters on the mouth or lips is typically HSV-1. However, HSV-1 can cause genital infections, too, and HSV-2 can cause oral lesions.

SIGNS/SYMPTOMS

With the initial outbreak, people often have flulike symptoms, such as fever and swollen glands. A female may have itching or burning in her vagina, pain, vaginal discharge, and tiny red bumps or blisters in the genital area, which turn into painful ulcers. These may be preceded by a tingling sensation. In the first outbreak, the sores usually disappear in a few weeks, but in subsequent outbreaks, the lesions often resolve within several days. The virus stays in the body for life, and sores recur from time to time. Sores can cause painful urination; they can open, ooze, bleed, and scab over.

A male with genital herpes may first experience testicle discomfort, followed by sores on the penis, anus, buttocks, scrotum, or thighs. He may have fever and swollen lymph nodes in the groin. Subtle signs are irritation around the anus, small skin slits, and skin redness. Sometimes a man may mistakenly think he has jock itch, acne, or irritation caused by sexual activity.

About five outbreaks a year is typical, but this may decrease to one or two annually as time passes. Some of the factors that can trigger new bouts of herpes are stress, illness, poor nutrition, and excessive activity or sunlight. Prodrome symptoms—an itchy feeling in the genital area, a burning feeling in the legs—signal that herpes is in an active stage.

TRANSMISSION

Most people get genital herpes when a partner has no visible symptoms. You contract genital herpes by having sex—oral, vaginal, or anal—with an infected individual. You cannot get genital herpes from toilet seats, towels, and so on. You can also get herpes (usually HSV-1) by kissing a person with a cold sore or by sharing razors or eating utensils and such.

TEST

Physical exam and viral culture of a sample that has been swabbed from a sore.

TREATMENT

Antiviral agents such as acyclovir (Zovirax) and valacyclovir (Valtrex) control outbreaks and minimize discomfort of outbreaks. Drugs can reduce symptoms and work especially well when taken within 24 hours of onset of symptoms. A person with genital herpes can choose either suppressive or episodic antiviral treatments that can help prevent or shorten the duration of outbreaks. In some cases, suppressive antiviral therapy tends to decrease the risk of transmission as well.

PREVENTION

Abstinence (no sexual activity at all) is the only surefire way to prevent getting genital herpes. If you are sexually active, use condoms and barriers (dental dams), but be aware that these should not be viewed as guarantees that you will not contract this disease. Using latex condoms provides some protection, but not 100 percent, because viral shedding can occur in an area that is not covered by a condom even when there is no visible herpes lesion. Herpes is contagious before and during an outbreak and also is contagious sometimes when no sores can be seen. Contact with a toilet seat or hot tub is very unlikely to spread the virus. If you kiss someone who has herpes around the mouth in the contagious stage or if you have sexual contact and the person is shedding virus in the genital area, you are likely to contract herpes from that individual. Do not have oral sex with someone who has oral herpes lesions. If you have herpes, even after sores are healed, wait several days before having sexual contact with anyone. Use condoms between

herpes recurrences. If you use long-term suppressive medication therapy, you will probably reduce the likelihood of transmitting herpes to a partner.

COMPLICATIONS

HSV makes people more susceptible to HIV and makes HIV-infected people more infectious. Psychological distress can occur because in many people this virus reactivates repeatedly over a lifetime, with discomfort and sores.

A newborn who contracts herpes from the mother may have meningitis and/or brain damage. A woman with active genital herpes at time of delivery probably should have a cesarean section, but in women with genital herpes, infecting an infant is actually very rare. An infant in the birth canal who has direct contact with herpes can contract the disease during delivery. Infection in a mother who has viral shedding at the time of delivery can cause serious damage to her baby, especially if she has only recently acquired the infection.

During pregnancy, a woman who has had herpes for a long time transmits protective antibodies to the fetus, which help protect the baby from infection even if some virus exists in the birth canal.

If you are pregnant and have a sex partner who has herpes, use condoms throughout the nine months and do not have intercourse at all the last trimester. If you are in your last months of pregnancy, avoid all forms of sex with a partner whose infection status is unknown or one you know has oral or genital herpes.

GENITAL WARTS

Also called venereal warts and condyloma acuminata, genital warts are caused by human papillomavirus (HPV) and infect about 1 million to 2 million people in the United States every year. This is probably the most common STD.

SIGNS/SYMPTOMS

About three weeks to three months after exposure, genital warts appear as small painless bumps on the penis, scrotum, anus, or vaginal area. Untreated, these can develop into larger cauliflowerlike growths. Some are too small to be seen. (Note: the warts that people have on hands and feet are not sexually transmitted.) Usually external genital warts (EGWs) are caused by types of HPV that are low-risk, meaning they do not lead to cervical cancer, but some strains of HPV can lead to cervical cancer. Occasionally genital warts occur in the mouth, after oral sex with an infected person.

TRANSMISSION

Sexual contact, including foreplay, anal intercourse, oral–genital sex, and vaginal intercourse. HPV can be present in an individual for some time without symptoms, so it can be difficult to pinpoint who transmitted it to you. You get genital warts from skin-to-skin contact with lesions (visible or not) that are shedding HPV DNA. Only rarely are genital warts transmitted by nonliving material such as surgical gloves, via a person's fingers or hand, or by an infected mother to a newborn during childbirth. You cannot contract genital warts by touching an inanimate object.

TEST

Physical examination. Sometimes, a woman first discovers that she has HPV through an abnormal Pap smear result. Your doctor may do a colposcopy to inspect the cervix and vagina and apply a solution to the cervix to highlight cellular changes caused by HPV. He or she may biopsy a small tissue sample(s).

TREATMENT

Your sex partners should be checked for genital warts and treated as needed. Genital warts may remain the same size, go away, or grow larger. Sometimes, left untreated, genital warts eventually go away. Often treatment includes a therapy the doctor administers and one that the patient uses at home. You can self-treat with podofilox gel (Condylox) or imiquimod (Aldara) cream. Use topical treatments only for external genital and perianal warts. A doctor can use a technique such as cryotherapy (freezing) or laser vaporization. If genital warts recur or are profuse in nature, your doctor may do interferon injections. Very large warts can be surgically removed. If you have a recurrence of warts, see your doctor as soon as possible for treatment; do not have sex until these are elim-

inated. Note: often HIV causes an abnormal Pap smear finding. After treatment, be sure to have follow-up Pap smears.

PREVENTION

Use condoms and barriers (dental dams). Be aware, however, that a condom definitely cannot cover the entire area that may have genital warts—those that are visible and those that are too small to be visible. The only sure way to prevent genital warts is not to have sex.

COMPLICATIONS

Throat warts in babies born to women with genital warts occur rarely but can be life-threatening. Certain high-risk HPV strains can cause cervical cancer in women, and these are also associated with vulvar cancer, anal cancer, and cancer of the penis.

GONORRHEA

Also called "the clap," gonorrhea is an ancient disease.

SIGNS/SYMPTOMS

Symptoms can appear from two to 30 days after infection. Some people do not show symptoms for months. In women, early symptoms can be mild or nonexistent, and a woman may have a yellow or bloody vaginal discharge and painful urination. Typically a person has discharge from the penis or vagina and burning with urination. An infected rectum can cause itching, discharge, and painful bowel movements. A woman's usual infection site is the endocervix or (less often) the rectum and urethra.

TRANSMISSION

Sexual intercourse—vaginal, oral, or anal. Also, touching infected genitals and then the eyes can result in an eye infection. Even when an infected individual is symptom-free, he or she can spread the infection to sex partners in cases of unprotected sex.

TEST

A small sample of discharge may be taken for lab analysis—Gram stain, culture, or detection of bacterial genes by using swabs. Often more than one test is needed to diagnose gonorrhea. For pharyngeal gonorrhea, a throat culture is used. A specific urine test can diagnose gonorrhea that is present in the genital tract.

TREATMENT

Antibiotics. For genital tract infections, drug combinations are used because people with gonorrhea infections are also routinely treated for chlamydia.

PREVENTION

Practice abstinence or limit the number of sex partners and use condoms consistently and barriers (dental dams). Condoms are not 100 percent effective because contact with bodily fluids or secretions is possible. Even if you have had gonorrhea, you contract it again if you have sexual contact with someone who has gonorrhea. A person whose only sexual activity is oral sex can contract gonorrhea in the throat and mouth.

COMPLICATIONS

Left untreated, gonorrhea can cause pelvic inflammatory disease. Having gonorrhea also gives someone a heightened chance of getting HIV if exposed to it. A woman who has gonorrhea can transmit the infection to her baby during delivery. The result can be an eye infection, blindness, joint infection, or a serious blood infection. Complications of gonorrhea for men include epididymitis, which can lead to infertility, and urethral scarring that makes urination difficult.

HEPATITIS A

SIGNS/SYMPTOMS

Vomiting, nausea, appetite loss, fever, yellow skin and eyes, dark urine, and abdominal pain. Adults usually have symptoms, but children rarely do. Hepatitis A can make you very sick, but it resolves within a few weeks.

TRANSMISSION

From contaminated food and water or from sexual contact. You contract hepatitis A from ingesting infected fecal matter. This disease can be transmitted by oral–anal sex ("rimming") or digital–anal contact. More common, though, is transmission by contaminated food and water. This means a food-preparation person had feces on the skin after failing to wash the hands well after a bowel movement. Someone can transmit the infection via stool two weeks before symptoms appear and before he or she is aware of being infected. In day care facilities, children occasionally spread hepatitis A to other children and adults.

TEST

Blood test.

TREATMENT

Rest, fluids, and medication for nausea. No alcoholic beverages should be consumed.

PREVENTION

The CDC recommends immunization for illegal drug users, travelers to developing countries, children in high-disease-incidence areas, homosexual men, and people with occupational risk factors, chronic liver disease, or clotting-factor disorders. If you have antibodies, these confer protection against reinfection with hepatitis A. Use condoms and barriers (dental dams).

HEPATITIS B

SIGNS/SYMPTOMS

You may be symptom-free, or you may have symptoms two to three months after you contract hepatitis B: fatigue, decreased appetite, nausea, vomiting, headache, fever, dark urine, abdominal pain, yellow eyes and skin, and a flulike feeling. Symptoms last about six weeks.

TRANSMISSION

Sexual contact, saliva, and blood to blood; often, hepatitis B is contracted via anal intercourse. Other means are needle sharing by drug addicts, needle sharing in a tattoo or body-piercing salon, needlestick injury, transfusion with infected blood or blood products, mother-to-child transmission, and health-care environment transmission. You do not get hepatitis B sharing bathroom facilities or having casual contact.

TEST

Blood test (but you may not test positive the first time if your infection is very recent). You may need a liver biopsy to allow the doctor to stage your disease.

TREATMENT

No treatment cures hepatitis B, but the body sometimes does so on its own. People with chronic hepatitis B may benefit from treatment with a combination of IV steroids and alpha-interferon, alpha-interferon alone, or the oral medications lamivudine or adefovir. A person who has hepatitis B should be blood-tested for hepatitis D as well. Hepatitis D (delta hepatitis) occurs only in someone who has hepatitis B; the combination can be serious.

PREVENTION

Use condoms and barriers (dental dams). Hepatitis B is transmitted more easily than is HIV, and you are at higher risk if you already have an STD. If you know your partner has hepatitis B, get immunized. Recommended for immunization are homosexual men, people diagnosed with STDs, those with several sex partners, infants born in the United States, a child age 11 to 12 who has not had the three-shot series, health care workers who may be exposed to contaminated body fluids, people who share a house with a person who has chronic hepatitis B, people who travel to countries that have a high prevalence of hepatitis B, prostitutes, and prisoners.

A small percentage of those with hepatitis B are lifelong chronic carriers. A child or HIV patient is likely to be a chronic carrier.

COMPLICATIONS

Hepatitis B can cause liver inflammation and damage. Liver destruction (cirrhosis) is a feared complication, as is liver cancer.

HEPATITIS C

SIGNS/SYMPTOMS

Symptoms that may show up in six to seven weeks include fatigue, yellow skin, diarrhea, nausea, and decreased appetite. Hepatitis C usually is not diagnosed initially and proceeds to the chronic state.

TRANSMISSION

Blood and sex. The most common ways that hepatitis C is spread are transfusions with contaminated blood and IV drug abuse. (In 1992, blood banks began screening for hepatitis C.) Sexual transmission can occur.

TEST

ELISA and RIBA. The latter is done to confirm the results of the ELISA. A blood test typically yields a positive result for hepatitis C six weeks after infection, but sometimes it takes months. You can use the Home Access Hepatitis C Check Test Service. Sometimes a liver biopsy is necessary.

TREATMENT

Forty-eight weeks of combination therapy with interferon and ribavarin. Get immunization against hepatitis A and B, do not drink alcohol, and avoid taking any medications that may damage the liver.

PREVENTION

You are at increased risk if you had a tattoo, organ transplantation, or nonautologous blood transfusion before 1992; you had a nonautologous clotting-factor transmission before 1987; you are an IV drug user; you work in a health care setting; you are on long-term hemodialysis; you were born to an infected mother; you have an infected partner or multiple sex partners; or you have a history of STDs. Because hepatitis C is infectious, do not donate blood or organs if you have this disease, and avoid sharing razors or toothbrushes. If you have a long-term sex partner who is infected, the risk of transmission is low. Use condoms and barriers (dental dams).

COMPLICATIONS

Hepatitis C is a common cause of chronic liver disease. Chronic hepatitis C can lead to cirrhosis and liver cancer after many years.

HEPATITIS D

Also called delta hepatitis, hepatitis D can only occur in someone who already has hepatitis B. Hepatitis D can be sexually transmitted, but blood exposure is a more likely means of getting it. You can be simultaneously infected with hepatitis D and B, or superinfected with D while carrying B.

HIV/AIDS

Half of the new HIV infections in the United States occur in people younger than 25; that means thousands of U.S. teens are infected with HIV every year. An HIV-positive person who is symptom-free can infect others. Acquired immunodeficiency syndrome (AIDS) is caused by the human immunodeficiency virus (HIV), which destroys the body's ability to fight infection. Today about 900,000 people in the United States have HIV.

SIGNS/SYMPTOMS

About six to eight weeks after exposure, some of the following symptoms occur in most people who are HIV-infected: weight loss, extreme weakness, persistent cough, white patches in the mouth, swollen lymph glands, hair loss, hives, chronic diarrhea, frequent fever, night sweats, skin rashes, and vaginal yeast infections that are unresponsive to treatment.

TRANSMISSION

HIV can be transmitted from someone who has the infection to another person by way of blood, semen, vaginal fluid, and breast milk. The virus enters the body via the lining of the vulva, vagina, penis, rectum, or mouth. If a woman has HIV and is pregnant, she can transmit the virus to her unborn child during pregnancy, delivery, or breast-feeding. Besides sexual activity, HIV is spread by needle sharing in the use of intravenous drugs and in tattooing. You can get HIV from a blood transfusion or organ transplantation, although this is unlikely because of stringent screening procedures. HIV transmission by a needlestick is rare, but it can happen. Biting that involves blood and tissue damage can spread HIV. Open-mouth kissing that exposed a person to contaminated blood is reported to have transmitted HIV in one case. You do not contract HIV through hugs, sneezes, toilet seats, towels, phones, or insects. In countries such as the United States, where blood is tested for HIV before it is used in transfusions, the blood supply is viewed as safe.

TEST

Blood tests ELISA or EIA, and for confirmation, the Western blot; or saliva and urine tests. The FDA has licensed a rapid test. Usually people have HIV antibodies that are detectable three months after contracting the disease, but six months may elapse from time of infection before a test can detect HIV. Hence, get tested and then retested six months after being exposed, but protect yourself against other exposure to HIV and protect others, too. Many advocate mandatory HIV testing of pregnant women.

TREATMENT

Drugs are used to slow the virus's invasion of your body after you contract HIV and to help you resist other infections; there is no cure for HIV or AIDS, but people now live much longer with this disease. A pregnant woman with HIV can be treated to prevent passing the virus to her unborn child.

PREVENTION

You can practice abstinence, or use latex condoms for all forms of sexual intercourse. Use of latex condoms for sex (oral, anal, and vaginal) and barriers (dental dams) can reduce the risk of contracting HIV. Avoid sexual practices that include oral–fecal exposure. Avoid all contact with body fluids, and do not share needles (for drugs or tattoos). Do not presume you can detect whether a sex partner is HIV-positive by his or her appearance; many people who have HIV appear perfectly healthy. Oral sex carries the risk of contracting HIV when you do not know the other person's HIV status, or he or she is HIV-positive or an IV drug user, or he or she is not monogamous. Oral sex can transmit HIV and other STDs. Factors that make oral sex extremely risky with a person who is (or could be) HIV-positive are oral ulcers, bleeding gums, and/or genital sores. Having another STD increases the likelihood of contracting HIV.

COMPLICATIONS

Although many people who have HIV and undergo treatment may look and feel healthy for a long time, most have AIDS in about 10 years. Opportunistic infections can present enormous problems for people with HIV and AIDS.

LYMPHOGRANULOMA VENEREUM

SIGNS/SYMPTOMS

An initial painless red bump, tiny blister, or ulcer in the anal or genital area that appears one to three weeks after exposure; this can occur in various locations such as the penis head or on the cervix or labia. It is often not noticed, but then, painful, one-sided enlarged lymph nodes develop. The enlarged inflamed lymph nodes may drain pus. Fever, chills, and/or a rash may occur. Oral sex performed on someone who is infected can result in mouth ulcers and lymph node enlargement in the neck. In some cases, a person may experience blockage of stool passage caused by rectal scarring. With this disease, men are more likely to have symptoms than women are.

TRANSMISSION

Sexually transmitted.

TEST

Blood test.

TREATMENT

Antibiotics (doxycycline or erythromycin).

PREVENTION

Safe sex practices. Use condoms and barriers (dental dams).

COMPLICATIONS

Some people have rectal scarring. When you have lymphogranuloma venereum and open sores in the genital area, you are more likely to contract HIV if you have sex with an infected person because the sores facilitate transmission.

MOLLUSCUM CONTAGIOSUM

SIGNS/SYMPTOMS

Often there are no noticeable symptoms. You may have painless, dome-shaped bumps that itch or become irritated. Located on genitals, lower abdomen, buttocks, or inner thighs, these dimpled bumps are shiny, are flesh-colored, and have a dent in the center. These bumps can merge and/or spread from the genital area to the stomach and thighs.

Usually the bumps recede in a month or two. Time from infection to appearance of bumps varies greatly—a week to a year.

TRANSMISSION

In adults, molluscum contagiosum is usually transmitted sexually. In general, transmission occurs via sexual activity or skin-to-skin contact (even if the infected person has no symptoms). Also, a person can spread the infection from one part of the body to another. Molluscum contagiosum may be transmitted by contact with an inanimate object such as a towel that has the virus on it.

TEST

Usually the diagnosis is easily reached by visual examination by a doctor. Occasionally other methods are necessary such as lesion biopsy to confirm diagnosis.

TREATMENT

Bumps often resolve spontaneously, or a doctor can scrape them off or treat them with a chemical irritant: liquid nitrogen, tricarboxylic acid (TCA), salicylic acid, and so on.

PREVENTION

Consistent use of latex condoms and barriers (dental dams), although these are not 100 percent effective.

PUBIC LICE

SIGNS/SYMPTOMS

Itching in pubic area or thigh hair caused by louse infestation (lice are very tiny insects that feed on human blood).

TRANSMISSION

Usually spread through sexual contact; in rare cases, people have contracted pubic lice from infested bedding, towels, or clothes.

TEST

Visual inspection can reveal the presence of pinhead-sized pubic lice that are oval and gray or red–brown when blood-filled. Tiny white eggs can be seen clinging to pubic hair.

TREATMENT

Over-the-counter shampoos or lotions, or a prescription product such as permethrin (Elimite) cream or lindane (Kwell) cream. Lindane has been associated with causing seizures in some people.

Do not use a product containing lindane if you are pregnant, and check with your doctor about using this on a child or baby. Use calamine lotion on irritated skin. If you have lice in your eyelashes, apply a prescription petrolatum ointment twice a day thickly for several days, or, with a cotton-tipped applicator, use ophthalmic ointment prescribed by your doctor. Within 24 hours of being separated from the human body, pubic lice die. Family and sex partners of an infected person need to be treated. Wash bedding and clothing in hot water and dry on high dryer heat. Eggs live about six days, so repeat the treatment as recommended by your doctor. Note that scratching can spread the infestation to other parts of your body.

PREVENTION

Use condoms and barriers (dental dams) consistently. Have no sexual contact with someone who has pubic lice (probably, if you look closely, you will see the infestation).

SCABIES

This is a fairly common skin infestation that is very contagious.

SIGNS/SYMPTOMS

About a month after exposure to scabies, small red bumps show up where the scabies mite has burrowed into the skin to lay eggs. Sometimes these appear in lines in the commonly affected areas—genitals, elbows, wrists, between fingers, on abdomen.

TRANSMISSION

Scabies, a highly contagious skin infestation with a tiny mite, is spread via close contact including sexual activity and can be transmitted before you are even aware you have scabies. It is also believed that scabies can be transmitted by contact with infested clothing, bedding, or towels.

TEST

A scraping of an irritated area is examined microscopically for the presence of mites.

TREATMENT

Permethrin cream (Elimite)—which is applied to skin below the chin—works well. Sometimes a second application in 14 days is needed. Occasionally lindane lotion is used. Do not use lindane if you are pregnant, and do not apply on young children. Precipitated sulfur in petrolatum is occasionally used, but it has the downside of being messy and smelly. Even after treatment, your skin may feel itchy because the irritated skin remains a problem. To soothe, use hydrocortisone cream. Wash clothing and bedding in hot water to eliminate mites. Have sex partners and family members treated.

PREVENTION

Do not have sex without condoms or barriers (dental dams), and watch for signs of scabies on sex partners.

SYPHILIS

SIGNS/SYMPTOMS

The classic first symptom of syphilis is a chancre—a painless open sore on the penis or in the vaginal area that appears within three days to three months of exposure (usually, two to six weeks). Other possible locations are the anus, hands, or mouth. Left untreated, syphilis can proceed to advanced stages, characterized by aches, low fever, patchy hair loss, sore throat, and itchless penny-sized brown sores that come and go and are often on the soles of the feet and on the palms of the hands. An infant who has congenital syphilis may show symptoms at birth or several weeks later; these can include rashes, fever, hoarse crying, skin sores, yellowish skin, anemia, and deformities.

TRANSMISSION

Sexual (vaginal, oral, and anal sex). It is almost always spread by sexual contact. Also, a pregnant woman can pass the syphilis infection to her unborn child, who may as a result be born with serious physical and/or mental problems. Antibodies, which sometimes stay in the body for years, do not protect against contracting a new syphilis infection. You do not contract syphilis from inanimate objects such as toilet seats or towels.

TEST

Microscopic identification of bacteria, blood test, or physical examination. Often two blood tests are required because false-positive results sometimes occur. Commonly used tests are the VDRL and RPR. Tests to confirm results are the FTA-ABS and TPHA.

TREATMENT

Penicillin injection. Make sure that your sex partners are checked for syphilis as soon as possible. Do not have sex with new partners until you are sure that all of your sores are healed and you have completed your course of treatment. (If you have had syphilis longer than one year, you will probably need additional doses of penicillin.)

PREVENTION

Use condoms, and have no contact with the open sores that are infectious during active stages of syphilis. Condoms do not provide total protection because an infected person can have sores that expose others to skin contact beyond the condom's coverage. Also, syphilis sores can be hidden in the rectum, mouth, and vagina. If you have had syphilis and have been treated, you need to have follow-up blood tests to confirm that the infectious agent has been eradicated completely. An untreated pregnant woman who has active syphilis is highly likely to pass the infection to her unborn child, so it is very important to seek testing and treatment early in pregnancy. This condition can also cause stillbirth.

COMPLICATIONS

If you leave the disease untreated, serious health problem can develop. In late stages, syphilis can cause heart and central nervous system deterioration, including blindness, mental disorders, heart abnormalities, paralysis, numbness, brain damage, and even death. Syphilis increases risk of contracting HIV because entry via sores is easier. Untreated syphilis can cause major birth defects in the infant of an infected mother.

TRICHOMONIASIS

Trichomonas vaginalis is a microscopic parasite that causes the very common STD trichomoniasis. About 2 million women become infected with trichomoniasis every year in the United States.

SIGNS/SYMPTOMS

Within six months of exposure, a woman may have a bad-smelling, frothy green vaginal discharge; itching; and vaginal or vulvar redness. Pain during intercourse, painful or frequent urination, and lower abdominal pain are other symptoms. Some people have no symptoms at all. Men rarely have symptoms, but if they do, these may include an urgent need to urinate, discharge from the urethra, and/or burning with urination.

TRANSMISSION

Sexual activity. Infection is most common in women who have multiple sex partners. You are very unlikely to get trichomoniasis via sitting on a toilet seat because the parasite cannot live long on objects, but there is a slight possibility of contracting trichomoniasis from contact with infected towels or bedding. In rare cases, a baby born to an infected mother can contract infection during delivery. Usually infection in a young child is a sign of sexual abuse. In a teen, a diagnosis of trichomoniasis suggests that she or he is sexually active or has been sexually abused. Even if you have had trichomoniasis, you can be infected again.

TEST

In women, a physical exam and collection of a vaginal sample for microscopic examination. A doctor evaluates a man for trichomoniasis with specimens collected from the urethra.

TREATMENT

Antimicrobial medication (all sex partners should be treated, too). Do not have unprotected intercourse while you are being treated. Typically, a single dose of metronidazole (Flagyl) is given (do not drink alcohol when you are taking this drug).

PREVENTION

You can practice abstinence, or you can limit sexual activity to one partner and use latex condoms every time you have intercourse to provide some protection, but remember that organisms can be in places not covered by a condom. If you are infected with trichomoniasis, be treated and make sure your partner is treated so that you do not become reinfected.

COMPLICATIONS

Increased risk of transmission of HIV; increased risk of a low-birth-weight baby or preterm delivery. Only rarely does a baby contract trichomoniasis from an infected mother during delivery.

THE CDC OFFERS SOME GENERAL GUIDELINES FOR PREVENTING STDS:

1. If you do not want to be abstinent, then have a mutually monogamous sexual relationship with one uninfected partner.

2. Use male latex condoms correctly and with each instance of sexual activity.

3. If you inject intravenous drugs, be sure to use clean needles.

4. Prevent and control STDs in order to decrease susceptibility to HIV (and if you have HIV already, to reduce your level of infectiousness).

5. Delay starting sexual activity. The younger a person is when he or she has sex for the first time, the more likely that individual is to get an STD. Your risk also increases with the number of partners you have.

6. If you are sexually active, have regular STD checkups, especially if you are having sex with someone new.

7. Know the symptoms of STDs, and if you have symptoms, seek medical evaluation as soon as possible.

8. Do not have sex during a menstrual period (this makes a woman more susceptible to STD infection).

9. Avoid having anal intercourse. If you do have intercourse anally, use a male condom each time.

10. Do not douche; this removes some of a woman's natural bacteria and therefore increases the risk of development of sexually associated problems such as bacterial vaginosis.

11. Do not be afraid to ask your doctor for help, treatment, or information. Chances are, if you have an STD, it can be treated successfully.

BIBLIOGRAPHY

BOOKS

Bartlett, John G., and Finkbeiner, Ann K. *The Guide to Living with HIV Infection,* 4th ed. Baltimore: The Johns Hopkins University Press, 1998.

Centers for Disease Control and Prevention. *Sexually Transmitted Disease Surveillance 2000: Chlamydia.* Atlanta, Ga.: Centers for Disease Control and Prevention, 2001.

Chandra, R. K., ed. *Primary and Secondary Immunodeficiency Disorders.* Edinburgh: Churchill Livingstone, 1983.

Curtis, Michele G., and Hopkins, Michael P. *Glass's Office Gynecology,* 5th ed. Baltimore: Williams & Wilkins, 1999.

Fitzpatrick, Thomas B. et al. *Color Atlas and Synopsis of Clinical Dermatology,* 3d ed. New York: McGraw-Hill, 1997.

Gallo, R. C. *Virus Hunting. AIDS, Cancer, and the Human Retrovirus: A Story of Scientific Discovery.* New York: HarperCollins, 1991.

Gilbert, David, Moellering, Robert, Jr., and Sande, Merle. *The Sanford Guide to HIV Antimicrobial Therapy 2001,* 31st ed. Hyde Park, Vt.: Antimicrobial Therapy, Inc., 2001.

Kelley, William N. *Textbook of Internal Medicine,* 3d ed. Philadelphia: Lippincott-Raven, 1997.

Marr, Lisa. *Sexually Transmitted Diseases.* Baltimore: The Johns Hopkins University Press, 1998.

McCloskey, Jenny. *Your Sexual Health.* San Francisco: Halo Books, 1993.

Princeton, Douglas C. *Manual of HIV/AIDS Therapy.* Laguna Hills, Calif: Current Clinical Strategies Publishing, 2003.

Sande, Merle, Gilbert, David, Moellering, Robert, Jr., *The Sanford Guide to HIV/AIDS Therapy 2001,* 10th ed. Hyde Park, Vt.: Antimicrobial Therapy, Inc., 2001.

Stanberry, Lawrence Raymond. *Understanding Herpes.* Jackson: University Press of Mississippi, 1998.

Update in Sexually Transmitted Diseases. Course booklet, November 2001. University of Texas Southwestern Medical Center, Dallas, Texas. Course directors James W. Smith and Gary Sinclair.

U.S. Department of Health and Human Services Centers for Disease Control and Prevention. *1998 Guidelines for Treatment of Sexually Transmitted Diseases.* McLean, Va.: International Medical Publishing, 1998.

Watstein, Sarah Barbara, and Chandler, Karen. *The AIDS Dictionary.* New York: Facts On File, 1998.

ARTICLES

"AAD: Common Skin Conditions in Women May Indicate HIV." Doctor's Guide Website. Available online. URL: http://www.docguide.com. Downloaded May 15, 2002.

Abedon, Stephen T. "Nosomial Infections." Supplemental lecture. Available online. URL: http://www.phage.org/biol2053.htm. Downloaded on October 10, 2001.

"About amfAR: Introduction and History." Available online. URL: //www.amfar.org/cgi-bin/iowa/amfar/index.html. Downloaded on September 1, 2002.

"AIDS Activist Invites the World to Live Webcasts from His Home." CNN Website. Available online. URL: http://www.cnn.com. Downloaded January 20, 2002.

"AIDS-Arts Timeline." The AIDS-Arts Forum Website. Available online. URL: http://www.artery:theaids-artsforum.com. Downloaded February 17, 2002.

"AIDS Drugs Help Even When Virus Is Resistant, Study Finds." Reuters. MSNBC Website. Available online. URL: http://www.msnbc.com. Downloaded April 5, 2002.

"AIDS Epidemic May Be Fed by High Levels of HIV in Primary Infection." Doctor's Guide Website. Available online. URL: http://www.docguide/news.com. Downloaded February 1, 2002.

"AIDS History." National Institute of Allergy and Infectious Diseases Website. Available online. URL: http://www.aidshistory.nih.gov.

"AIDS-Related KS." American Cancer Society Website. Available online. URL: http://www.cancer.org. Downloaded July 2, 2002.

"AIDS Timeline." AIDS Project Los Angeles Website. Available online. URL: http://www.apla.org/apla/ed/timeline.htm. Downloaded October 1, 2001.

"AIDS Tips for Teens." Dr. Koop Website. Available online. URL: http://www.drkoop.com. Updated October 23, 2000.

"AIDS: Will Any HIV Nonprogressor Be Spared?" *Physician's Weekly* 15, no. 31 (August 17, 1998). Available online. URL: http://www.physweekly.com.

"Alarm at Spread of Drug-Resistant AIDS." AVERT Website. *The Guardian,* December 20, 2001. Available online. URL: http://www.avert.org.

AMA (American Medical Association), Council on Scientific Affairs. "The Acquired Immunodeficiency Syndrome (Commentary)." *Journal of the American Medical Association* 252, no. 15 (1984): 2037–2047.

Amann, A. J. et al. "Acquired Immunodeficiency in an Infant: Possible Transmission by Means of Blood Products." *Lancet* 1, no. 8331 (1983): 956–958.

"About amfAR." amfAR Website. Available online. URL: http://www.amfar.org/td. Downloaded January 20, 2002.

"Alcohol Researchers Show 'Friendly' Virus Slows HIV Cell Growth." Available online. URL: http://www.nih.gov. Downloaded September 5, 2002.

"The amfAR Treatment Insider." amfAR Website. Available online. URL: http://www.amfar.org/td. Downloaded February 16, 2002.

Ammann, A. J. et al. "Acquired Immune Dysfunction in Homosexual Men: Immunologic Profiles." *Clin Immunology Immunopathology* 27, no. 3 (1983): 315–325.

"Amphlicor CT/NG Test for Chlamydia and Gonorrhea Gives Same-Day Results." Doctor's Guide Website. Available online. URL: http//www.docguide/news.com. Downloaded February 1, 2002.

"Anal Cancer Screening for Gay and Bisexual Men Saves Lives." Doctor's Guide Website. Available online. URL: http://www.docguide/news.com. Downloaded on February 1, 2002.

Andiman, W. A. et al. "Rate of Transmission of Human Immunodeficiency Virus Type 1 Infection from Mother to Child and Short-Term Outcome of Neonatal Infection." *American Journal of Diseases of Children* 144 (1990): 758–766.

Artery: The AIDS-Arts Forum Website. Information for timeline in Introduction. Available online. URL: http://www.artistswithaids.org/artery. Downloaded November 30, 2001.

Ascher, M. S. et al. "Does Drug Use Cause AIDS?" *Nature* 362 (1993): 103–104.

Ascher, M. S. et al. "Aetiology of AIDS." *Lancet* 341 (1993): 1223.

Association of Professors of Gynecology and Obstetrics. "Diagnosis of Vaginitis." APGO Educational Series in Women's Health Issues. Washington, D.C.: Association of Professors of Gynecology and Obstetrics, 1996.

Auerbach, D. M. et al. "Cluster of Cases of the Acquired Immune Deficiency Syndrome: Patients Linked by Sexual Contact." *American Journal of Medicine* 76, no. 3 (1984): 487–492.

Ault, Alicia. "Monkey Virus in Humans May Trigger Cancer." Reuters Health. Medline Website. National Library of Medicine. Available online. URL: http://www.medline.com. Downloaded August 29, 2002.

AVERT Website. Information for timeline in Introduction. Available online. URL: http://www.avert.org. E-mail: info@avert.org. Downloaded November 30, 2001.

Bagasra, O. et al. "Detection of Human Immunodeficiency Virus Type 1 Provirus in Mononuclear Cells by In Situ Polymerase Chain Reaction." *New England Journal of Medicine* 326, no. 21 (1992): 1385–1391.

Bagnarelli, P. et al. "Molecular Profile of Human Immunodeficiency Virus Type 1 Infection in Symptomless Patients and in Patients with AIDS." *Journal of Virology* 66, no. 12 (1992): 7328–7335.

Baldwin, H. E. "STD Update: Screening and Therapeutic Options." *International Journal of Fertility and Women's Medicine* on the Web. 46, no. 2 (March–April): 79–88. Available online. URL: http://www.pubmedcentral.gov.nih. Downloaded on October 1, 2001.

Balter, Michael. "Virus From 1959 Sample Marks Early Years of HIV." *JAMA* HIV/AIDS Resource Center Website. *Science Magazine* 279 (February 6, 1998). Available online. URL: http://www.amaassn.org/special/hiv/newsline/special/science/sci801.htm. Downloaded on December 15, 2001.

Berger, Edward A., Moss, Bernard, and Pastan, Ira. "Reconsidering Target Toxins to Eliminate HIV Infection: You Gotta Have HAART." *Proceedings of the National Academy of Sciences of the United States of America* 95, no. 20 (September 1998). Available online. URL: http://www.pubmedcentral.gov.nih. Downloaded on October 1, 2001.

Bethea, Lesa. "Primary Prevention of Child Abuse." *American Family Physician* Website. Available online. URL: http://www.aafp.org.afp/990315ap/1577.html. Downloaded May 1, 2002.

"Bill on Medical Privacy Proposed." Alive & Kicking!'s FastFax Website. Available online. URL: http://www.peoplewithaids.org/fastfax/ff227.htm.

Blanche, S. et al. "Relation of the Course of HIV Infection in Children to the Severity of the Disease in Their Mothers at Delivery." *New England Journal of Medicine* 330, no. 5 (1994): 308–312.

Blattner, W., Gallo, R. C., and Temin, H. M. "HIV Causes AIDS." *Science* 241, no. 4865 (1988): 515–516.

Blattner, W. et al. "Blattner and Colleagues Respond to Duesberg." *Science* 241, no. 514 (1988): 517.

Blattner, W. et al. "HIV/AIDS in Laboratory Workers Infected With HTLV-IIIB." Ninth International Conference on AIDS (abstract no. PO-B01-0876), Berlin, Germany: June 6–11, 1993.

Blower, Sally, Gershengorn, H. B., and Grant, R. M. "A Tale of Two Futures: HIV and Antiretroviral Therapy in San Francisco." *Science Magazine* 287 (January 28, 2000): 650–654. PubMed Website. National Library of Medicine. Available online. URL: http://www.ncbi.com.

Boulos, R. et al. "Effect of Maternal HIV Status on Infant Growth and Survival." Tenth International Conference on AIDS (abstract no. 054B), Yokohama, Japan: August 7–12, 1994.

Boulton, Mary et al. "General Practice and the Care of Children with HIV Infection: Six-Month Prospective Interview Study." *British Medical Journal 1999.* Available online. URL: http://www.pubmedcentral.nih.gov.bmj.

Breitkopf, Daniel M. "A Review of Genital Chlamydial Infections." *Hospital Physician* 36, no. 2 (February 2000).

"Britain Examines Success of Drug 'Shooting Galleries.'" AVERT Website. *The Independent.* Available online. URL: http://www.avert.org.

British Cooperative Clinical Group. "Homosexuality and Venereal Disease in the United Kingdom." *British Journal of Venereal Disease* 49 (1973): 329–334. Available online. URL: http://www.pubmedcentral.nih.gov.

Brown, Janelle. "High Noon for the Morning-After Pill." Salon.com Website. Available online. URL: http://www.salonmag.com/mwt/feature/2001/06/20/pill/index.html.

Buchbinder, S. P. et al. "Long-term HIV-1 Infection Without Immunologic Suppression." *AIDS* 8, no. 8 (1994): 1123–1128.

"Bulgaria Presses Libya on HIV Case." AVERT Website. News item from *NAM AIDS Treatment Update* 108 (December 2001). Web news from BBC News Online, December 19, 2001. Available online. URL: http://www.avert. org.

Burk, Robert D. "Human Papillomavirus and the Risk of Cervical Cancer." *Hospital Practice* 34, no. 12 (November 15, 1999).

Bushman, Frederic, Landau, Nathaniel R., and Emini, Emilio A. "New Developments in the Biology and Treatment of HIV." *Proceedings of the National Academy of Sciences of the United States of America* 95, no. 19 (September 1998). Available online. URL: http://www.

pubmedcentral.gov.nih. Downloaded on January 20, 2002.

Cao, Y. et al. "Virologic and Immunologic Characterization of Long-Term Survivors of Human Immunodeficiency Virus Type 1 Infection." *New England Journal of Medicine* 332, no. 4 (1995): 201–208.

"Caring for Someone with AIDS at Home." Centers for Disease Control and Prevention. From WebMD Website. Available online. URL: http://mg.webmd.com/content/article. Downloaded July 10, 2002.

Catalina, Gabriel, and Navarro, Victor. "Hepatitis C: A Challenge for the Generalist." *Hospital Practice* 35, no. 1 (January 15, 2000).

Catchpole, Michael A. et al. "Serosurveillance of Prevalence of Undiagnosed HIV-1 Infection in Homosexual Men With Acute Sexually Transmitted Infection." *British Medical Journal* 2000. Available online. URL: http://www.pubmedcentral.nih.gov.bmj.com.

CDC. "Are Health Care Workers at Risk of Getting HIV on the Job?" CDC Website. Available online. URL: http://www.cdc.gov/hiv/pubs/faq/faq28.htm. Downloaded on September 18, 2001.

CDC. "Are Patients in a Dentist's or Doctor's Office at Risk of Getting HIV?" CDC Website. Available online. URL: http://www.cdc.gov/hiv/pubs/faq/faq29.htm. Downloaded on September 18, 2001.

CDC. "Are There Other Tests Available?" Available online. URL: http://www.cdc.gov/hiv/pubs/faq/faq8.htm. Updated November 30, 1998.

CDC. "Are These Stories True?" CDC Website. Available online. URL: http://www.cdc.gov/hiv/pubs/faq. faq5a.htm. Updated March 28, 2001.

CDC. "Bacterial Vaginosis (BV)." Available online. URL: http://www.cdc.gov/od/oc/media/pressrel. Updated September 2000.

CDC. "Basic Statistics." Available online. URL: http://www.cdc.gov. Downloaded June 1, 2002.

CDC. "Can I Get HIV from Anal Sex?" CDC Website. Available online. URL: http://www.cdc.gov/hiv/pubs/faq/faq22.htm. Downloaded on September 18, 2001.

CDC. "Can I Get HIV from Casual Contact?" CDC Website. Available online. URL: http://www.cdc.gov/hiv/pubs/faq/faq31.htm.

CDC. "Can I Get HIV from Getting a Tattoo or Through Body Piercing?" CDC Website. Available online. URL: http://www.cdc.gov/hiv/pubs/faq/faq27.htm. Downloaded on September 18, 2001.

CDC. "Can I Get HIV from Open-Mouth Kissing?" CDC Website. Available online. URL: http://www.cdc.gov/hiv/pubs/faq/faq18.htm. Downloaded September 18, 2001.

CDC. "Can I Get HIV from Performing Oral Sex?" CDC Website. Available online. URL: http://www.cdc.gov/hiv/pubs/faq/faq19.htm. Downloaded on September 18, 2001.

CDC. "Can I Get Infected with HIV from Mosquitoes?" CDC Website. Available online. URL: http://www.cdc.gov/hiv/pubs/faq/faq32.htm.

CDC. "CDC Expands Global AIDS Program to the Caribbean and Latin America." Available online. URL: http://www.cdc.gov/od/oc/media/pressrel. Updated June 7, 2001.

CDC. "CDC Issues New Report on STD Epidemics." Available online. URL: http://www.cdc.gov. Updated December 5, 2000.

CDC. "CDC Issues Major New Report on STD Epidemics: Gonorrhea Rates Increase From 1997 to 1999, Suggesting Possible Reversal of Two-Decade Decline: Syphilis Rates at All-Time Low: First-of-Its-Kind Research on HPV Also Released." CDC Website. Available online. URL: http://www.cdc.gov. Updated on December 11, 2001.

CDC. "CDC's International Activities Support Global HIV Prevention Efforts." Available online. URL: http://www.cdc.gov/od/oc/media/pressrel. Updated November 1999.

CDC. "Chlamydia: Disease Information." CDC Website. Available online. URL: http://www.cdc/gov. Updated May 2001.

CDC. "Classification for Human Immunodeficiency Virus (HIV) Infection in Children Under 13 Years of Age." *Morbidity and Mortality Weekly Report* 35 (1987): 224–235.

CDC. "Condoms and Their Use in Preventing HIV Infections and Other STDs." Available online. URL: http://www.cdc.gov/od/oc/media/pressrel. Updated September 1999.

CDC. "The Deadly Intersection between TB and HIV." Available online. URL: http://www.cdc.gov/od/oc/media/pressrel. Updated November 1999.

CDC. "Does HIV Cause AIDS?" Available online. URL: http://www.cdc.gov/hiv/pubs/faq.faq2.htm. Downloaded November 30, 2001.

CDC. "Eighth Conference on Retroviruses and Opportunistic Infections, Chicago, February 4–7, 2001." Available online. URL: http://www.cdc.gov/od/oc/media/pressrel/fs010205.htm. Updated September 18, 2001.

CDC. "Facts about Drug-Resistant Gonorrhea." Available online. URL: http://www.cdc.gov/od/oc/media/pressrel/fs2k0922a.htm. Updated on September 22, 2000.

CDC. "Facts About Youth Risk Behavior Surveillance—United States 1999." Available online. URL: http://www.cdc.gov. Updated June 9, 2000.

CDC. "False Report: HIV Can Be Transmitted by Contact with Unused Feminine (Sanitary) Pads." CDC Website. Available online. URL: http://www.cdc.gov/hiv/pubs/faq/hoax2.htm.

CDC. "Family Adolescent Risk Behavior and Communication Study." Available online. URL: http://www.cdc.gov/od/oc/media/pressrel. Updated October 1998.

CDC. "Genital HPV Infection." CDC Website. Available online. URL: http://www.cdc/gov. Updated May 2001.

CDC. "Gonorrhea." Available online. URL: http://www.cdc.gov/od/media/pressrel. Updated May 2001.

CDC. "HIV/AIDS among African Americans in the U.S." Available online. URL: http://www.cdc.gov/od/oc/media/pressrel. Updated September 2000.

CDC. "HIV/AIDS among Hispanics in the U.S." Available online. URL: http://www.cdc.gov/od/oc/media/pressrel. Updated September 2000.

CDC. "HIV/AIDS among U.S. Women: Minority and Young Women at Continuing Risk." Available online. URL: http://www.cdc.gov/od/oc/media/pressrel. Updated September 2000.

CDC. "HIV/AIDS and U.S. Women Who Have Sex With Women (WSW)." Available online. URL: http://www.cdc.gov/od/oc/media/pressrel. Updated August 1999.

CDC. "HIV and Its Transmission." Available online. URL: http://www.cdc.gov/od/oc/media/pressrel. Updated July 1999.

CDC. "HIV Prevalence Trends in Selected Populations in the United States: Results from National Serosurveillance, 1993–1997." Available online. URL: http://www.cdc.gov/hiv/pubs/hivprevalence/hivprevalence.htm. Downloaded December 2001.

CDC. "How Is HIV Passed from One Person to Another?" CDC Website. Available online. URL: http://www.cdc.gov/hiv/pubs/faq/faq16.htm. Downloaded September 18, 2001.

CDC. "How Long after a Possible Exposure Should I Wait to Get Tested for HIV?" Available online. URL: http://www.cdc.gov/hiv/pubs/faq. Updated November 30, 1998.

CDC. "How Many People Have HIV and AIDS?" Available online. URL: http://www.cdc.gov/hiv/pubs/faq/faq13.htm. Downloaded December 10, 2001.

CDC. "Human Immunodeficiency Virus Type 2." Available online. URL: http://www.cdc.gov/od/oc/media/pressrel. Updated October 1998.

CDC. "I'm HIV Positive. Where Can I Get Information about Treatments?" Available online. URL: http://www:cdc/gov/hiv/pubs/faq/faq12.htm. Updated September 18, 2001.

CDC. "Immunodeficiency among Female Sex Partners of Males with Acquired Immunodeficiency Syndrome (AIDS)—New York." *Morbidity and Mortality Weekly Report* 31 (1998): 697–698.

CDC. "Milestones in the U.S. HIV Epidemic." Available online. URL: http://www.cdc.gov.

CDC. "Mortality Declines for Several Leading Causes of Death in 1999." Available online. URL: http://www.cdc.gov/od/oc/media/pressrel. Updated June 26, 2001.

CDC. "Need for Sustained HIV Prevention among Men Who Have Sex with Men." Available online. URL: http://www.cdc.gov/od/oc/media/pressrel. Updated September 2000.

CDC. "New CDC Treatment Guidelines Critical to Preventing Health Consequences of Sexually Transmitted Diseases." Available online. CDC Website. URL: http://www.cdc.gov/od/oc/media/pressrel. Downloaded June 5, 2002.

CDC. "New Data Show AIDS Patients Less Likely to Be Hospitalized." Available online. URL: http://www.cdc.gov/od/oc/media/pressrel. Updated February 25, 2000.

CDC. "NIH Researchers Recall the Early Years of AIDS." Information for timeline in Introduction. Available online. URL: http://www.cdc.gov. Downloaded December 12, 2001.

CDC. "Opportunistic Infections and Kaposi's Sarcoma among Haitians in the United States." *Morbidity and Mortality Weekly Report* 31 (1982): 353–361.

CDC. "Oral Polio Vaccine and HIV/AIDS." Available online. URL: http://www.cdc.gov. Downloaded July 15, 2002.

CDC. "Pelvic Inflammatory Disease." CDC Website. Available online. URL: http://www.cdc/gov. Updated May 2001.

CDC. "Preventing Occupational HIV Transmission to Health Care Workers." Available online. URL: http://www.cdc.gov/od/oc/media/pressrel. Updated June 1999.

CDC. "Primary HIV Infection Associated with Oral Transmission." Available online. URL: http://www.cdc.gov. Updated on March 2000.

CDC. "Revision of the Case Definition of Acquired Immunodeficiency Syndrome for National Reporting-United States." *Morbidity and Mortality Weekly Report* 34 (1985): 373–375.

CDC. "Rumor: *Weekly World News* Story Made Claims That CDC Had Discovered a Mutated Version of HIV That Is Transmitted through the Air. Is This True? Response: This Story Is Not True." CDC Website. Available online. URL: http://www.cdc.gov/hiv/pubs/faq/hoax1.htm.

CDC. "Scabies." Available online. URL: http:www.cdc.gov. Updated September 18, 2001.

CDC. "Scabies in the Child Care Setting." Available online. URL: http://www.cdc.gov. Updated January 1997.

CDC. "Should I Be Concerned about Getting Infected with HIV While Playing Sports?" CDC Website. Available online. URL: http:www.cdc.gov/hiv/pubs/faq/faq30.htm. Downloaded on September 18, 2001.

CDC. "Status of Perinatal HIV Prevention: U.S. Declines Continue." Available online. URL: http://www.cdc.gov/od/oc/media/pressrel. Updated November 1999.

CDC. "Syphilis among Infants Down More than Half in Three Years." Available online. URL: http://www.cdc. Updated July 12, 2001.

CDC. "Syphilis Elimination: History in the Making." CDC Website. Available online. URL: http://www.cdc.gov. Updated May 2001.

CDC. "Take Action on HEDIS." Available online. URL: http://www.cdc.gov. Downloaded October 1, 2001.

CDC. "Testing a Vaccine Designed to Help Curb the Devastating Toll of HIV in the Developing World." Available online. URL: http://www.cdc.gov/nchstp/htv_aids/dhap.htm. Updated February 1999.

CDC. "Trichomoniasis." Available online. URL: http://www.cdc.gov/od/oc/media/pressrel. Updated September 2000.

CDC. "Trichomonas Infection." Available online. URL: http://www.cdc.gov. Updated February 22, 1999.

CDC. "Tracking the Hidden Epidemics: Trends in STDs in the United States 2000." Available online. URL: http://www.cdc.gov/nchstp/htv_aids/dhap.htm. Downloaded February 10, 2002.

CDC. "20 Years of AIDS: 450,000 Americans Dead, Over 1 Million Have Been Infected." Available online. URL: http://www.cdc.gov/od/oc/media/pressrel. Updated May 31, 2001.

CDC. "What If I Test Positive for HIV?" Available online. URL: http://www.cdc.gov/hiv/pubs/faq. Updated November 30, 1998.

CDC. "What Is AIDS? What Causes AIDS?" Available online. URL: http://www.cdc.gov/hiv/pubs/faq. faq2.htm. Updated November 30, 1998.

CDC. "What Are Rapid HIV Tests?" Available online. URL: http://www.cdc.gov/hiv/pubs/faq. Updated November 30, 1998.

CDC. "Where Can I Get Tested for HIV Infection?" CDC Website. Available online. URL: http://www.cdc/hiv/pubs/faq/faq6.htm. Downloaded on September 18, 2001.

CDC. "You Can Prevent PCP: A Guide for People with HIV Infection." Available online. URL: http://www.cdc/hiv/pubs. Downloaded on September 5, 2002.

CDC. "Young People at Risk: HIV/AIDS among America's Youth." Available online. URL: http://www.cdc.gov/hiv. Updated September 2000.

CDC Update. "CDC Guidelines for Improved Data on U.S. HIV Epidemic." Available online. URL: http://www.cdc.gov.nchstp/hiv_aids/dhap.htm. Updated December 1999.

CDC Update. "CDC Statement in Response to Presentation on Origin of HIV-1 at 6th Conference on Retroviruses and Opportunistic Infections." Available online. URL: http://www.cdc.gov. Updated January 31, 1999.

CDC Update. "Combating Complacency in HIV Prevention." Available online. URL: http://www.cdc.gov. Updated June 1998.

CDC Update. "Comprehensive HIV Prevention Messages for Young People." Available online. URL: http://www.cdc.gov. Downloaded June 2, 2002.

CDC Update. "Draft Guidelines for National HIV Case Surveillance, Including Monitoring for HIV Infection and Acquired Immunodeficiency Syndrome (AIDS)." Available online. URL: http://www.cdc.gov. Downloaded October 1, 2001.

CDC Update. "HIV Complacency Could Threaten Progress." Available online. URL: http://www.cdc.gov. Downloaded February 1, 2002.

CDC Update. "HIV Prevention Community Planning: Successes and Challenges." Available online. URL: http://www.cdc.gov. Updated January 1998.

CDC Update. "Multi-State Study on Impact of New Treatment on HIV Risk Behavior." Available online. URL: http://www.cdc.gov. Downloaded August 15, 2002.

CDC Update. "National Data on HIV Prevalence among Disadvantaged Youth in the 1990s." Available online. URL: http://www.cdc.gov. Updated September 1998.

CDC Update. "Need for Sustained HIV Prevention for Gay and Bisexual Men." Available online. URL: http://www.cdc.gov/nchstp/hiv_aids/dhap.htm. Updated January 2000.

CDC Update. "New Treatment Guidelines for HIV Patients Suggest Drug Treatment Can Be Delayed," by Lindsey Tanner (Associated Press). URL: http://www.cdc.gov. Updated July 8, 2002.

CDC Update. "Oral Sex Contributes Significantly to HIV Transmission." Available online. URL: http://www.cdc.gov. Downloaded August 25, 2002.

CDC Update. "Patterns of Condom Use among Adolescents." American Journal of Public Health, October 1, 1998. Available online. URL: http://www.cdc.gov. Updated October 1998.

CDC Update. "PHS Report Summarizes Current Scientific Knowledge on the Use of Post-Exposure Antiretroviral Therapy for Non-Occupational Exposures." Available online. URL: http://www.cdc.gov. Downloaded October 15, 2001.

CDC Update. "Preventing the Sexual Transmission of HIV, the Virus That Causes AIDS." Available online. URL: http://www.cdc.gov. Downloaded September 20, 2001.

CDC Update. "Questions and Answers on the Thailand Phase III Vaccine Study and CDC's Collaboration." Available online. URL: http://www.cdc.gov. Downloaded September 20, 2001.

CDC Update. "Recent HIV/AIDS Treatment Advances and the Implications for Prevention." Available online. URL: http://www.cdc.gov. Updated June 1998.

Chase, Marilyn. "Sexually Transmitted Diseases Appear Sharply Underreported." The Wall Street Journal February 13, 2002.

Cheingsong-Popov, R. et al. "Prevalence of Antibody to Human T-Lymphotropic Virus Type III in AIDS and AIDS-Risk Patients in Britain." Lancet 2, no. 8401 (1984): 477–480.

Cheng, A. C. et al. "Psychosocial Factors Are Associated with Prolonged Hospitalization in a Population with Advanced HIV." PubMed Website. Available online. URL: http://www.ncbi.nlm.nih.gov/entrez/query.fcgi. Downloaded on October 30, 2001.

Chin, J., and Mann, J. M. "The Global Patterns and Prevalence of AIDS and HIV Infection." AIDS 2 (suppl 1) (1988): S247–S252.

"China Finally Tackles Ignorance of AIDS." AVERT Website. The Guardian, March 12, 2001. Available online. URL: http://www.avert.org.

"Chlamydia Infection." JAMA Women's Health Website. Available online. URL: http://www.ama-assn.org/special/std/support/educate/stdclam.htm. Downloaded on August 6, 2001.

"Chlamydia's Quick Cure." WebMD. Available online. URL: http://www.wedmd.com. Updated on June 6, 2001.

"Chlamydia Screening Study: Most MDs Disregard CDC Recommendations." Dr. Koop Sexual Health Website. Available online. URL: http://www.drkoop.com.

Clay, D. "Mental Health and Psychosocial Issues in HIV Care." PubMed Website. Lippincott's Primary Care Practice 4, no. 1 (January–February 2000). Available online. URL: http://www.ncbi.nlm.nih.gov/entrez/query. Updated August 22, 2001.

Cleghorn, F. R. et al. "A Distinctive Clade B HIV Type 1 Is Heterosexually Transmitted in Trinidad and Tobago." Proceedings of the National Academy of Sciences of the United States of America 97, no. 19 (September 2000). Available online. URL: http://www.pubmedcentral.nih.gov.bmj.com.

"Clinton Aide Gives Bush Unwelcome Advice on Sex." AVERT Website. The Guardian, June 30, 2001. Available online. URL: http://www.avert.org.

Cohen, D., Dent, C., and MacKinnon, D. "Condom Skills Education and Sexually Transmitted Disease Reinfection." Journal of Sex Research 28, no. 1 (1991).

Cohen, J. "Could Drugs, Rather Than a Virus Be the Cause of AIDS?" *Science* 266, no. 5191 (1994): 1648–1649.

Cohen, J. "The Duesberg Phenomenon." *Science* 266, no. 5191 (1994): 1642–1644.

Cohen, Mark. "Psychiatric Complications and Psychosocial Issues in HIV Disease." Available online. URL: http://www.medical-library.org/index.htm.

"Colombian Rebels Expel HIV Victims from Town." AVERT Website. *The Guardian,* October 23, 2001. Available online. URL: http:/www.avert.org.

"Colombian Rebels Force AIDS Test." AVERT Website. *Daily Telegraph* Online, December 10, 2001. Available online. URL: http://www.avert.org.

Conant, Eve. "A Social Neutron Bomb." *Newsweek,* September 17, 2001. Available online. Downloaded October 1, 2001.

Concorde Coordinating Committee. "MRC/ANRS Randomised Double-Blind Controlled Trial of Immediate and Deferred Zidovudine in Symptom-Free HIV Infection." *Lancet* 343, no. 8902 (1994): 871–881.

"Condoms Do Prevent HIV, Gonorrhea: U.S. Panel." Medline Plus. Reuters. Available online. URL: http://www.medline.com. Downloaded on November 27, 2001.

"Condom Use by Adolescents." PubMed Website. *Pediatrics* 107, no. 6 (June 2001): 1463–1469. Available online. URL: http://www.ncbi.nlm.nih.gov/entrez. Downloaded June 6, 2001.

"Congress May Extend Medicaid to HIV+ People." Alive & Kicking!'s FastFax Website. Available online. URL: http://www.peoplewithaids.org/fastfax/ff227.htm. Downloaded on December 12, 2001.

Connor, R. I., and Ho, D. D. "Transmission and Pathogenesis of Human Immunodeficiency Virus Type 1." *AIDS Research and Human Retroviruses* 10, no. 4 (1994): 321–323.

Connor, R. J. et al. "Increased Viral Burden and Cytopathicity Correlate Temporally With CD4+ T-lymphocyte Decline and Clinical Progression in Human Immunodeficiency Virus Type 1-Infected Individuals." *Journal of Virology* 67, no. 4 (1993): 1772–1777.

Corbitt, G., Bailey, A. S., and Williams, G. "HIV Infection in Manchester, 1959." *Lancet* 336, no. 8706 (1990): 51.

"Counseling Can Help Correct Misconceptions about Sexually Transmitted Diseases." Doctor's Guide Website. Available online. URL: http://www.docguide.news. Downloaded February 1, 2002.

Curran, J. W. et al. "Acquired Immunodeficiency Syndrome (AIDS) Associated with Transfusions." *New England Journal of Medicine* 310, no. 2 (1984): 69–75.

Curran, J. W. et al. "Epidemiology of HIV Infection and AIDS in the United States." *Science* 239, no. 4840 (1988): 610–616.

"Current Newborn Screening by State." Available online. URL: http://www.aboutnewbornscreening.com/stats.htm.

Da Costa, Xavier J., Jones, Cheryl A., and Knipe, David M. "Immunization against Genital Herpes with a Vaccine Virus That Has Defects in Productive and Latent Infection." *Proceedings of the National Academy of Sciences of the United States of America* 96, no. 12 (June 8, 1999). Available online. URL: http://www.pubmedcentral.gov.nih.

Davachi, F. "Pediatric HIV Infection in Africa." In: M. Essex et al, eds. *AIDS in Africa.* New York: Raven Press, 1994, pp. 439–62.

Davis, Michael A. "Aspergillosis." Medical Library Website. Available online. URL: http://www.medical-library.org/index.htm. Downloaded May 1, 2002.

Davis, Michael A. "HIV Pathogenesis." Medical Library Website. Available online. URL: http://www.medical-library.org/index.htm. Downloaded May 5, 2002.

Davis, Michael A. "Primary HIV Infection." Medical Library Website. Available online. URL: http://www.medical-library.org/index.htm. Downloaded on May 5, 2002.

DeCock, Kevin. "CDC Statement in Response to Presentation on Origin of HIV-1 at 6th Conference on Retroviruses and Opportunistic Infections." CDC Update. Available online. URL: http://www.cdc.gov. Updated January 31, 1999.

Defino, Theresa. "Twice Yearly Chlamydia Tests Recommended for Young Women." WebMD Medical News. MSN Website. Available online. URL: http://content.health.msn.com/content/article/1728.72062.

Desrosiers, R. C. "The Simian Immunodeficiency Viruses." *Annual Review of Immunology* 8 (1990): 557–578.

Dewhurst, S. et al. "Sequence Analysis and Acute Pathogenicity of Molecularly Cloned SIVSMM-PBj14." *Nature* 345, no. 6276 (1990): 636–640.

"Diagnosing Depression." Mayo Clinic Website. Available online. URL: http://www.MayoClinic.com. Downloaded August 10, 2002.

"Diagnosing Genital Herpes." Health Advice Company Website. Available online. URL: http://www.advicecenter.com/diag.html.

Dillion, Beth, et al. "Oral Sex Contributes Significantly to HIV Transmission." CDC Update. (Key findings from CDC, 7th Conference on Retroviruses and Opportunistic Infections, San Francisco, Calif., January 30–February 2, 2000). Poster presentation. Available online. URL: http://www.cdc.gov. Downloaded on November 28, 2001.

Dobkin, Jay F. "New Insights into Nonprogressive HIV Infection." Medscape Website. *Infections in Medicine* 15, no. 2 (1998): 82. Available online. URL: http://www.

medscape.com/SCP/IIM/1998/v15.n02/m4088.dobkin/m4088.dobkin.html. Downloaded on December 15, 2001.

"Doctors: It's Your Responsibility." Health Care Financing Administration. Available online. URL: http://www.hcfa.gov/hiv. Downloaded November 28, 2001.

Drew, W. L. et al. "Prevalence of Cytomegalovirus Infection in Homosexual Men." *Journal of Infectious Diseases* 143 (1981): 188–192.

Duesberg, P. "HIV Is Not the Cause of AIDS." *Science* 241, no. 4865 (1988): 514, 517.

Duesberg, P. H. "Human Immunodeficiency Virus and Acquired Immunodeficiency Syndrome: Correlation but Not Causation." *Proceedings of the National Academy of Science of the United States of America* 86, no. 3 (1989): 755–764. Available online. URL: http://www.pubmedcentral.gov.nih.

Duesberg, P. H. "AIDS Epidemiology: Inconsistencies with Human Immunodeficiency Virus and with Infectious Disease." *Proceedings of the National Academy of Sciences of the United States of America* 88, no. 4 (1991): 1575–1579. Available online. URL: http://www.pubmedcentral.gov.nih.

Duncan, Barbara et al. "Qualitative Analysis of Psychosocial Impact of Diagnosis of Chlamydia Trachomatis: Implications for Screening." PubMed Site. *British Medical Journal* 322 (2001): 195–199. Available online. URL: http://www.pubmedcentral.gov.bmj.

Durack, D. T. "Opportunistic Infections and Kaposi's Sarcoma in Homosexual Men." *New England Journal of Medicine* 305, no. 24 (1981): 1465–1467.

Ebel, Charles. "Scientists Put Condom Report in Perspective." SexHealth Website. Available online. URL: http://www.SexHealth.com. Downloaded August 22, 2001.

"Effect of HIV Reporting by Name on Use of HIV Testing in Publicly Funded Counseling and Testing Programs." *JAMA* HIV/AIDS Resource Center Website. Available online. URL: http://www.ama-assn.org/special/hiv/library/readroom/jama98/joc80227.htm. Downloaded on December 12, 2001.

"E History of AIDS." AVERT Website. Available online. URL: http://www.avert.org.

Eighth Conference on Retroviruses and Opportunistic Infections. Chicago. February 4–7, 2001. Centers for Disease Control and Prevention. URL: http://www.retroconference.org/2001/info.htm.

Erbelding, Emily J. et al. "The Hopkins HIV Report 2002." Johns Hopkins AIDS Service Website. Available online. URL: http://hopkins-aids.edu/publications. Downloaded July 9, 2002.

Essex, M. et al. "Naturally Occurring Persistent Feline Oncornavirus Infections in the Absence of Disease." *Infection and Immunity* 11, no. 3 (1975): 470–475.

Essex, M. "The Etiology of AIDS." In: M. Essex et al., eds. *AIDS in Africa.* New York: Raven Press, 1994, pp. 1–20.

European Collaborative Study. "Children Born to Women with HIV-1 Infection: Natural History and Risk of Transmission." *Lancet* 337 (1991): 253–260.

Evans, A. S. "Causation and Disease: The Henle-Koch Postulates Revisited." *Yale Journal of Biology and Medicine* 49, no. 2 (1976): 175–195.

Evans, A. S. "Does HIV Cause AIDS? An Historical Perspective." *Journal of Acquired Immune Deficiency Syndrome* 2, no. 2 (1989): 107–113.

Evans, A. S. "AIDS: The Alternative View." *Lancet* 339, no. 8808 (1992): 1547.

Evans, Barry et al. "Exposure of Healthcare Workers in England, Wales, and Northern Ireland to Bloodborne Viruses between July 1997 and June 2000: Analysis of Surveillance Data." *British Medical Journal* 322 (February 2001). Available online. URL: http://www.pubmedcentral.nih.gov/articlerender.fcgi. Updated August 3, 2001.

Evatt, B. L. et al. "Coincidental Appearance of LAV/HTLV-III Antibodies in Hemophiliacs and the Onset of the AIDS Epidemic." *New England Journal of Medicine* 312, no. 8 (1985): 483–486.

"Everything Government Says about AIDS Is False." 1992 Flyer with 1999 introduction. Available online. URL: http://www.members.aol.com/_ht_a/MrGayPride/AIDS.html. Downloaded October 4, 2001.

"Evidence HIV Causes AIDS." AVERT Website. Available online. URL: http://www.avert.org.

"Evidence That HIV Causes AIDS." Fact Sheet. Available online. URL: http://www.nih.gov. Downloaded August 15, 2002.

"Facts about HIV and AIDS." American Academy of Pediatrics. Medem Website. Available online. URL: http://www.medem.com. Downloaded November 30, 2001.

"FAQ about HPV." Health Advice Company Website. Available online. URL: http://www.advicecenter.com/hpv/hpvtreat.html.

Fauci, A. S. "The Human Immunodeficiency Virus: Infectivity and Mechanisms of Pathogenesis." *Science* 239 no. 4840 (1988): 617–622.

Fauci, Anthony S. et al. Guidelines for the Use of Antiretroviral Agents in HIV-Infected Adults and Adolescents. A booklet developed by the Panel on Clinical Practices for Treatment of HIV Infection, convened by the Department of Health and Human Services and the Henry J. Kaiser Family Foundation. An educational service from Merck, 2001.

"FDA OKs HIV Drug-Resistance Test." MSNBC Website. Available online. URL: http://www.msnbc.com. Downloaded on May 5, 2002.

Forman, Sara Frim, and Emans, S. Jean. "Current Goals for Adolescent Health Care." *Hospital Physician* 36, no. 1 (January 2000).

Fox, Maggie. "Clues for Creating Chemical Condoms." Reuters. MSNBC Website. Available online. URL: http://www.msnbc.com. Downloaded January 20, 2002.

Franchini, G. et al. "Sequence of Simian Immunodeficiency Virus and Its Relationship to the Human Immunodeficiency Viruses." *Nature* 328, no. 6130 (1987): 539–543.

Francis, D. P., Curran, J. W., and Essex, M. "Epidemic Acquired Immune Deficiency Syndrome: Epidemiologic Evidence for a Transmissible Agent." *Journal of the National Cancer Institute* 71, no. 1 (1983): 1–4.

"Frequently Asked Questions about Newborn Screening." Available online. URL: http://www.aboutnewbornscreening.com/faq.htm.

Friedman-Kien, A. E. "Disseminated Kaposi's Sarcoma Syndrome in Young Homosexual Men." *Journal of the American Academy of Dermatology* 5, no. 4 (1981): 468–471.

Gallo, R. C. et al. "Frequent Detection and Isolation of Cytopathic Retroviruses (HTLV-III) from Patients with AIDS and at Risk for AIDS." *Science* no. 4648 (1984): 500–503.

Gallo, R. C., and Montagnier, L. "The Chronology of AIDS Research." *Nature* 326, no. 6112 (1987): 435–436.

"Garlic Supplements Can Impede HIV Medication." National Institute of Allergy and Infectious Disease Website. Available online. URL: http://www.nih.gov/news/pr/dec2001/niaid-05.htm. Downloaded on December 12, 2001.

Garrett, Laurie. "STD Prevention in Societies under Stress: A Global Perspective." A presentation at the 2002 National STD Prevention Conference, sponsored by the CDC and American Social Health Association, San Diego, California. Available online. URL: http://www.kaisernetwork.org/health.

"Genital Herpes." *JAMA* Women's Health Website. Available online. URL: http://www.ama-assn.org/special/std/support/educate/stdherp.htm. Downloaded on August 6, 2001.

"Getting Tested for HIV." Health Care Financing Administration Website. Available online. URL: http://www.hcfa.gov/hiv/subpg2.htm. Downloaded October 15, 2001.

Gilden, Dave. "NCI Conference Considers Specter of Widespread Drug Resistance." amfAR Website. Available online. URL: http://www.amfar.org/td. Updated January 2002.

Ginsberg, H. D. (moderator). "Scientific Forum on AIDS: A Summary: Does HIV Cause AIDS?" *Journal of Acquired Immune Deficiency Syndrome* 1, no. 2 (1998): 165–172.

"GlaxoSmithKline to Extend Cheaper AIDS Drugs." AVERT Website. *The Financial Times,* November 6, 2001. Available online. URL: http://www.avert.org.

"The Global Infectious Disease Threat and Its Implications for the United States." Available online. URL: http://www.cia.gov/nic/pubs/other_products/inf_diseases_paper.html.

Gonda, M. A. et al. "Sequence Homology and Morphologic Similarity of HTLV-III and Visna Virus, a Pathogenic Lentivirus." *Science* 227, no. 4683 (1985): 173–177.

"Gonorrhea." JAMA Women's Health Website. Available online. URL: http://www.ama-assn.org/special/std/support/educate/stdgon.htm. Downloaded on August 6, 2001.

"Gonorrhea." New York City Department of Health Website. Available online. URL: http://www.ci.nyc.ny.us/htm/doh/html/std/stdg3.html. Downloaded on December 14, 2001.

Gordon, David F. "The Global Infectious Disease Threat and Its Implications for the United States." January 2000. National Intelligence Council. From an unclassified version of a National Intelligence Estimate on the reemergence of the threat from infectious diseases worldwide and its implications for the U.S. Available online. URL: http://www.cdc.gov.globalinfectiousdiseasethreat.

Goudsmit, J. "Alternative View on AIDS." *Lancet,* 339, no. 8804 (1992): 1289–1290.

Goudsmit, Jaap, et al. "Human Herpesvirus 8 Infections in the Amsterdam Cohort Studies (1984–1997): Analysis of Seroconversions to ORF65 and ORF73." *Proceedings of the National Academy of Sciences of the United States of America* 97, no. 9 (April 25, 2000). Available online. URL: http://www.pubmedcentral.gov.nih. Downloaded on September 1, 2001.

Graber, Mark A., and Martinez-Bianchi, Viviana. "Genitourinary and Renal Disease: Sexually Transmitted Diseases." Virtual Hospital Website, University of Iowa Family Practice Handbook, 3d ed, Chapter 14. Available online. URL: http://www.vh.org/Providers/ClinRef/FPHandbook/Chapter11/05-11.html. Downloaded on December 14, 2001.

Graham, N. M. et al. "The Effects on Survival of Early Treatment of Human Immunodeficiency Virus Infection." *New England Journal of Medicine* 326, no. 16 (1992): 1037–1042.

Greiger-Zanlungo, Paola. "HIV and Women: An Update." *The Female Patient* 26, no. 3 (March 2001).

Greene, W. C. "AIDS and the Immune System." *Scientific American* 269, no. 3 (1993): 98–105.

Greener, Mark. "Pap Smears Alone Prove Unreliable for Diagnosing Sexually Transmitted Diseases." Doctor's Guide Website. Available online. URL: http://www.docguide.com.

"Guidelines for National Human Immunodeficiency Virus Case Surveillance, Including Monitoring for Human Immunodeficiency Virus Infection and Acquired Immunodeficiency Syndrome." *Morbidity and Mortality Weekly Reports Recommendations and Reports* December 10, 1999. CDC Website. Available online. URL: http://www.cdc.gov. Downloaded February 1, 2002.

Guidelines for the Management of Occupational Exposures to HBV, HCV, and HIV and Recommendations for Postexposure Prophylaxis (booklet). From the CDC's *Morbidity and Mortality Weekly Report Recommendations and Reports* 50 (June 29, 2001).

Guidelines for the Treatment of Sexually Transmitted Diseases (booklet). From the CDC's *Morbidity and Mortality Weekly Report Recommendations and Reports* 47 (January 23, 1998).

Guidelines for the Use of Antiretroviral Agents in HIV-Infected Adults and Adolescents (booklet). Developed by the Panel on Clinical Practices for Treatment of HIV Infection, convened by the Department of Health and Human Services and the Henry J. Kaiser Family Foundation. Panel leadership: Anthony Fauci, National Institutes of Health; John G. Bartlett, Johns Hopkins University; Eric P. Goosby, DHHS; Jennifer Kates, Henry J. Kaiser Foundation.

Haas, Elson M. "Nutritional Program for Yeast Syndrome." Health Forum online. Available online. URL: http://www.healthy.net/asp/templates/article.html. Posted on October 23, 2001.

Hahn, B. et al. "AIDS as a Zoonosis: Scientific and Public Health Implications." *Science* 200, no. 287: 607–614.

Hamilton, Jon. "Human Papillomavirus a Threat when Infection Lingers." WebMD Website. Available online. URL: http://www.webmd.com. Updated June 6, 2001.

Harden, Victoria A. "Koch's Postulates and the Etiology of AIDS: An Historical Perspective." *History and Philosophy of the Life Sciences* 14, no. 2 (1992): 249–269.

Harris, S. B. "The AIDS Heresies: A Case Study of Skepticism Taken Too Far." *Skeptic* 3, no. 2 (1995): 42–79.

Hauschildt, Elda. "Self-Obtained Vaginal Swabs Could Control Sexually Transmitted Diseases." Doctor's Guide channels. *Archives of Pediatrics and Adolescent Medicine* (June 19, 2001). Available online. URL: http://www.docguide.com. Downloaded February 1, 2002.

"Having Sex Is about Making Choices." Planned Parenthood Website. URL: http://www.plannedparenthood.org/teenissues/bcchoices/html. Downloaded October 1, 2002.

Heimer, Robert, and Abdala, Nadia. "Viability of HIV-1 in Syringes: Implications for Interventions among Injec-

tion Drug Users." *The AIDS Reader.* Available online. URL: http://www.medscape.com/SCP/TAR/2000/v10.n07/a1007.01.heim-01.html.

Henry, Keith. "Immune Responses in Long-Term Nonprogressors." The Body Website. Available online. URL: http://www.thebody.com/basics.html.

"Hepatitis A: New Focus for Immunization Guidelines." *Consultant* 40, no. 1 (January 2000): 54–57.

"Hepatitis." Fact sheet. *JAMA* Women's Health Website. URL: http://www.ama-assn.org/special/std/support/educate/stdhep.htm. Downloaded January 20, 2002.

"Herpes in Pregnancy." Health Advice Company Website. Available online. URL: http://www.advicecenter.com/pregnancy.html.

"Helping Women to Cope with AIDS in Rwanda." AVERT Website. News item from *The Guardian,* with editing by AVERT, May 12, 2001. URL: http://www.avert.org. Downloaded June 1, 2002.

Herting, Robert L, Jr., and Frohberg, Nora R. "Neurology: Peripheral Neuropathy." Virtual Hospital Website, University of Iowa Family Practice Handbook, 3d ed. Chapter 14. Available online. URL: http://www.vh.org/Providers/ClinRef/FPHandbook/Chapter14/10-14.html. Downloaded on December 14, 2001.

Hickling, Lee. "Privacy and HIV Testing: What's in a Name?" Dr. Koop Website. Available online. URL: http://www.askdrkoop.com/news/specialreports/hiv_testing/privacy.html. Downloaded on December 12, 2001.

Highfield, Roger. "AIDS Link with Polio Vaccine Finally Rejected," *Daily Telegraph,* April 26, 2001.

"High Levels of Infection in Rwandan Women." AVERT Website. *Positive Nation,* November 2001. Available online. URL: http://www.avert.org.

"High Noon for the Morning-After Pill." *SalonMag* Website. Available online. URL: http://www.salonmag.com/mwt/feature/2001/06/20/pill/index.html. Downloaded on December 12, 2001.

Hirsch, V. M. et al. "An African Primate Lentivirus (SIVsm) Closely Related to HIV-2." *Nature* 321, no. 24 (1989): 1621–1625.

Hirschler, Ben. "New 'Fusion Inhibitor' Drug Offers AIDS Lifeline." Reuters. Medline Website. Available online. URL: http://www.medlineplus.com. Downloaded August 25, 2002.

"The HIV/AIDS Epidemic: 20 Years in the U.S." White House Website. Summary Fact Sheet on HIV/AIDS. Available online. URL: http://www.whitehouse.gov. Downloaded on February 17, 2002.

"HIV/AIDS Hotlines." Johns Hopkins AIDS Service Website. Available online. URL: http://www.thebody.com. Downloaded June 5, 2002.

"HIV/AIDS Milestones 1981–1990." U.S. Food and Drug Administration Website. Last revised in June 1996. URL: http://www.fda.gov/oashi/aids/miles81.html.

"HIV/AIDS Milestones 1991–1994." U.S. Food and Drug Administration Website. Last revised in June 1996. URL: http://www.fda.gov/oashi/aids/miles91.html.

"HIV/AIDS Milestones 1995–1999." U.S. Food and Drug Administration Website. Last revised on September 11, 2001. URL: http://www.fda.gov/oashi/aids/miles95.html.

"HIV/AIDS Milestones 2000–2001." U.S. Food and Drug Administration Website. Last revised in December 2001. URL: http://www.fda.gov/oashi/aids/miles00.html.

HIV/AIDS Update. December 2000. "Preventing the Sexual Transmission of HIV, the Virus That Causes AIDS: What You Should Know about Oral Sex." Available online. URL: http://www.cdc.gov.

"HIV and AIDS-Related News as Reported in England." AVERT Website. Available online. URL: http://www.avert.org. Downloaded June 1, 2002.

"HIV ELISA/Western Blot." Medline Website. Available online. URL: http://www.medline.com. Downloaded September 22, 2002.

"HIV Infection and AIDS." *JAMA* Women's Health Website. Available online. URL: http://www.ama-assn.org/special/std/support/educate/hivinf.htm. Updated on August 6, 2001.

"The HIV Postexposure Prophylaxis Registry." *JAMA* HIV/AIDS Resource Center Website. Available online. URL: http://www.ama-assn.org/special/hiv/preventn/pepflybw.htm. Downloaded on December 12, 2001.

"HIV Prevention through Early Detection and Treatment of Other Sexually Transmitted Diseases—United States." *Morbidity and Mortality Weekly Report* 47, no. RR-12 (July 31, 1998).

"HIV 'Rides' into Cells on Membrane Rafts, NIAID Scientists Determine." Available online. URL: http://www.NIAID.gov. Downloaded September 5, 2002.

"HIV Testing Delays May Be Fueling AIDS Crisis." MSNBC Website. Available online. URL: http://www.msnbc.com. Downloaded on February 10, 2002.

"HIV Vaccine Promising in Monkeys." Alive & Kicking!'s FastFax Website. Available online. URL: http://www.peoplewithaids.org/fastfax/ff227.htm. Downloaded on December 12, 2001.

Ho, D. D., Pomerantz, R. J., and Kaplan, J. C. "Pathogenesis of Infection with Human Immunodeficiency Virus." *New England Journal of Medicine* 317, no. 5 (1987): 278–286.

Hodgkinson, Neville. "AIDS: Is Anyone Positive?" *The European,* June 22, 1998. Available online. URL: http://www.virusmyth.net/aids. Downloaded on November 10, 2001.

Hogg, Robert S. et al. "Rates of Disease Progression by Baseline CD4 Cell Count and Viral Load after Initiating Triple-Drug Therapy." *JAMA* Website. (2001). Available online. URL: http://www.jama.ama.org. Downloaded on May 5, 2002.

Holzman, Robert, and Mertz, David. "Is HIV the Cause of AIDS?" Sci.med.aids Website. Available online. URL: http://www.aids.wustl.edu/aids/sci.med.aids.faq6.html.

"Hopes for the Global Health Fund." AVERT Website. *The Guardian.* Available online. URL: http://www.avert.org.

Horowitz, Leonard G., Kyle, Walter, and Cantwell, Alan R. "A New Theory on the Iatrogenic Origin of AIDS." Available online. URL: http://www.inx.net/~carolynv/vaccines/horowitz.htm. Downloaded on December 15, 2001.

"Human Immunodeficiency Virus Infections in the Child-Care Setting." Medem Website. Available online. URL: http://www.medem.com. Downloaded January 18, 2002.

"Human Immunodeficiency Virus Infection Is Rare from Receptive Oral Sex with a Man." Doctor's Guide Website. Available online. URL: http://www.docguide.com.

"Human Immunodeficiency Virus Can Be Transmitted to Others within a Week of Infection." Doctor's Guide Website. Available online. URL: http://www.docguide.com. Downloaded on February 17, 2002.

"Human Papillomavirus and Genital Warts." *JAMA* Women's Health Website. Available online. URL: http://www.ama-assn.org/special/std/support/educate/stdhpv.htm. Downloaded on August 8, 2001.

"Human Papillomavirus Linked to Head and Neck Cancer." Doctor's Guide Website. Available online. URL: http://www.docguide/news.com. Downloaded on February 1, 2002.

"Human Papillomavirus Testing Highly Valuable in Cervical Cancer Screening." Doctor's Guide Website. Available online. URL: http://www.docguide.com. Downloaded August 2, 2002.

Iglesias, Elba A., Alderman, Elizabeth, and Fox, Amy S. "Use of Wet Smears to Screen for Sexually Transmitted Diseases." *Infections in Medicine.* Available online. URL: http://www.medscape.com. Downloaded on November 1, 2001.

"Immunization against Genital Herpes with a Vaccine Virus That Has Defects in Productive and Latent Infection." *Proceedings of the National Academy of Sciences of the United States of America* 96, no. 12. Available online. URL: http://www.pubmedcentral.gov.nih. Downloaded on November 3, 2001.

"Immunodeficiency Disorders." Medline website. National Library of Medicine. Available online. URL: http://www.medline.com. Downloaded on August 25, 2002.

Imrie, John et al. "A Cognitive Behavioural Intervention to Reduce Sexually Transmitted Infections among Gay Men: Randomized Trial." *British Medical Journal* 322 (June 16, 2001). Available online. URL: http://www.pubmedcentral.gov.bmj. Downloaded on November 1, 2001.

"An Introduction to Sexually Transmitted Diseases." *JAMA* Women's Health Website. Available online. URL: http://www.ama.assn.org/special/std/support/educate/stdinfo.htm. Downloaded on August 6, 2001.

"An Introduction to Sexually Transmitted Diseases." July 1999. Fact Sheet, National Institute of Allergy and Infectious Diseases, U.S. National Institutes of Health. Available online. URL: http://www.nih.gov. Downloaded December 2001.

"IPC: Trial Supports Human Papillomavirus Testing as Primary Cancer Screen." Doctor's Guide Website. Available online. URL: http://www.docguide.com. Downloaded on February 1, 2002.

"Is the Pap Smear Obsolete?" SexHealth Website. Available online. URL: http://www.sexhealth.com/sexhealth/user/display.cfm. Updated October 1, 2001.

"IVF Clinics 'Shun' HIV Patients." AVERT Website. BBC News Online. Available online. URL: http://www.avert.org. Downloaded on February 12, 2001.

Jacobs, E. "Anal Infections Caused by Herpes Simplex Virus." *Diseases of the Colon and Rectum* 19, no. 2 (1976): 151–157.

Jaffe, H. W. et al. "The Acquired Immunodeficiency Syndrome in a Cohort of Homosexual Men: A Six-Year Follow-up Study." *Annals of Internal Medicine* 103, no. 2 (1985): 210–214.

JAMA Women's Health Sexually Transmitted Disease Information Center. "Hepatitis." Fact sheet. Available online. URL: http://www.ama-assn.org/stdinfo.htm. Updated August 1992.

JAMA Women's Health STD Information Center. "Vaginal Infections and Vaginitis." Fact sheet. Available online. URL: http://www.ama.org/stdinfo.htm. Updated January 2000.

JAMA Women's Health STD Information Center. "Other Important STDs." Fact sheet. Available online. URL: http://www.ama-org/stdinfo.htm. Updated January 2000.

"Japanese Official Guilty in 'Bad Blood' Scandal." AVERT Website. *Positive Nation,* November 2001. URL: http://www.avert.org.

Jefferiss, F. J. G. "Venereal Disease and the Homosexual." *British Journal of Venereal Disease* 32 (1956): 17–20.

Johnson, J. P. et al. "Natural History and Serologic Diagnosis of Infants Born to Human Immunodeficiency Virus-Infected Women." *American Journal of Diseases of Children* 143, no. 10 (1989): 1147–1153.

Johnson, Margaret. "Epidemiology of HIV/AIDS." Medical Library Website. Available online. URL: http://www.medical-library.org/index.htm. Downloaded May 5, 2002.

Johnson, R. A. "Diagnosis and Treatment of Common Sexually Transmitted Diseases in Women." *Clinical Cornerstone* 3, no. 1 (2000): 1–11.

Johnston, Cameron. "DG Dispatch-ICAAC: Valacylovir Superior to Episodic Therapy for Patients with Recurring Genital Herpes." Doctor's Guide Website. Available online. URL: http://www.docguide/news. Downloaded February 1, 2002.

Judge, D. E. "STD Risks from Multiple Sex Partners." *Journal Watch Women's Health* 4, no. 12 (December 1999).

Judge, D. E. "Syphilis in the U.S. Down but Not Out." *Journal Watch Women's Health* 4, no. 12 (December 1999).

Kaiser Daily HIV/AIDS Report Website. "Media and Society: Magic Johnson Tells '60 Minutes' He's 'Healed,' Not 'Cured.'" Available online. URL: http://report.kff.org/archive/aids/1998/05/kh980511.5.html. Downloaded October 4, 2001.

Kanabus, Annabel, and Allen, Sarah. "The Origin of AIDS and HIV." AVERT Website. Available online. URL: http://avert.org. Updated January 9, 2002.

Kaslow, R. A. et al. "No Evidence for a Role of Alcohol or Other Psychoactive Drugs in Accelerating Immunodeficiency in HIV-1-Positive Individuals: A Report from the Multicenter AIDS Cohort Study." *Journal of the American Medical Association* 261, no. 23 (1989): 3424–3429.

Keet, I. P. et al. "Predictors of Rapid Progression to AIDS in HIV-1 Seroconverters." *AIDS* 7, no. 1 (1993): 1236–1243.

"Know Your COBRA Rights." Insure.com Website. Available online. URL: http://www.insure.com.

Koenig, S. et al. "Group-Specific, Major Histocompatibility Complex Class-I Restricted Cytotoxic Responses to Human Immunodeficiency Virus I (HIV-1) Envelope Proteins by Cloned Peripheral Blood T Cells from an HIV-1 Infected Individual." *Proceedings of the National Academy of Science of the United States of America* 85, no. 22 (1988): 8638–8642. Available online. URL: http://www.pubmedcentral.gov.nih. Downloaded on November 1, 2001.

Kornreich, Jennifer. "The Risks of Young Love." MSNBC Website. Available online. URL: http://www.msnbc.com. Downloaded September 5, 2002.

Kovacs, Joseph A. et al. "New Insights into Transmission, Diagnosis, and Drug Treatment of Pneumocystis Carinii Pneumonia." *JAMA* 286, no. 19 (November 21, 2001): 2450–2459.

Kurth, R. "Does HIV Cause AIDS? An Updated Response to Duesberg's Theories." *Intervirology* 31, no. 6 (1990): 301–314.

Lang, D. J., and Kummer, J. F. "Cytomegalovirus in Semen: Observations in Selected Populations." *Journal of Infectious Diseases* 132 (1975): 472–473.

"'Latent' HIV Lasts a Lifetime: Study." *Alive & Kicking!'s FastFax Website*. Available online. URL: http://www.peoplewithaids.org/fastfax/ff227.htm. Downloaded on December 12, 2001.

Lauritsen, John. "Petruschka Was Poisoned: Did AZT Contribute to Nureyev's Untimely Death?" Virus Myth Homepage. *New York Native,* February 1, 1993. Available online. URL: http://www.virusmyth.net/aids/data/jlpetruschka.htm.

"Legal Ruling May Lead to Massive Rise in HIV Cases." AVERT Website. *British Medical Journal* and AVERT. Available online. URL: http://www.avert.org. Downloaded May 1, 2002.

Lehman, Stan et al. "Are At-Risk Populations Less Concerned about HIV Infection in the HAART Era?" CDC Update Website. Available online. URL: http://www.cdc.gov. Downloaded November 1, 2001.

Leishman, Katie. "Controversy and Need for Study on Condoms." Medline Plus. *UPI Science News.* Available online. URL: http://www.nlm.nih.gov/medlineplus/news/fullstory_2976.html. Downloaded August 3, 2001.

Leu, Melanie, Welker, Mary Jo, and Haines, Danell J. "A Perspective on Lesbian Health Care for the Primary Care Physician." *Family Practice Recertification* 21, no. 13 (November 1999).

Leung, Alexander K. C., and Pinto-Rojas, Alfredo. "Infectious Mononucleosis." *Consultant* 40, no. 1 (January 2000): 134–136.

Levy, J. A. "Pathogenesis of Human Immunodeficiency Virus Infection." *Microbiological Reviews* 57, no. 1 (1993): 183–289.

"Limiting Exposure to Opportunistic Pathogens: Latest Recommendations for HIV-Infected Patients." *Consultant* (Primary Care Update) 39 (November 1999): 3023–3026.

Little, Susan J. et al. "Antiretroviral-Drug Resistance among Patients Recently Infected with HIV." *New England Journal of Medicine* 347, no. 6 (August 8, 2002). From the New England Journal of Medicine Website. Available online. URL: http://content.nejm.org/cgi/content/abstract/347/6/385.

Lori, Franco, and Lisziewicz, Julianna. "Structured Treatment Interruptions for the Management of HIV Infection." *Journal of the American Medical Association* 286, no. 23 (December 19, 2001).

Loshak, David. "Difficulties Confront Development of Vaccines for Sexually Transmitted Diseases." A Doctor's Guide Website review of "Progress Slow for Vaccines Against HPV, HIV and Other Viruses" (*Infectious Disease News*). Available online. URL: http://www.docguide/news.com. Downloaded February 1, 2002.

"Low Blood HIV Levels Reduce Risk of Heterosexual Transmission." Doctor's Guide Website. Available online. URL: http://www.docguide/news.com. Downloaded February 10, 2002.

Lowenstein, J. M. "Is AIDS a Myth?" California Academy of Sciences: *Pacific Discovery Magazine,* fall 1994.

MacLennan, Anne. "Female Genital Ulcers May Enhance HIV Transmission." Doctor's Guide Website. *Journal of Infectious Diseases* 181 (2000): 1950–1956. Available online. URL: http://www.docguide/news.com. Downloaded February 1, 2002.

"MACS History." StatePI Website. Available online. URL: http://www.statepi.jhsph.educ/macs/macs.html. Downloaded on December 12, 2001.

"MACS Public Data Set." StatePI Website. Available online. URL: http://www.statepi.jhsph.edu/macs/pdt.html. Downloaded on December 17, 2001.

Mann, J. M. "AIDS—the Second Decade: A Global Perspective." *Journal of Infectious Diseases* 165, no. 2 (1992): 245–250.

"Maternal HIV Consumer Information Project." Health Care Financing Administration. Available online. URL: http://www.hcfa.gov/hiv/hivcipct.htm. Downloaded November 28, 2001.

Mavligit, G. M. et al. "Chronic Immune Stimulation by Sperm Alloantigens: Support for the Hypothesis That Spermatozoa Induce Immune Dysregulation in Homosexual Males." *Journal of the American Medical Association* 251, no. 2 (1984): 237–241.

Mayeaux, E. J., Jr. "Workup of Bacterial Vaginosis." *The Female Patient* 26, no. 3 (March 2001).

"Mbeki Regime in Court for Barring AIDS Drug." AVERT Website. *The Guardian.* Available online. URL: http://www.avert.org.

Mbori-Ngacha, Dorothy et al. "Morbidity and Mortality in Breastfed and Formula-Fed Infants of HIV-1-Infected Women: A Randomized Clinical Trial." *JAMA* 286, no. 19 (November 21, 2001).

McConnell, Harvey. "Urine Screen May Find Most Sexually Transmitted Diseases in Young Women." Doctor's Guide Website. *Western Medical Journal* 173 (2000):

292–293. Available online. URL: http://www. docguide/news. Downloaded February 1, 2002.

McQueen, Anjetta. "Study Finds Condoms Mostly Effective against HIV, Gonorrhea, but Evidence Lacking for Other Diseases." MedlinePlus. Associated Press, July 19, 2001. Available online. URL: http://www.pubmed. Downloaded November 28, 2001.

"Medicaid and Acquired Immunodeficiency Syndrome (AIDS) and Human Immunodeficiency Virus (HIV) Infection." Health Care Financing Administration fact sheet. Available online. URL: http://www.hcfa.gov. Updated February 2001.

"Medicaid and Acquired Immunodeficiency Syndrome (AIDS) and Human Immunodeficiency Virus (HIV) Infection." Health Care Financing Administration Website. Available online. URL: http://www.hcfa.gov/ Medicaid/obs11.htm. Updated on September 17, 2001.

Mirken, Bruce. "Answering the AIDS Denialists: CD4 (T Cells) Counts, and Viral Load." AIDS Treatment News Archive, April 21, 2000. Available online. URL: http://www.aids.org.

Mitka, Mike. "Syphilis Rates at All-Time Low." JAMA Website. *JAMA* 286 (2001). Available online. URL: http://jama.ama-assn.org.

"Mixed Messages Cause Confusion." *Queer News Aotearoa* (New Zealand) Website. Available online. URL: http://nz.com/NZ/Queer/QNA/1997/1997 April27.html. Downloaded on December 14, 2001.

Montagnier, L. et al. "A New Lymphotropic Retrovirus: Characterization and Possible Role in Lymphadenopathy and Acquired Immune Deficiency Syndromes." In: R. C. Gallo et al., eds. *Human T-Cell Leukemia/Lymphoma Virus.* Cold Spring Harbor, N.Y.: Cold Spring Harbor Laboratory, 1984, pp. 363–379.

Moore, R. Andrew et al. "Imiquimod for the Treatment of Genital Warts: A Quantitative Systematic Review." *BMC Infectious Diseases* 1 (June 2001): 3.

Morelli, Jim. "On the Horizon: A New Way to Rein in Sexually Transmitted Disease." WebMD. Available online. URL: http://www.webmd.com. Updated June 6, 2001.

Morse, S. A. "New Tests for Bacterial Sexually Transmitted Diseases." *Current Opinion in Infectious Diseases* 10 (February 14, 2001): 45–51. Available online. URL: http://www.pubmed.com.

My Counsel. "Same-Sex Parenting: Overview." Available online. URL: http://www.mycounsel.com. Downloaded on October 24, 2001.

"Myelosuppression." Oncology Services Website. Available online. URL: http://www.pagesz.net/~miriamr/ca/ drug200.htm. Downloaded on December 12, 2001.

Myers, G., MacInnes, K., and Korber, B. "The Emergence of Simian/Human Immunodeficiency Viruses." *AIDS Research and Human Retroviruses* 8, no. 3 (1992): 373–386.

Nahmias, A. J. et al. "Evidence for Human Infection with an HTLV III/LAV-like Virus in Central Africa." 1959 (letter). *Lancet* 31 (1986): 1279–1280.

Nakashima, Allyn K. et al. "Effect of HIV Reporting by Name on Use of HIV Testing in Publicly Funded Counseling and Testing Programs." JAMA HIV/AIDS Website. Available online. URL: http://www.ama-assn.org/ special/hiv/library/readroom/jama98/joc80227.htm.

"Names Reporting Condemned at Philadelphia Hearing." Alive & Kicking!'s FastFax Website. Available online. URL: http://www.peoplewithaids.org/fastfax/ ff227.htm. Downloaded on December 12, 2001.

National AIDS Hotlines. HIV Positive Website. Available online. URL: http://www.hivpositive.com/index.html. Downloaded February 1, 2002.

"National Institutes of Health: An Overview." National Institutes of Health Website. Available online. URL: http://www.nih.gov/about/NIHoverview.html. Downloaded on December 12, 2001.

Neal, Rosa Mae. "Hispanic Group's Aim: AIDS Awareness." *Miami Herald.* Available online. URL: http://www.aegis.com/news/mh/2001/MH010908. html. Downloaded January 25, 2002.

"Needle Exchange Programs: Part of a Comprehensive HIV Prevention Strategy." Health and Human Services Website. Available online. URL: http://www.hhs.gov/ news/press.html. Downloaded on December 12, 2001.

"Needle Exchange Programs." Human Rights Campaign Website. URL: http://www.org/issues/hiv_aids/ background/exchange.asp.

"Newborn Screening Tests." PageWise, Inc. Website. Available online. URL: http://gaga.essortment.com/ newbornscreenin_ohe.htm. Downloaded on December 14, 2001.

"New HIV/AIDS Developments in Tanzania and the United States." AVERT Website. News item from '+ve,' November 2001. Available online. URL: http://www.avert.org.

"New Research Identifies Effective Teen Pregnancy Prevention Programs." The National Campaign to Prevent Teen Pregnancy Website. Available online. URL: http://www.teenpregnancy.org./054001/eaprrls.htm. Downloaded on December 12, 2001.

"NIAID Phase III HIV Vaccine Trial to Determine Correlates of Protection Will Not Proceed." Available online. URL: http://www.nih.gov. Downloaded on May 5, 2002.

"NIAID Renews Funding for Multicenter AIDS Cohort Study." National Institutes of Health Website. Available online. URL: http://www.nih.gov.news/pr/apr99/ niaid20.htm. Downloaded on December 12, 2001.

Nicoll, Angus et al. "Sexual Health of Teenagers in England and Wales: Analysis of National Data." *British Medical Journal* 318 (May 15, 1999). Available online. URL: http://www.bbc.co.uk.

"Nigeria to Import Cheap Copies of HIV Drugs." AVERT Website. *The Guardian,* November 12, 2001. Available online. URL: http://www.avert.org.

"NIH Researchers Recall the Early Years of AIDS." National Institutes of Health Website. Available online. URL: http://www.nih.gov. Updated on June 4, 2001.

"Non-Hodgkin's Lymphoma." Medline Website. National Library of Medicine. Available online. URL: http://www.medline.com.

"Norwegian Scabies." Available online. URL: http://www.safe2use.com/pests/scabies/Norwegian.htm. Downloaded on December 15, 2001.

"Notes and News: Transmission of HIV by Human Bite." *Lancet* 2 (1987): 522.

Novick, B. E., and Rubinstein, A. "AIDS—the Pediatric Perspective." *AIDS* 1, no. 1 (1987): 3–7.

"New Research Identifies Effective Teen Pregnancy Prevention Programs." Available online. URL: http://www.teenpregnancy.org/053001/easprrls.htm. Downloaded December 28, 2001.

Olkon, Sara. "Starting to ACT Up Again." CDC Website. *Miami Herald* February 3, 2002. Available online. URL: http://www.cdc.gov. Downloaded February 18, 2002.

Ono, A., and Freed, E. O. "Plasma Membrane Rafts Play a Critical Role in HIV-1 Assembly and Release." *Proceedings of the National Academy of Sciences of the United States of America* 98 (2001): 13925–13930.

"One-Fifth of People with STDs Unaware of Infection." Doctor's Guide Website. Available online. URL: http://www.docguide.com.

"Other Important STDs." Fact Sheet, National Institute of Allergy and Infectious Diseases, National Institutes of Health. June 1998.

"Overview of WHO." World Health Organization Website. Available online. URL: http://www.who.org. Downloaded December 1, 2001.

Owens, Jay. "AIDS 2002: PMMA Facial Implants for Lipodystrophy Correction Found Safe and Well Tolerated." Doctor's Guide Website. Available online. URL: http://www.docguide.com.

Padget, David A. et al. "Social Stress and the Reactivation of Latent Herpes Simplex Virus Type 1." *Proceedings of the National Academy of Sciences of the United States of America* 95, no. 12 (June 9, 1998). Available online. URL: http://www.pubmedcentral.gov.nih. Downloaded on November 1, 2001.

Padian, N., and Glass, S. "Transmission of HIV Possibly Associated with Exposure of Mucous Membranes to Contaminated Blood." *Morbidity and Mortality Weekly Report,* July 11, 1997. National Center for HIV, STD, and TB Prevention, CDC.

Pantaleo, G., Graziosi, C., and Fauci, A. S. "The Immunopathogenesis of Human Immunodeficiency Virus Infection." *New England Journal of Medicine* 328, no. 5 (1993): 327–335.

Pantaleo, G. et al. "HIV Infection Is Active and Progressive in Lymphoid Tissue during the Clinically Latent Stage of Disease." *Nature* 362, no. 6418 (1993): 355–358.

Pantaleo, G., and Fauci, A. S. "Apoptosis in HIV Infection." *Nature Medicine* 1, no. 2 (1995): 118–120.

Pape, J., and Johnson, W. D., Jr. "AIDS in Haiti: 1982–1992." *Clinical Infectious Diseases* 17 (suppl 2) (1993): S341–S345.

Patten-Hitt, Emma. "U.S. Congenital Syphilis Cases Halved in Three Years." Medline Plus. Reuters. Available online. URL: http://www.pubmed. Downloaded November 28, 2001.

Pauk, John et al. "Mucosal Shedding of Human Herpesvirus 8 in Men." *New England Journal of Medicine* 343, no. 19 (November 9, 2000): 1369–1377. Available online. URL: http://nejm.com.

"PCP Treatment Can Stop If HAART Is Effective: Study." Alive & Kicking!'s FastFax Website. Available online. URL: http://www.peoplewithaids.org/fastfax/ff227.htm. Downloaded on December 12, 2001.

Peck, Peggy. "New Guidelines Include Screening High-Risk Women for Hepatitis C." WebMD. Available online. URL: http://www.webmd.com. Updated June 6, 2001.

Peck, Peggy. "Women Are Never Too Old for Sex—or for Sexually Transmitted Disease." WebMD. Reviewed by Tonya Wynn Hampton. Available online. URL: http://www.webmd.com. Updated on May 8, 2001.

"Pelvic Inflammatory Disease." JAMA Women's Health Website. Available online. URL: http://www.ama-assn.org/special/std/support/educate/stdpid.htm. Downloaded on August 6, 2001.

"Peripheral Neuropathy." Medline Plus Website. National Library of Medicine. URL: http://www.medline.com. Downloaded August 10, 2002.

Peters, Michael (reviewer). "Warning as Britain's Specialty Clinics Struggle to Cope with Demand." MSN Website. Available online. URL: http://content.health.msn.com/content/article.

"Pharmaceutical Giants Defeated over AIDS Drugs." AVERT Website. AVERT, April 23, 2001. Available online. URL: http://www.avert.org.

Phillips, Andrew et al. "HIV Viral Load Response to Antiretroviral Therapy according to the Baseline CD4 Cell Count and Viral Load." JAMA Website. *JAMA* 286 (2001). Available online. URL: http://www.jama.ama.org.

Physicians' Research Network Website. Available online. Resource links and related sites-New York, NY. URL: http://www.prn.org. Updated June 21, 2001.

Pincock, Stephen. "Experts Call Attention to HIV Risk from Oral Sex." Medline Plus, July 5, 2001. Reuters.

Available online. URL: http://www.nlm.nih.gov/med-lineplus/news/fullstory_2589.html. Downloaded on November 1, 2001.

Piot, P. et al. "AIDS: An International Perspective." *Science* 239, no. 4840 (1988): 573–579.

Popovic, M. et al. "Detection, Isolation, and Continuous Production of Cytopathic Retroviruses (HTLV-III) from Patients with AIDS and Pre-AIDS." *Science* 224, no. 4648 (1984): 497–500.

"Prophylaxis of Venereal Disease." *Journal of the American Medical Association* 286, no. 21 (December 5, 2001). Available online. URL: http://www.jama.ama.org.

"Protection of Cervix Very Important in Preventing Human Immunodeficiency Infection." Doctor's Guide Channels Website. Available online. URL: http://www.docguide.com. Downloaded January 15, 2002.

"Protein May Be Key to Treating Kaposi's." Alive & Kicking!'s FastFax Website. Available online. URL: http://www.peoplewithaids.org/fastfax/ff227.htm. Downloaded on December 12, 2001.

"Questions about Crusted Norwegian Scabies." Available online. URL: http://www.safe2use.com/pests/scabies/norwegian.htm. Downloaded on May 28, 2001.

Quigley, M. A., Weiss, H. A., and Hayes, R. J. "Male Circumcision as a Measure to Control HIV Infection and Other Sexually Transmitted Diseases." *Current Opinion in Infectious Diseases* 14, no. 1 (February 14, 2001): 71–75. Available online. URL: http://www.pubmed.com. Downloaded on November 1, 2001.

Quinn, T. C. "Population Migration and the Spread of Types 1 and 2 Human Immunodeficiency Viruses." *Proceedings of the National Academy of Sciences of the United States of America* 91, no. 7 (1994): 2407–2414. Available online. URL: http://www.pubmedcentral.gov.nih. Downloaded on November 1, 2001.

Ramrakha, Sandhya et al. "Psychiatric Disorders and Risky Sexual Behaviour in Young Adulthood: Cross Sectional Study in Birth Cohort." *British Medical Journal* 321 (2000): 263–266. Available online. URL: http://www.pubmedcentral.gov.bmj. Downloaded on November 1, 2001.

Rana-Mukkavilli, Gopi. "Yogurt for Vaginal Candidiasis." *Hospital Medicine* 35, no. 6 (June 1999).

Ratner, L., Gallo, R. C., and Wong-Staal, F. "HTLV-III, LAV, ARV Are Variants of Same AIDS Virus." *Nature* 313, no. 6004 (1985): 636.

"Reducing HIV Transmission: The Maternal HIV Consumer Information Project." Health Care Financing Administration Website. Available online. URL: http://www.hcfa.gov/hiv/subpg6.htm. Downloaded on September 15, 2001.

Regan, Fiona A. M. et al. "Prospective Investigation of Transfusion Transmitted Infection in Recipients of Over 20,000 Units of Blood." *British Medical Journal* 320 (February 2000). Available online. URL: http://www.pubmedcentral.gov.bmj. Downloaded on February 1, 2002.

"The Relationship between the Human Immunodeficiency Virus and the Acquired Immunodeficiency Syndrome." National Institute of Allergy and Infectious Diseases, National Institutes of Health. Available online. URL: http://www.aids.wustl.edu/aids.faq.html.

Report from CDC National AIDS Clearinghouse. "Transmission of HIV Possibly Associated with Exposure of Mucous Membrane to Contaminated Blood." July 11, 1997. Available online. URL: http://www.cdc.gov/hiv/pubs. Downloaded October 1, 2001.

Reuters. "Viral Load in Women Strongly Related to HIV Risk." Medline Plus, National Library of Medicine. Available online. URL: http://www.nlm.nih.gov/medlineplus. Downloaded on October 20, 2001.

Ries, Kristen. "HIV Infection and AIDS: A Diagnostic Consideration in Every Patient." *Consultant* 39 (1999): 3027–3035.

Rinaldo, C. R., Jr., Black, P. H., and Hirsch, M. S. "Interaction of Cytomegalovirus with Leukocytes from Patients with Mononucleosis Due to Cytomegalovirus." *Journal of Infectious Diseases* 136 (1977): 667–678.

Rinaldo, C. R., Jr. et al. "Mechanisms of Immunosuppression in Cytomegaloviral Mononucleosis." *Journal of Infectious Diseases* 141 (1980): 488–495.

Ringel, Marcia. "HIV Disease in the New Century." *Patient Care*, October 15, 1999.

Rodrigo, Allen G. "HIV Evolutionary Genetics." PubMed Central. *Proceedings of the National Academy of Sciences of the United States of America*. Available online. URL: http://www.pubmedcentral.nih.gov. Downloaded on October 30, 2001.

Rosenblatt, Jane. "AIDS: Two Decades Later." Available online. URL: http://www.drkoop.com. Downloaded on January 14, 2002.

Rosenfeld, W. D. "Sexually Transmitted Diseases in Adolescents: Update 1991." *Pediatric Annals* 20, no. 6 (June 1991): 303–312. Available online. URL: http://www.pubmed. Downloaded on January 12, 2001.

Rubeiro, Ruy M., and Bonhoeffer, Sebastian. "Production of Resistant HIV Mutants during Antiretroviral Therapy." PubMed Central Website. *Proceedings of the National Academy of Sciences of the United States of America* 97, no. 14 (July 2000). Available online. URL: http://www.pubmedcentral.gov.nih. Downloaded on November 10, 2001.

"Salvage Strategies and STI at the 10th Annual Retrovirus Conference." Gay Men's Health Crisis Website. Available online. URL: http://www.gmhc.org. Downloaded March 5, 2003.

Satcher, David. "Global HIV/AIDS Revisited." JAMA Website. *Journal of the American Medical Association* 286, no. 20 (November 28, 2001). Available online. URL: http://www.jama.ama-assn.org.

Saunders, Carol S. "Healthy People 2010 to Track Indicators." *Patient Care* 34, no. 6 (March 2000).

Saunders, Carol S. Article consultants Schaffner, William, Sedlacek, Thomas A., and Steller, Michael A. "Monitoring HPV Infection." *Patient Care* 34, no. 5 (March 15, 2000).

Schechter, M. T. et al. "Aetiology of AIDS." *Lancet* 341, no. 8854 (1993): 1222–1223.

Scherzer, Mark. "Life and Disability Insurance." Body Positive Website. Available online. URL: http://www.bodypositive.com. Downloaded August 12, 2002.

Schorr, Melissa. "HIV-Infected Moms Likely to Pass along Syphilis." Medline Website. Reuters. Available online. URL: http://www.nlm.nih.gov/medlineplus/news/fullstory_2662.html.

Schlecht, Nicolas et al. "Persistent Human Papillomavirus Infection as a Predictor of Cervical Intraepithelial Neoplasia." JAMA Website. *Journal of the American Medical Association* 286 (2001): 3106–3114. Available online. URL: http://www.jama.ama-assn.org.

"Scientists Put Condom Report in Perspective." Sexhealth Website. Available online. URL: http://www.sexhealth.com/sexhealth/user/display. Downloaded October 1, 2001.

Seidman, S. N., and Rieder, R. O. "A Review of Sexual Behavior in the United States." *American Journal of Psychiatry* 151, no. 3 (1994): 330–341.

"Seven-Day-On, Seven-Day-Off Regimen Could Reduce Cost, Toxicities of HIV Therapy." National Institute of Allergy and Infectious Disease Website. Available online. URL: http://www.nih.gov/news/pr/dec2001/niaid-03.htm. Downloaded on December 12, 2001.

SexHealth. "Chlamydia Screening Study: Most MDs Disregard CDC Recommendations." Available online. URL: http://www.DrKoop.com. Updated September 19, 2001.

SexHealth. "Is the Pap Smear Obsolete?" Available online. URL: http://www.sexhealth.com.

"Sexually Transmitted Diseases Treatment Guide—2002." Centers for Disease Control and Prevention *MMWR* Website, May 10, 2002. URL: http://www.cdc.gov/mmwr/previous/mmwrhtml/n5106A1.htm.

Shirriff, Ken. "What Are Strecker and Segal's Theories That HIV Is Manmade?" sci.med.aids, a USENet newsgroup. Available online. URL: http://www.aids.wustl.edu/aids/streck.html.

Siegal, F. P. et al. "Severe Acquired Immunodeficiency in Male Homosexuals, Manifested by Chronic Perianal Ulcerative Herpes Simplex Lesions." *New England Journal of Medicine* 305, no. 24 (1981): 1439–1444.

Simanski, J. W. "The Birds and the Bees: An Analysis of Advice Given to Parents through the Popular Press." PubMed Website. Available online. URL: http://www.ncbi.nlm.nih.gov/entrez/query.fcgi. Downloaded November 1, 2001.

Slim, Jihad, series editor of AIDS Update. "Mechanisms of Virologic Failure in HIV-Infected Patients." *Hospital Physician* 36, no. 3 (March 2000).

Slim, Jihad, series editor of AIDS Update. "Cervical Shedding of Herpes Simplex Virus in HIV-Infected Women." *Hospital Physician* 36, no. 3 (March 2000).

Slim, Jihad, series editor of AIDS Update. "Hepatotoxicity Associated with Antiretroviral Therapy and Hepatitis Virus Infection." *Hospital Physician* 36, no. 3 (March 2000).

Slim, Jihad, series editor of AIDS Update. "Vertical Transmission of HIV-1." *Hospital Physician* 35, no. 6 (June 1999).

Slim, Jihad, series editor of AIDS Update. "Prevalence of Lower Genital Tract Infections." *Hospital Physician* 36, no. 1 (January 2000).

Smith, Kendall A., et al. "Restoration of Immunity with Interleukin-2 Therapy." *The AIDS Reader.* Available online. URL: http://www.medscape.com/SCP/TAR/1999/v09.n08/a6812.smit/a6812.smit-01.html.

Smoots, Elizabeth. "Contracting Chlamydia." WebMD Website. Available online. URL: http://www.webmd.com. Updated June 4, 2001.

"Social Security Benefits for People Living With HIV/AIDS." Fact sheet from Social Security Administration. SSA Publication No. 05-10019, May 1995.

"South African Men Accused of Raping Baby as Cure for AIDS." AVERT Website. *The Sunday Telegraph*, November 11, 2001. Available online. URL: http://www.avert.org.

"Special Medicaid Coverage for Pregnant Women." Health Care Financing Administration Website. Available online. URL: http://www.hcfa.gov/hiv/subpg4.htm. Updated on September 17, 2001.

Spitzer, Roger. "Living with HIV: Genotyping." Living With HIV Website. Updated January 15, 2003. Available online. URL: http://www.ourworld.compuserve.com/homepages/bugdoc/livhiv2.htm. Downloaded October 15, 2001.

"State Health Facts Online." The Henry Kaiser Foundation Website. Available online. URL: http://www.

statehealthfacts.kff.org/cgi-bin/healthfacts. "Cumulative AIDS Cases, through June 2000."

"State Health Facts Online." The Henry Kaiser Foundation Website. Available online. URL: http://www.statehealthfacts.kff.org/cgi-bin/healthfacts. "Minors' Right to Consent to HIV/STD Services, as of July 2000."

"State Health Facts Online." The Henry Kaiser Foundation Website. Available online. URL: http://www.statehealthfacts.kff.org/cgi-bin/healthfacts. "State Requirements: STD/HIV/AIDS Education Curriculum as of July 2000."

"Statements/Resolutions/Policies on Increased Access to Clean Needles and Syringes." SFAF HIV Prevention Project (Needle Exchange) Website. Available online. URL: http://www.sfaf.org/prevention/needleexchange/statements.html. Downloaded on December 12, 2001.

"Statscript Installs New HIV Management System." Alive & Kicking!'s FastFax Website. Available online. URL: http://www.peoplewithaids.org/fastfax/ff227.htm. Downloaded April 25, 2002.

Steele, Robert. "What Are the Special Needs of Adolescent Patients with HIV/AIDS?" 2000 American Academy of Pediatrics Annual Meeting, October 28, 2000. Available online. URL: http://www.pediatricsmedscape.com. Downloaded November 28, 2001.

Stephenson, Joan. "Can a Common Medical Practice Transform Candida Infections from Benign to Deadly?" JAMA Website. *Journal of the American Medical Association* 286 (2001). Available online. URL: http://www.jama.ama-assn.org. Downloaded on May 5, 2002.

Stranford, Sharon A. et al. "Lack of Infection in HIV-Exposed Individuals Is Associated with a Strong CD8+ Cell Noncytotoxic Anti-HIV Response." *Proceedings of the National Academy of Sciences of the United States of America* 96, no. 3 (February 1999). Available online. URL: http://www.pubmedcentral.gov.nih. Downloaded on January 10, 2002.

"Study: HIV Not Tied to Polio Vaccine." MSNBC Website. Available online. URL: http://www.msnbc.com. Downloaded January 15, 2002.

"Study Points to Possible Route for AIDS Vaccine." CNN Website. Available online. URL: http://www.cnn.com. Downloaded January 15, 2002.

"Surgeon General's Call to Action to Promote Sexual Health and Responsible Sexual Behavior." Available online. URL: http://www.surgeongeneral.gov/library/sexualhealth. Downloaded August 20, 2002.

Susman, Ed. "AIDS—a Case of Casual Contact?" MSNBC Website. Available online. URL: http://www.msnbc.com.

Susman, Ed. "AIDS 2002: Lidocaine Patch Treats HIV-Associated Peripheral Neuropathy." Doctor's Guide Website.

Available online. URL: http://www.docguide.com. Downloaded on August 6, 2002.

"Syphilis." *JAMA* Women's Health Website. Available online. URL: http://www.ama-assn.org/special/std/support/educate/stdsyph.htm. Downloaded on August 6, 2001.

Szucs, Thomas D. et al. "The Estimated Economic Burden of Genital Herpes in the United States: An Analysis Using Two Cost Approaches." PubMed Website. Taken from *BMC Infectious Diseases* 1, no. 5 (June 2001). Available online. URL: http://www.pubmedcentral.nih.gov/articlerender.fcgi. Downloaded on August 3, 2001.

"T-20 Open Label Study Announced." AVERT Website. *NAM AIDS Treatment Update* 108 (December 2001). Available online. URL: http://www.avert.org.

Taylor, Maida. "Barrier and Nonhormonal Contraception: What's New, What's Next." *Consultant Magazine* 39, no. 11 (November 1999).

Temin, H. M. "Is HIV Unique or Merely Different?" *Journal of Acquired Immune Deficiency Syndrome* 2, no. 1 (1989): 1–9.

Thorne, C., Newell, M. L., and Peckham C. S. "Disclosure of Diagnosis and Planning for the Future in HIV-Affected Families in Europe." PubMed Website. *Child Care Health Development* 26, no. 1 (January 2000). Available online. URL: http://www.ncbi.nlm.gov/entrez/query.fcgi. Updated August 22, 2001.

"Transmission of HIV Possibly Associated with Exposure of Mucous Membrane to Contaminated Blood." *Morbidity and Mortality Weekly Report* 30 (July 11, 1997).

Turner, B. J. et al. "Survival Experience of 789 Children with the Acquired Immunodeficiency Syndrome." *Journal of Pediatric Infectious Diseases* 12, no. 4 (1993): 310–320.

"Types of Depression." Mayo Clinic Website. Available online. URL: http://www.MayoClinic.com. Downloaded August 10, 2002.

U.S. Department of Justice, Civil Rights Division. "A Guide to Disability Rights Laws." Available online. URL: http://www.pueblo.gsa.gov/cic. Downloaded on October 24, 2001.

"U.S. FDA Warning to Manufacturers of AIDS Drugs." News item from *British Medical Journal* (December 5, 2001). AVERT Website. URL: http://www.avert.org.

"Vaccines." National Institutes of Health Fiscal Years 2003, Plan for HIV-Related Research. Prepared by the Office of AIDS Research. Available online. URL: http://www.nih.gov. Downloaded on October 1, 2002.

"Vaginal Bacteria Imbalance Might Increase AIDS Risk." Doctor's Guide Website. Available online. URL: http://www.docguide.com.

Varmus, H. "Retroviruses." *Science* 240, no. 4858 (1988): 1427–1435.

Vastag, Brian. "Chlamydia Toxin and Chronic Illness." JAMA Website. Health Agencies Update. *Journal of the American Medical Association* 286, no. 23 (December 19, 2001).

"VDRL." Medline Website. Available online. URL: http://www.medline.com. Downloaded August 20, 2002.

Vidmar, L. et al. "Transmission of HIV-1 by Human Bite." *Lancet* 347 (1996): 1762–1763.

"Virus 'Blips' May Not Always Signal Failure of AIDS Drugs." MSNBC Website. Available online. URL: http://www.msnbc.com.

Wagner, Wynn. "HIV: Day One." Available online. URL: http://www.aegis.com/topics/dayone/html. Updated September 17, 2001.

Wald, N. J. et al. "Chlamydia Pneumoniae Infection and Mortality from Ischaemic Heart Disease: Large Prospective Study." *British Medical Journal* 321 (July 22, 2000): 204–207. Available online. URL: http://www.pubmed.

Walzer, P. D. et al. "Pneumocystis Carinii Pneumonia in the United States: Epidemiologic, Diagnostic, and Clinical Features." *Annals of Internal Medicine* 80 (1974): 83–93.

Wasserheit, Judy. "Talking Points: Congenital Syphilis Media Telebriefing." CDC STD Prevention. Available online. URL: http://www.cdc.gov. Downloaded on October 15, 2001.

WebMD. "HIV-AIDS Update for the New Millennium." Available online. URL: http://www.content.health.msn.com. Downloaded on June 6, 2001.

WebMD. "Counseling to Prevent HIV Infection and Other Sexually Transmitted Diseases." Available online. URL: http://www.content.health.msn.com. Updated June 6, 2001.

WebMD. "Sexually Transmitted Diseases Statistics." Available online. URL: http://www.content.health.msn.com. Updated on June 6, 2001.

Wei, X. et al. "Viral Dynamics in Human Immunodeficiency Virus Type 1 Infection." *Nature* 373 (1995): 117–122.

Weiner, H. Richard. "Chlamydia Infection: The Hidden Epidemic." *Emergency Medicine* 31, no. 11 (November 1999): 88–95.

Weiss, R. A. "How Does HIV Cause AIDS?" *Science* 260, no. 5112 (1993): 1273–1279.

Weiss, R. A., and Jaffe, H. W. "Duesberg, HIV and AIDS (commentary)." *Nature* 345 (1990): 659–660.

"West Blames 'Lustful' Blacks for AIDS, Says Mbeki." AVERT Website. *The Daily Telegraph,* October 27, 2001. Available online. URL: http://www.avert.org.

"What Is Bipolar Disorder?" Mayo Clinic Website. Available online. URL: http://www.mayoclinic.com. Downloaded August 20, 2002.

"What You Need to Know about This Dangerous Sexually Transmitted Disease." MSN Website. Available online. URL: http://content.health.msn.com/content/article.

WHO (World Health Organization). "AIDS: Images of the Epidemic." Geneva, 1994.

Wiesenfeld, H. C. et al. "Self-Collection of Vaginal Swabs for the Detection of Chlamydia, Gonorrhea, and Trichomoniasis: Opportunity to Encourage Sexually Transmitted Disease Testing among Adolescents." PubMed Website. National Library of Medicine. *Sexually Transmitted Diseases* 28, no. 6 (June 2001): 321–325. Available online. URL: http://www.pubmed.com.

"Will Any HIV Nonprogressor Be Spared?" Physician's Weekly Website. *Physician's Weekly* 15, no. 31 (August 17, 1998). Available online. URL: http://www.physweekly.com/archive.html. Downloaded on December 15, 2001.

Witkin, Steven S., and Giraldo, Paulo C. "The Quandary of Recurrent Vaginal Candidiasis." *Patient Care* 34, no. 2 (January 2000).

Wodarz, Dominik, and Nowak, Martin A. "HIV Therapy: Managing Resistance." *Proceedings of the National Academy of Sciences of the United States of America* 97, no. 15 (July 2000). Available online. URL: http://www.pubmedcentral.gov.nih. Downloaded on January 12, 2002.

Wofsy, C. B. et al. "Isolation of AIDS-Associated Retrovirus from Genital Secretions of Women with Antibodies to the Virus." *Lancet* 8, no. 8480 (1986): 527–529.

"Woman Infected With HIV Through Artificial Insemination." Available online. URL: http://www.docguide.com.

"World AIDS Conference: Drug Use, Being Uncircumcised Found as Risk Factors for Gay/Bisexual Men." Doctor's Guide Website. Available online. URL: http://www.docguide.com.

"WTO Relaxes Rule on Drug Patents." AVERT Website. *The Guardian.* Available online. URL: http://www.avert.org. Downloaded May 5, 2002.

Wyatt, Gail. "HIV-AIDS Update for the New Millennium." MSN Health with Web MD Website. Available online. URL: http://content.health.msn.com/content/article.

Yeung, S. C. et al. "Patients Infected with HIV Type 1 Have Low Levels of Virus in Saliva Even in the Presence of Periodontal Disease." *Journal of Infectious Diseases* 167 (1993): 803–809.

"You Can Prevent MAC: A Guide for People with HIV Infection." Medem Website. Available online. URL:

http://www.medem.com. Downloaded November 30, 2001.

"You Can Prevent PCP in Children: A Guide for People with HIV Infection." Medem Website. Available online. URL: http://www.medem.com. Downloaded September 1, 2002.

Younai, Fariba S. "Recognizing and Managing Common Oral Mucosal Lesions." *Family Practice Recertification* 21, no. 9 (August 1999): 33–53.

INDEX

Page numbers in **boldface** indicate extensive treatment of a topic.